Perspectives in Veterinary Toxicology and Pharmacology

Guest Editors

Maria Vittoria Varoni
Department of Veterinary Medicine
University of Sassari
Sassari
Italy

Elena Baralla
Department of Veterinary Medicine
University of Sassari
Sassari
Italy

Valeria Pasciu
Department of Veterinary Medicine
University of Sassari
Sassari
Italy

Editorial Office

MDPI AG
Grosspeteranlage 5
4052 Basel, Switzerland

This is a reprint of the Special Issue, published open access by the journal *Animals* (ISSN 2076-2615), freely accessible at: https://www.mdpi.com/journal/animals/special_issues/DQUI017PN3.

For citation purposes, cite each article independently as indicated on the article page online and as indicated below:

Lastname, A.A.; Lastname, B.B. Article Title. *Journal Name* **Year**, *Volume Number*, Page Range.

ISBN 978-3-7258-6352-5 (Hbk)
ISBN 978-3-7258-6353-2 (PDF)
https://doi.org/10.3390/books978-3-7258-6353-2

Cover image courtesy of Elena Baralla

Contents

Preface

We are pleased to present the Reprint of the Special Issue titled "Perspectives in Veterinary Toxicology and Pharmacology". This represents a collection of seven original research articles, a review, and a brief report that provide valuable insights into the emerging disciplines of veterinary pharmacology and toxicology. In the present day, the study of these disciplines is of great concern for evaluating the well-being of people, animals, and the environment from a One Health perspective.

This Reprint, together with the study of the therapeutic effect of drugs and other natural products against several diseases, explores the impact of emerging contaminants and their industrial applications, demonstrated on different animal models, and analyzes the risks related to the consumption of contaminated food.

We believe this Reprint will be of particular interest to academics, researchers, and scientists interested in the "One Health" paradigm.

We want to thank all of the contributing authors from around the world for their high-quality work, the reviewers for their valuable efforts in reviewing these scientific papers, and all of the editorial staff.

We hope you enjoy reading and find inspiration from this Reprint.

Maria Vittoria Varoni, Elena Baralla, and Valeria Pasciu
Guest Editors

animals

MDPI

Article

The Effects of Aflatoxin B1 Intake in Assaf Dairy Ewes on Aflatoxin M1 Excretion, Milk Yield, Haematology and Biochemical Profile

Raúl Bodas [1,*], F. Javier Giráldez [2], Sara Olmedo [1], Marta Herrera [3], Susana Lorán [3], Agustín Ariño [3], Secundino López [2], Alberto Benito [1] and Teresa Juan [3,4]

1 Agrarian Technological Institute of Castile and Leon (ITACyL), Ctra. Burgos, Km 119, 47071 Valladolid, Spain
2 Instituto de Ganadería de Montaña (CSIC-Universidad De León), Finca Marzanas s/n, 24346 Grulleros, Spain
3 Facultad de Veterinaria, Instituto Agroalimentario de Aragón-IA2 (Universidad de Zaragoza-CITA), 50013 Zaragoza, Spain
4 Centro de Investigación y Tecnología Agroalimentaria de Aragón (CITA), Avda. Montañana 930, 50059 Zaragoza, Spain
* Correspondence: bodrodra@itacyl.es

Simple Summary: Aflatoxin B1 is a mycotoxin produced by toxigenic moulds that contaminate feedstuffs. If aflatoxin B1 is ingested by ewes, they can get sick and aflatoxin M1 can be found in milk. The objective of this work was to study the transfer of different moderate doses of aflatoxin B1 ingested by Assaf ewes (40 or 80 µg aflatoxin B1/day) into milk (aflatoxin M1) and its effect on animals' health and performance. There is a clear transfer of aflatoxin B1 (feed) into aflatoxin M1 (milk). The transfer rate depends on the aflatoxin B1 dose (the lower the dose, the higher the transfer rate) and milk yield (high-producing animals show higher transfer rates than low-producing ones). Ewes' milk yield and health were not visibly affected.

Abstract: The aim of this study was to investigate the in vivo transfer of aflatoxin B1 (AFB1) to Assaf ewes' milk (aflatoxin M1, AFM1) and its effect on animal performance and health. Thirty Assaf ewes were allocated to three groups (C, L, H), and received a different individual daily dose of AFB1 (0, 40 and 80 µg) for 13 days. Milk (days 1, 2, 3, 4, 7, 14, 16 and 18) and blood (days 1, 7, 14 and 18) samples were collected. Milk yield, composition (except protein) and somatic cell counts (SCC) were not affected by AFB1 intake ($p > 0.05$). Haemoglobin concentration increased ($p < 0.05$) and haematocrit and alanine aminotransferase levels tended to increase ($p < 0.10$) in group H on day 14. AFM1 excretion was highly variable and detected in L and H animals from days 1 to 16 (3 days increase, 10 days steady-state, 3 days clearance). Carry-over rate (0.23%) was significantly higher in L (0.22–0.34%) than in H (0.16–0.19%) animals ($p < 0.05$). AFB1 daily doses of 40 to 80 µg do not impair milk yield; however, it may start affecting animals' health. Milk AFM1 depends mainly on the AFB1 intake whereas carryover rate is positively influenced by the level of milk production.

Keywords: aflatoxin B1; aflatoxin M1; milk; dairy ewes; Assaf; carryover; haematology; blood biochemical parameters

1. Introduction

Aflatoxins are mycotoxins produced by toxigenic strains of *Aspergillus flavus* and *A. parasiticus* that may contaminate foodstuffs. Aflatoxin M1 (AFM1) is the hydroxylated metabolite of aflatoxin B1 (AFB1) and can be found in milk and derived products obtained from livestock that have ingested contaminated feed. The contamination of food and feed with mycotoxins is a global threat to food safety and has great public health and economic significance. The European Food Safety Authority (EFSA) is continuously updating its risk assessment to advise the EU Commission about the need for new limits and/or modifications to the existing maximum contents in food and feed.

The presence of AFM1 in milk in the EU should not be considered a major public health concern as there are strict regulations in place to protect the health of consumers. Furthermore, several screenings carried out on milk and dairy products [1–4] have shown that levels are controlled. Thus, although AFB1, which is the precursor of AFM1, is present in up to 30% of cattle feed, the amounts are below the maximum limit established in the legislation, with very few positive cases [2,4–6].

However, outside the EU, the number of AFB1-positive feed samples can be much higher [7]. In this regard, the import of feedstuffs from third countries in a food shortage scenario may increase the frequency of AFB1-positives. In this regard, the impact of the Russia–Ukraine conflict on agri-food products trade has been immediate, inducing critical shortages of animal feed that may be addressed by securing imports from other origins [8].

Aflatoxins possess a high acute and chronic toxicity, including genotoxic and carcinogenic effects on animal and human health [9]. Ruminants have a higher resistance to aflatoxicosis than other animals; however, their ability to inactivate AFB1 is severely limited [9], and this mycotoxin can affect the animals' biochemical profile. For example, increases in aspartame transaminase (AST), alanine transaminase (ALT), alkaline phosphatase (ALP), malondialdehyde (MDA) and lipid peroxidation as well as decreases in gamma-glutamyl transferase (GGT) have been reported in response to mycotoxin intake [10,11].

The main target organ of aflatoxins in animals is the liver, whose adverse effects have been reported in the form of acute intoxication characterized by severe liver damage, anorexia, jaundice, weight loss, gastrointestinal disorders, haemorrhage, oedema and even death. Chronic sublethal exposure leads to immunosuppression, nutritional dysfunctions and cancer. Several studies on AFM1 occurring in milk reported carcinogenic and immunosuppressive effects similar to those of AFB1, both in humans and in other animals, although with a less potent effect [12]. AFM1 is the only mycotoxin for which maximum levels in milk have been established. Lactocytes also have some ability to transform AFB1 into AFM1, which transports both by passive diffusion and via an active xenobiotic transporter into the lumen of the mammary alveolus, allowing high concentrations to be reached in short periods of time [9]. Moreover, a recent study has shown that, depending on the concentration of spores and fungi present in the feed, aflatoxin production may be also possible in the rumen of the animals [13].

The transfer rate of AFB1 from feeds to AFM1 in milk is highly variable, with values ranging from 0.6 to 6% in cows [6]. The transfer rate in sheep is generally lower, with values ranging from 0.08 to 0.33% in Sarda ewes [14,15] to 0.54% in Lacaune ewes [16]. Nevertheless, the transfer rate is influenced by various pathophysiological factors, including feeding regime, health status, individual biotransformation capacity and volume of milk production. In this regard, the expression of the BCRP/ABCG2 transporter, present in the luminal part of the lactocytes and contributing to the excretion of AFM1 in milk, seems to increase with the production potential of the animal [9].

Sheep milk production is typical in the Mediterranean region, and Spain is one of the main producers with an approximate production of 536,000 t/yr [17]. Almost 45% of the Spanish dairy industry is located in in Castile and Leon (northwest Spain), which produces 54% of the total ewe milk production of Spain [17,18]. Spanish Assaf is currently the most important dairy sheep breed in Spain. This breed has undergone a process of adaptation and selection over the last 35 years to achieve sustained high levels of production over time [19]. These animals are heavier and with higher milk production potentials than the Sarda [14,15] and Lacaune ewes [16]. However, there are no available data in the literature concerning the rate of transfer of AFB1 to AFM1 or the average excretion of AFM1 in milk in Assaf ewes.

Therefore, the aim of the present work was to study the in vivo transfer of AFB1 ingested by Assaf ewes into milk (detected as AFM1) and its effect on the productive performance and biochemical profile and haematic parameters.

2. Material and Methods

2.1. Animal Ethics

The experiment was compliant with the Directive 2010/63/EU of the European Parliament and of the Council of 22 September 2010 on the protection of animals used for scientific purposes. The experimental procedures were approved by the Institutional Animal Care and Use Committee of the Agrarian Technological Institute of Castilla y León (ITACyL, Spain) and the competent authority (Directive 2010/63/EU) under the protocol number 2017/25/OH.

2.2. Animals and Diets

Thirty lactating Assaf ewes in week 4 of lactation were used (average body weight $\pm$ standard deviation = 80.0 $\pm$ 8.23 kg). Animals were allocated to three experimental groups balanced by body weight and milk yield at the experimental farm of the Instituto de Ganadería de Montaña (CSIC-Universidad de León) located in the northwest of Spain (Castilla y León). The ewes were individually housed, fed and milked, and were able to hear and see other sheep. All the animals received during the whole experimental period the same total mixed ration (TMR) comprised of 472 g of dehydrated alfalfa, 147 g of maize, 134 g of soybean meal, 76 g of barley, 53 g of beet pulp, 50 g of cereal straw, 42 g of molasses, 11 g of mineral vitamin corrector, 10 g of sodium bicarbonate and 5 g of sodium chloride per kg of mix. The chemical composition of the TMR was as follows (per kg): 909 g of dry matter, 116 g of ash, 154 g of crude protein, 2.3 g of ether extract, 328 g of neutral detergent fibre and 214 g of acid detergent fibre. Individual feed consumption was measured daily. The TMR was supplied once a day after milking; the amount of feed offered was adjusted daily on the basis of the previous day's intake, allowing refusals of 20% of feed offered. The ewes were weighed (Magriña 102, Barcelona, Spain) on days 1 and 18 of the experimental period immediately after milking and before TMR supply.

AFB1 was purchased from Sigma-Aldrich (Merck, Rahway, NJ, USA). The mycotoxin was suspended in methanol and doses prepared by pipetting onto a wheat flour matrix contained in an oral gelatine capsule. The capsule was offered to the animals and ingested by them immediately after daily milking and before supplying the TMR, and was administered ensuring that each ewe received the correct dose of AFB1. The ewes of each group were orally supplemented from day 1 to 13 of the experimental period with different amounts of aflatoxin B1: no addition (control group C, only the amount naturally present in the ration and one capsule without AFB1 added), 40 µg aflatoxin B1 in one capsule per day (group L, low dose, 0.5 µg/kg body weight per day) and 80 µg aflatoxin B1 in one capsule per day (group H, high dose, 1.0 µg/kg body weight per day).

2.3. Milking

Ewes were machine-milked once a day (at 08:00) in a 1 $\times$ 10 low-line Casse system milking parlour (120 pulsations/min, 50:50 pulsation ratio, 36 kPa vacuum). Milk yield was recorded daily, and milk samples were taken on days 1, 2, 3, 4, 7 and 14. To assess AFM1 excretion after cessation of AFB1 intake, samples were taken on days 16 and 18. Two subsamples of milk were taken: one was immediately stored at -20 °C until used for AFM1 analysis and the other one was preserved (Bronopol, Broad Spectrum Micro-tabs II, D&F Control Systems, Inc., Norwood, MA, USA) and kept at 4 °C until analysed for chemical composition, which was performed within the following 24 h.

2.4. Blood Samples and Analyses

Blood sampling by jugular venepuncture took place on days 1, 7, 14 and 18 before offering the daily TMR. Blood samples were collected into Vacutainer tubes (10 mL; Becton Dickinson, Franklin Lakes, NJ, USA) containing either no anticoagulant or sodium heparin. Blood samples in sodium-heparin tubes were processed immediately using the automated haematology cell analyser Dymind DF50 Vet (Dymind, Shenchen, Guangdong, China) to determinate the following haematological parameters: haematocrit, haemoglobin, red blood cells, mean corpuscular volume, mean corpuscular haemoglobin, leukocytes, segmented leukocytes, eosinophils, lymphocytes and monocytes. Blood samples in tubes with no anticoagulant were allowed to clot for 30 min at room temperature and centrifuged at 2000× *g* for 15 min at 4 °C. The serum was stored at −20 °C until used to measure the metabolic profile (Analítica Veterinaria, Mungia, Spain), which consisted of: aspartate aminotransferase (AST), alanine aminotransferase (ALT), gamma glutamyl transferase (GGT), alkaline phosphatase (ALP), total protein, albumin, urea and creatinine.

2.5. Physicochemical Analysis

Feed samples were analysed for dry matter [20], ash [21], crude protein [22], neutral and acid detergent fibre [23,24] and ether extract [25]. Milk samples were assayed for fat, protein and lactose concentration by automatic infrared spectrophotometry [26] using a MilkoScan 255 A/S N (Foss Electric A/S, Hillerrød, Denmark), while somatic cell counts (SCC) were assayed by a fluoro-opto-electronic technique using a Fossomatic 90 A/S N (Foss Electric A/S, Hillerrød, Denmark)).

2.6. Aflatoxin Analysis

Aflatoxin M1 in milk was analysed by method ISO 14501:2007 with some modifications. Milk samples were thawed, then 100 mL was warmed to 37 °C for ten minutes and then centrifuged at 4200 rpm for 30 min to separate the fat layer. The extract (lower phase) was filtered through Whatman No. 4 filter paper. About 50 mL of the filtrate was transferred into a syringe barrel attached to an immunoaffinity clean-up column (IAC Afla M1, VICAM, Watertown, MA, USA) and passed at 1–2 drops per second. The column was rinsed with 20 mL of milli-Q water for impurities removal. After that, 1.25 mL of acetonitrile/methanol (3:2 *v/v*) and 1.25 mL of milli-Q water were passed through the column to elute aflatoxin M1. The eluate was filtered with a 0.45 µm filter, placed in autosampler vials and analysed by UPLC with fluorescence detection.

The chromatographic system consisted of an Acquity UPLC H-Class system (Waters Corp., Milford, MA, USA) coupled to a fluorescence detector (2475 Multi λ Fluorescence Detector, Waters Corp., Milford, MA, USA) and controlled by Empower 3 software (Waters Corp., Milford, MA, USA). Separation was carried out on an Acquity UPLC HSS T3 column (150 mm × 2.1 mm × 1.8 µm, Waters Corp., Milford, MA, USA), with a mobile phase consisting of water/acetonitrile/methanol (68:24:8, *v/v/v*) acidified with formic acid up to pH 2.0, pumped at a flow rate of 0.2 mL/min in isocratic mode. The samples and the column were kept at 5 °C and 35 °C, respectively. The injection volume was 15 µL and the total running time was 10 min. The retention time of AFM1 was approximately 6.25 min. The wavelength of the detector was set at 360 nm (excitation) and 440 nm (emission). The detection limit was 0.92 ng/L of AFM1.

Aflatoxins in the TMR were analysed by method EN 17375:2006 with some modifications, as described by Bervis et al. [6]. Briefly, a 25 g sample was extracted with a solvent solution, filtered and diluted with water. The assay portion was passed through an immunoaffinity column, eluted with methanol, and then quantified by reversed-phase high-performance liquid chromatography (RP-HPLC) with photochemical derivatization (PHRED) followed by fluorescence detection (FLD).

2.7. Calculations and Statistical Analysis

Data of daily milk yield and composition, AFM1 concentration and carryover, feed intake and blood parameters were analysed using a mixed model with the fixed effects of diet, sampling day and their interaction, and the random effect of the animal nested within the treatment and the residual error. Fat- and protein-corrected milk [27] on day 0 (before the commencement of the trial) was used as a covariate in the analyses of milk yield and composition. Different covariance matrices were evaluated based on Schwarz's Bayesian information model fit criteria. The linear mixed-effects model was performed using the lmerTest package [28] of the statistical software R version 3.3.3 [29].

The daily carryover of AFM1 in milk was calculated as the ratio between the AFM1 excreted in milk and the intake of AFB1 the previous day. Average carryover of AFM1 was calculated for the steady state (from day 4 to 13 of the experimental period). Clearance rate was calculated as the difference between AFM1 excretion on days 16 and 14 divided by that of day 14.

A stepwise regression analysis was performed (stats package of R) to select those independent parameters that helped to explain the variation in AFM1 excretion (dry matter intake, fat- and protein-corrected milk yield and AFB1 intake) and carryover rate (dry matter intake, fat- and protein-corrected milk yield, AFB1 intake and AFM1 excretion).

3. Results and Discussion

3.1. Feed Intake, Body Weight and Milk Yield and Composition

Table 1 shows that the ingestion of AFB1 (G) only affected the protein milk content ($p < 0.05$). The day of experiment (D) affected milk production and components ($p < 0.001$), but did not affect feed intake and udder health status (SCC). The G × D interaction was not significative in any case.

Table 1. Mean values of feed intake, milk yield and composition for animals receiving no AFB1 or 40 and 80 μg AFB1/day (groups C, L and H, respectively) throughout the experimental period.

	G	Days					s.e.d.			*p*-Value		
		D 1 *	D 4 *	D 7 *	D 14	D 18	G	D	G × D	G	D	G × D
Feed intake (kg/animal and day)	C	3.22	3.21	3.27	3.20	3.18	0.147	0.117	0.166	0.110	0.351	0.341
	L	3.13	3.04	2.92	3.15	3.01						
	H	2.92	3.03	3.04	3.14	2.77						
Milk yield (kg/animal and day)	C	2.38	2.00	1.93	1.95	1.79	0.139	0.095	0.136	0.987	<0.001	0.977
	L	2.39	1.95	2.01	1.90	1.84						
	H	2.38	1.85	2.02	1.89	1.88						
Fat (%)	C	5.80	5.94	5.50	5.66	5.75	0.351	0.208	0.294	0.792	<0.001	0.612
	L	5.90	5.70	5.84	5.48	5.67						
	H	5.89	5.82	5.78	5.70	5.80						
Protein (%)	C	4.90	5.03 ^{a}	5.07 ^{a}	4.88 ^{a}	4.92 ^{a}	0.156	0.066	0.093	0.010	<0.001	0.565
	L	4.93	5.20 ^{ab}	5.19 ^{ab}	5.11 ^{ab}	5.08 ^{ab}						
	H	5.20	5.54 ^{b}	5.53 ^{b}	5.40 ^{b}	5.37 ^{b}						
Lactose (%)	C	4.81	4.83	4.78	4.73	4.79	0.065	0.030	0.043	0.357	<0.001	0.528
	L	4.83	4.88	4.80	4.78	4.85						
	H	4.75	4.82	4.71	4.73	4.74						
Total solids (%)	C	16.50	16.60	16.20	16.20	16.50	0.431	0.228	0.322	0.228	<0.001	0.692
	L	16.70	16.60	16.70	16.30	16.60						
	H	16.90	17.00	16.90	16.80	17.00						
Somatic cell counts (log cells/mL)	C	4.88	4.79	4.78	4.80	4.76	0.160	0.062	0.089	0.724	0.169	0.689
	L	4.85	4.81	4.91	4.87	4.88						
	H	4.99	4.92	4.94	4.94	4.85						
Total solids (g/animal per day)	C	394	331	313	316	294	20.4	15.2	21.8	0.655	<0.001	0.846
	L	398	324	335	309	304						
	H	402	314	338	315	320						
Fat and protein corrected milk (kg/animal per day)	C	2.16	1.85	1.74	1.76	1.62	0.111	0.083	0.119	0.738	<0.001	0.687
	L	2.19	1.79	1.86	1.69	1.66						
	H	2.21	1.72	1.87	1.73	1.75						

s.e.d. = standard error of the difference; G = Group; D = Day; * = Animals in groups L and H received 40 and 80 μg AFB1/day, respectively, from D 1 to D 13. ^{a,b} Different letters within the same day indicate significant differences ($p < 0.05$) between groups.

A decrease in milk production was observed as the experimental period progressed, although this occurred for all three experimental groups. Variations over time in milk production and composition are common in sheep and have already been described in experiments carried out under similar conditions to those described in the present study [30]. Ewes in the H group (i.e., receiving the highest dose of AFB1) had a higher protein percentage than control ewes from day 4 until the end of the experimental period ($p < 0.05$). Changes in protein percentage due to AFB1 intake are not a common effect in dairy animals. Indeed, neither sheep [14,16,31], goats [32] nor cattle [33] have suffered modifications in milk protein content in response to AFB1 administration. Therefore, this is an unexpected finding because impaired microbial protein synthesis and total protein balance in dairy animals have been previously reported [9,11]. In any case, this increased milk protein content might be also partially explained by the fact that animals in the H group exhibited numerically higher protein contents from the beginning of the experiment (6% in day 1, which become significant from day 4 onwards, with increments of 10, 9, 11 and 9% on days 4, 7, 14 and 18, respectively).

According to previous reports [14–16,31], AFB1 intake did not affect milk production or composition. In the experiment carried out with Lacaune ewes [16], these even received doses of AFB1 much higher than in the present work, as they were given an average of 210 μg AFB1/animal/day for 4 weeks. On the other hand, the AFB1 doses tested in Sarda sheep without effects on productivity ranged from 2 mg in a single acute dose [14], through to 32 to 128 μg/animal per day for 1 week [15], and up to 7 μg/animal per day for 2 weeks [31].

In addition, no changes were observed in feed intake and body weight ($p > 0.05$), with mean body weight values being 79.8, 80.3 and 79.9 kg at the beginning and 82.3, 82.6 and 81.1 kg at the end of the experimental period for groups C, L and H, respectively. Previous reports [14–16,31] have also described no changes in these parameters in response to varying doses of AFB1 in the diet.

3.2. Haematological and Biochemical Parameters

AFB1 ingestion only affected the level of haemoglobin in the blood ($p < 0.05$). The day of the experiment affected most of the haematological parameters ($p < 0.05$–$p < 0.001$) and a great part of them presented significant G $\times$ D interactions ($p < 0.001$). In general, haematological and biochemical parameters except for blood urea remained within expected reference values for sheep [14,30,34,35]. The intake of AFB1 did not cause statistically significant changes ($p > 0.05$) in most of the analysed parameters throughout the experimental period (Tables 2 and 3). Blood urea stood out for its high value in relation to what has been referenced (20–53 mg/dl, [34,35]). However, studies on the Lacaune breed [36] showed that this parameter is usually higher in lactating animals (69.1 mg/dl).

Haematological parameters were affected by the day of sampling; however, changes that could be detected throughout the experiment were observed in all groups of animals. No significant differences were observed between groups in white blood cells counts and distribution, as well red blood cells' mean corpuscular volume and mean corpuscular haemoglobin ($p > 0.10$). The only effect that could be observed was a slight but significant increase in blood haemoglobin concentration ($p < 0.05$) and a tendency to increase haematocrit ($p < 0.10$) in group H animals at the end of the AFB1 ingestion period (day 14). This effect could be due to the cumulative effects of consecutive daily AFB1 intake, because the differences between groups disappeared after the clearance period (day 18). In any case, the values are within the normal range for sheep. The only recent study on this regard reported a reduction in this parameter in cows [37], whereas no changes have been reported in sheep [14] or goats [32]. This variability in response would seem to indicate that the effect would be dose- and species-dependent.

Table 2. Mean values of haematological parameters for animals receiving no AFB1 or 40 and 80 µg AFB1/day (groups C, L and H, respectively) throughout the experimental period.

	G	Days				s.e.d.			*p*-Value		
		D 1 *	D 7 *	D 14	D 18	G	D	G × D	G	D	G × D
	C	28.7	28.6	29.2	29.3	1.21	0.64	0.90	0.083	0.021	0.030
Hematocrit (%)	L	29.4	29.1	28.7	29.8						
	H	30.8	30.0	32.7	31.7						
	C	10.0	10.0	10.1 ^{a}	10.2	0.36	0.21	0.29	0.032	0.231	0.001
Haemoglobin (g/dL)	L	10.4	10.3	10.0 ^{a}	10.4						
	H	10.8	10.6	11.5 ^{b}	10.7						
	C	8.99	9.01	9.17	9.31	0.409	0.191	0.270	0.289	0.027	0.004
Red blood cells (10^6 cells/µL)	L	8.92	8.92	8.78	9.13						
	H	9.39	9.22	10.07	9.42						
	C	32.2	32.0	32.0	31.7	1.24	0.20	0.28	0.704	0.012	<0.001
Mean corpuscular volume (fl)	L	33.0	32.7	32.7	32.7						
	H	32.9	32.6	32.6	33.7						
	C	11.2	11.1	11.0	11.0	0.34	0.06	0.08	0.386	<0.001	0.533
Mean corpuscular haemoglobin (pg)	L	11.6	11.5	11.4	11.4						
	H	11.5	11.5	11.5	11.4						
	C	34.8	35.0	34.7	35.0	0.88	0.23	0.33	0.957	<0.001	<0.001
Mean corpuscular haemoglobin (g/dL)	L	35.3	35.3	34.9	34.8						
	H	35.1	35.4	35.1	33.8						
	C	7.69	7.63	8.20	7.79	0.957	0.398	0.563	0.993	0.007	0.723
Leukocytes (10^3 cells /µL)	L	7.36	8.06	8.21	8.11						
	H	7.33	8.04	8.46	7.77						
	C	30.4	36.9	28.0	31.2	4.13	3.34	4.72	0.832	<0.001	<0.001
Segmented leukocytes (%)	L	27.4	36.1	23.4	32.6						
	H	25.2	34.4	38.2	23.8						
	C	2.20	5.70	1.00	3.50	1.132	1.030	1.456	0.576	<0.001	0.281
Eosinophils (%)	L	2.60	7.30	1.20	1.60						
	H	2.60	5.60	0.60	1.20						
Lymphocytes (%)	C	58.2	49.7	63.2	56.2	3.90	3.21	4.54	0.704	<0.001	0.001
Lymphocytes (%)	L	60.6	49.1	66.2	58.0						
	H	62.4	52.6	54.6	66.6						
Monocytes (%)	C	9.20	7.70	7.80	9.40	1.442	1.342	1.897	0.813	0.067	0.568
Monocytes (%)	L	9.40	7.50	9.20	7.80						
Segmented leukocytes	H	9.80	7.30	6.60	8.40						
(10^3 cells /µL)	C	2.12	2.83	2.32	2.47	0.475	0.321	0.453	0.994	<0.001	0.001
Segmented leukocytes	L	2.00	2.98	1.93	2.67						
(10^3 cells /µL)	H	1.87	2.77	3.19	1.77						
Eosinophils (10^3 cells /µL)	C	0.171	0.447	0.067	0.236	0.0985	0.0922	0.1304	0.550	<0.001	0.554
	L	0.208	0.607	0.085	0.129						
Eosinophils (10^3 cells /µL)	H	0.182	0.447	0.051	0.096						
Lymphocytes (10^3 cells /µL)	C	4.41	3.76	5.17	4.31	0.606	0.317	0.449	0.888	<0.001	0.029
	L	4.46	3.87	5.44	4.68						
Lymphocytes (10^3 cells /µL)	H	4.53	4.23	4.64	5.24						
Monocytes (10^3 cells /µL)	C	0.670	0.595	0.644	0.749	0.1404	0.1095	0.1548	0.961	0.351	0.627
Monocytes (10^3 cells /µL)	L	0.705	0.597	0.750	0.614						
	H	0.736	0.588	0.569	0.668						

s.e.d. = standard error of the difference; G = Group; D = Day; * = Animals in groups L and H received 40 and 80 µg AFB1/day, respectively, from D 1 to D 13. [a,b] Different letters within the same day indicate significant differences ($p < 0.05$) between groups.

Regarding effects on blood biochemistry, most of the parameters were affected by the day of sampling, indicating an evolution over time of some of them throughout the course of the experiment in all groups of animals. Some authors have pointed out that high acute doses of AFB1 (2 mg, single dose) can lead to liver damage, usually manifested by alterations in ALP in sheep [11,14] or AST in cattle [38]. However, Battacone et al. [31] showed that low doses (up to 7 µg AFB1/day) did not lead to alterations in blood biochemistry. The animals in the present experiment received between 40 and 80 µg AFB1/day, giving a total cumulative dose of 600 and 1200 µg AFB1, which is much lower than the acute dose used by Battacone et al. [14]. Thus, the only remarkable differences were the tendency to increase in alanine aminotransferase (ALT) and total protein concentrations on day 14 ($p < 0.10$), which disappeared on day 18. This brief temporal increase could be attributable to the potential damage caused by the cumulative effects of AFB1 on liver metabolism that disappeared after the clearance period [10,11,37–39].

Table 3. Mean values of serum biochemical parameters for animals receiving no AFB1 or 40 and 80 µg AFB1/day (groups C, L and H, respectively) throughout the experimental period.

		Days				s.e.d.			*p*-Value		
	G	D 1 *	D 7 *	D 14	D 18	G	D	G × D	G	D	G × D
Aspartate aminotransferase (AST, IU/L)	C	116	140	145	139	21.3	8.7	12.3	0.964	<0.001	0.958
	L	116	131	135	136						
	H	114	131	140	140						
Alanine aminotransferase (ALT, IU/L)	C	28.7	28.6	29.2	29.3	1.213	0.639	0.903	0.083	0.021	0.030
	L	29.4	29.1	28.7	29.8						
	H	30.8	29.9	32.7	31.7						
Gamma glutamyl transferase (GGT, IU/L)	C	48.1	69.2	65.9	59.7	8.13	5.06	7.15	0.573	0.004	0.224
	L	50.9	56.8	56.3	54.9						
	H	51.2	54.7	54.7	55.8						
Alkaline phosphatase (ALP, IU/L)	C	185	245	229	200	51.6	15.0	21.2	0.988	0.020	0.010
	L	230	227	215	218						
	H	235	233	206	206						
Total protein (g/dl)	C	6.68	6.29	6.76	7.01	0.217	0.143	0.202	0.096	<0.001	0.061
	L	6.59	6.14	6.87	6.91						
	H	6.93	6.47	7.49	7.11						
Albumin (g/dl)	C	3.39	3.28	3.49	3.52	0.163	0.092	0.130	0.575	<0.001	0.931
	L	3.46	3.31	3.60	3.67						
	H	3.47	3.42	3.68	3.72						
Urea (mg/dl)	C	66.5	59.3	60.8	59.5	3.35	2.19	3.09	0.625	<0.001	0.127
	L	66.6	61.1	61.9	64.8						
	H	71.5	62.2	62.6	59.9						
Creatinine (mg/dl)	C	0.780	0.740	0.750	0.780	0.0468	0.0351	0.0497	0.999	0.132	0.339
	L	0.740	0.760	0.770	0.780						
	H	0.800	0.700	0.780	0.770						

s.e.d. = standard error of the difference; G = Group; D = Day; * = Animals in groups L and H received 40 and 80 µg AFB1/day, respectively, from D 1 to D 13.

3.3. AFM1 Excretion

Both the ingestion of AFB1 (G) and the day of the experiment (D) affected the excretion of AFM1 ($p < 0.001$), and a significant G×D interaction ($p < 0.001$) was also observed (Tables 4 and 5). No differences between groups were observed in the present study on day 1, coinciding with the start of AFB1 supplementation ($p > 0.10$). The increase in AFM1 concentration observed in the supplemented groups (L, H) compared to the control group was already significant ($p < 0.001$) on day 2 (first milk sampling after AFB1 supplementation), reaching a mean AFM1 concentration of 45.6 ng/L in group L, and

68.6 ng/L in group H, which confirms that the toxin ingested orally is easily absorbed in the gastrointestinal tract and rapidly metabolised [9], as observed in previous studies in sheep supplemented with AFB1 [14–16,31].

It should be noted that AFM1 excretion was highly variable both between animals of the same group within each day and between days for the same animal. The presence of AFM1 was detected in all milk samples from the control group, with a mean concentration of 3.33 ng/L. The presence of AFM1 at residual concentrations was expected, since AFB1 (0.06 μg/kg), as well as aflatoxins B2 and G1 (0.03 and 0.05 μg/kg, respectively) were detected in the basal rations of the experiment.

Table 4. Mean values of AFM1 excretion in milk (ng AFM1/L milk) for animals receiving no AFB1 or 40 and 80 μg AFB1/day (groups C, L and H, respectively) throughout the experimental period.

	ng AFM1/L Milk											
	D 1 *	D 2 *	D 3 *	D 4 *	D 7 *	D 14	D 16	D 18		G	D	G × D
C	2.9	2.9 ^{x}	5.7 ^{x}	3.3 ^{x}	3.6 ^{x}	3.1 ^{x}	2.7	3	s.e.d.	10.16	9.14	12.92
L	2.7 ^{a}	45.6 ^{b,y}	55.9 ^{b,y}	71.9 ^{b,y}	56.2 ^{b,y}	57.2 ^{b,y}	8.3 ^{a}	2.4 ^{a}	*p*-value	<0.001	<0.001	<0.001
H	2.9 ^{a}	68.6 ^{b,z}	61.1 ^{b,y}	79.3 ^{b,y}	71.4 ^{b,y}	64.7 ^{b,y}	8.9 ^{a}	3.3 ^{a}				

s.e.d. = standard error of the difference; G = Group; D = Day; * = Animals in groups L and H received 40 and 80 μg AFB1/day, respectively, from D 1 to D 13. ^{a,b} Different letters within the same group indicate significant differences ($p < 0.001$) between days for a given parameter. ^{x,y} Different letters within the same day indicate significant differences ($p < 0.001$) between groups for a given parameter.

Table 5. Mean values of AFM1 excretion in milk (ng AFM1/animal and day) for animals receiving no AFB1 or 40 and 80 μg AFB1/day (groups C, L and H, respectively) throughout the experimental period.

	ng AFM1/Animal and Day											
	D 1 *	D 2 *	D 3 *	D 4 *	D 7 *	D 14	D 16	D 18		G	D	G × D
C	10.2	9.1 ^{x}	13.5 ^{x}	10.0 ^{x}	10.5 ^{x}	9.3 ^{x}	8.3	8.8	s.e.d.	21.54	18.47	26.51
L	6.4 ^{a}	90.2 ^{b,y}	104.8 ^{b,y}	136.4 ^{b,y}	106.8 ^{b,y}	108.9 ^{b,y}	15.4 ^{a}	4.2 ^{a}	*p*-value	<0.001	<0.001	<0.001
H	3.5 ^{a}	151.6 ^{b,z}	123.7 ^{b,y}	149.2 ^{b,y}	150.1 ^{b,y}	124.0 ^{b,y}	13.2 ^{a}	3.0 ^{a}				

s.e.d. = standard error of the difference; G = Group; D = Day; * = Animals in groups L and H received 40 and 80 μg AFB1/day, respectively, from D 1 to D 13. ^{a,b} Different letters within the same group indicate significant differences ($p < 0.001$) between days for a given parameter. ^{x,y} Different letters within the same day indicate significant differences ($p < 0.001$) between groups for a given parameter.

In the period of toxin supplementation, no statistically significant differences were observed within the same group between days 3 and 14, which could be considered a steady-state phase. This phase starts with an upward trend, reaching the maximum concentration on day 4 (79.3 and 71.9 ng/L in groups H and L, respectively). Once this maximum was reached, a downward trend was observed, with mean concentrations of 64.7 ng/L in group H and 57.2 ng/L in group L on day 14 (the first day after cessation of AFB1 supply). This kinetics, which has been described also in cattle [9,10,37] and goats [32], is very similar to those reported in sheep supplemented with doses of 23 μg, 64 μg and 128 μg of AFB1 [15]. Zhang et al. [40], in an in vitro assay, observed an increase AFM1 transporter protein gene expression followed by a gradual decrease with AFM1 incubation time. In addition, the decrease in milk yield during the experimental period may entail a reduction in the number of epithelial mammary cells and, therefore, a decrease in the transport of AFM1 to milk.

From days 14 to 16 (two days after AFB1 supply was stopped), the AFM1 concentration decreased rapidly to 8.9 and 8.3 ng/L for groups H and L, respectively, with the average clearance rates being 86 and 90% per day (3.8 and 5.1 ng/h). Clearance rates are highly variable between experiments; however, these values are within the wide range reported by other authors for dairy cattle [33,37,41]. On day 16, no statistically significant differences in AFM1 concentration in milk were observed between control and L and H groups. Likewise, the decrease in AFM1 concentration continued on day 18, as expected, when the mean concentrations were 3.27 ng/L (H group) and 2.36 ng/L (L group). These results agree with those obtained by Battacone et al. [31] in ewes fed with naturally contaminated feed, resulting in AFB1 intakes of 1.58, 3.22 and 7.07 µg/day. In ewes supplemented with 32, 64 and 128 µg of AFB1, Battacone et al. [14,15] reported that slightly longer periods (between 3 and 4 days) were needed for the disappearance of AFM1 in milk (restoration to the baseline situation).

The analysis of the regression of AFM1 concentration in milk versus AFB1 intake, milk yield and dry matter intake on the steady-state phase (once the plateau has been reached, days 2 to 14) allowed us to express AFM1 concentration in milk according to the following Equation (1):

$$\text{AFM1 (ng/L milk)} = 6.67 + 0.88 \times \text{AFB1 } (\mu\text{g/day}) \quad (1)$$

Residual standard error (RSE) = 23.57, R-square = 0.589, $p < 0.001$.

This means that the presence of AFM1 in milk, under the conditions of the present experiment, depends mainly on the amount of AFB1 ingested, and is not affected by the total dry matter intake or milk production. Furthermore, our results show that there may be a small amount of excretion of AFM1 in milk without being detected in the feed, something that has already been suggested by other authors [2].

Although the dose of AFB1 given to group H (80 µg) was twice that given to group L (40 µg), the excretion of AFM1 was only slightly higher in group H, and no statistically significant differences in AFM1 concentration were observed between the two groups within the same day of treatment in the plateau phase. This lack of difference is related to the carryover rate from AFB1 to AFM1, as discussed below.

3.4. *AFM1/AFB1 Carryover*

The carryover rate of AFB1 ingested orally to AFM1 excreted in milk was calculated. In so doing, the amount of AFB1 given to each animal, the individual milk production data and the concentration of AFM1 in milk was taken into consideration (Table 6). Overall, the carryover rate was around 0.23% (AFM1/AFB1) considering the average of both, L and H groups, during the steady-state phase (days 2 to 14 of the experimental period).

Table 6. Mean values of AFM1 carry over (AFM1/AFB1, %) for animals receiving 40 and 80 µg AFB1/day (groups L and H, respectively) throughout the experimental period.

	D 2 *	D 3 *	D 4 *	D 7 *	D 14	D 16		G	D	G × D
L	0.224 ^{b}	0.262 ^{b,y}	0.341 ^{b,y}	0.267 ^{b}	0.270 ^{b,y}	0.039 ^{a}	s.e.d.	0.0529	0.0424	0.0590
H	0.194 ^{b}	0.159 ^{b,x}	0.191 ^{b,x}	0.192 ^{b}	0.160 ^{b,x}	0.021 ^{a}	*p*-value	0.035	<0.001	0.193

s.e.d. = standard error of the difference; G = Group; D = Day; * = Animals in groups L and H received 40 and 80 µg AFB1/day, respectively, from D 1 to D 13. ^{a,b} Different letters within the same group indicate significant differences ($p < 0.001$) between days. ^{x,y} Different letters within the same day indicate significant differences ($p < 0.001$) between groups.

Both AFB1 ingestion (G) and the day of experiment affected ($p < 0.05$ and $p < 0.001$, respectively) AFM1 carry over, but the G × D interaction was not significant ($p > 0.10$, Table 6). From day 3 until the withdrawal of the AFB1 supplementation, the transfer rate was significantly higher ($p < 0.05$) in animals given 40 µg (0.22–0.34%) compared to those receiving 80 µg (0.16–0.19%). A similar dose-response in carryover rate has been already reported in dairy cows [10]. The results obtained are also in line with those reported by Battacone et al. [15] in ewes supplemented with 32, 64 and 128 µg AFB1 (0.33%, 0.29% and 0.26%, respectively). These authors observed a decreasing trend in carryover rate, without statistical significance between groups, as the AFB1 intake increased. Further research on sheep fed with naturally contaminated feeds (AFB1 intake of 1.58, 3.22 and 7.07 µg/day), revealed higher carryover rates (2.9, 1.9 and 1.3%, respectively) than those obtained in our study. These values also differed significantly depending on the dose ingested: the higher the AFB1 intake, the lower the carryover rate [31]. Carryover rates observed for Assaf ewes are somewhat lower than those reported for Lacaune ewes (0.24–0.54% [16]), even though the latter received higher doses (up to 160 μg/day) than those in the present study. Therefore, carryover rate in sheep depends not only on the dose and the individual; the breed also seems to have a clear influence.

The observed inverse relationship between AFM1 transfer and amount of AFB1 ingested could be related to the biotransformation processes of this mycotoxin in different animal tissues. Thus, AFB1 is metabolised through complex metabolic pathways involving different enzyme systems whose activity would be modified by increasing doses of AFB1, which would eventually be metabolised and secreted by other pathways. In fact, several studies have shown that the extensive variability in the expression and catalytic activity of liver enzymes involved in the biotransformation and detoxification of AFB1 (such as cytochrome P450 and glutathione transferases) are considered to be the main cause of the differences in AFM1/AFB1 transfer found between species [9–11,32].

Regression analysis shows that the carryover rate (AFM1/AFB1, %) in the steady-state phase (once the plateau was reached, from days 2 to 14) can be expressed as a function of AFM1 concentration in milk, AFB1 intake and milk yield according to the following Equation (2):

$$\text{AFM1/AFB1 (\%)} = 0.049 + 0.091 \times \text{Milk yield (L/day)} + 0.003 \times \text{AFM1 (ng/L)} - 0.003 \times \text{AFB1 } (\mu\text{g/d}) \quad (2)$$

RSE = 0.045, R-square = 0.887; $p < 0.001$.

Therefore, carryover rate is positively influenced by the level of milk production (probably due to increased numbers of mammary epithelial cells or AFM1 transporter proteins). Likewise, the negative influence of AFB1 may be explained by the limited AFM1 transport capacity [40].

4. Conclusions

In Assaf ewes that receive a daily dose of AFB1 (40 or 80 μg) for 13 days, the excretion of AFM1 in milk from starts 24 h after the first intake and depends on the dose. AFM1/AFB1 carryover is higher in animals supplemented with 40 μg AFB1 (0.22–0.34%) than in those receiving 80 μg AFB1 (0.16–0.19%). Likewise, carryover rate is positively influenced by milk yield. Once AFB1 intake has ceased, AFM1 decreases sharply, with a clearance rate of nearly 90% in the first 24 h. At the levels tested in the present study, AFB1 intake does not impair milk yield; however, it might affect animals' health since changes in haemoglobin, ALT and total proteins were observed after 13 days AFB1 supplementation.

Author Contributions: Conceptualization, R.B., F.J.G., M.H., A.A. and T.J.; methodology, R.B., F.J.G., S.O., M.H., S.L. (Susana Lorán), A.A., S.L. (Secundino López), A.B. and T.J.; formal analysis, R.B., F.J.G., S.O., M.H., S.L. (Susana Lorán), A.A., S.L. (Secundino López), A.B. and T.J.; investigation, R.B., F.J.G., M.H., S.L. (Susana Lorán), A.A. and T.J.; resources, R.B., F.J.G., A.A. and T.J.; data curation, R.B. and T.J.; writing—original draft preparation, R.B., M.H. and T.J.; writing—review and editing, F.J.G., S.O., S.L. (Susana Lorán) and A.A.; project administration, R.B., S.O., A.A. and T.J.; funding acquisition, R.B., S.O., A.A., S.L. (Secundino López) and T.J. All authors have read and agreed to the published version of the manuscript.

Funding: This research was funded by the Spanish Agencia Estatal de Investigación (grant number INIA RTA 2017-00085), and the Government of Aragón (grant Grupo A06-20R).

Institutional Review Board Statement: The study was conducted according to the guidelines of the Directive 2010/63/EU on the protection of animals used for scientific purposes, and approved by the Institutional Animal Care and Use Committee of the Agrarian Technological Institute of Castilla y León (ITACyL, Spain) and the competent authority (Directive 2010/63/EU) under the protocol number 2017/25/OH.

Informed Consent Statement: Not applicable.

Data Availability Statement: The data presented in this study are available on request from the corresponding author.

Acknowledgments: Raúl Carbajo and Juan Ramón Bertolín for his technical support.

Conflicts of Interest: The authors declare no conflict of interest.

References

1. De Roma, A.; Rossini, C.; Ritieni, A.; Gallo, P.; Esposito, M. A Survey on the Aflatoxin M1 Occurrence and Seasonal Variation in Buffalo and Cow Milk from Southern Italy. *Food Control* **2017**, *81*, 30–33. [CrossRef]
2. Rodríguez-Blanco, M.; Ramos, A.J.; Prim, M.; Sanchis, V.; Marín, S. Usefulness of the Analytical Control of Aflatoxins in Feedstuffs for Dairy Cows for the Prevention of Aflatoxin M1 in Milk. *Mycotoxin Res.* **2020**, *36*, 11–22. [CrossRef] [PubMed]
3. Rodríguez-Blanco, M.; Ramos, A.J.; Sanchis, V.; Marín, S. Mycotoxins Occurrence and Fungal Populations in Different Types of Silages for Dairy Cows in Spain. *Fungal Biol.* **2021**, *125*, 103–114. [CrossRef] [PubMed]
4. Rubio, R.; Licón, C.C.; Berruga, M.I.; Molina, M.P.; Molina, A. Short Communication: Occurrence of Aflatoxin M1 in the Manchego Cheese Supply Chain. *J. Dairy Sci.* **2011**, *94*, 2775–2778. [CrossRef] [PubMed]
5. Ogunade, I.M.; Martinez-Tuppia, C.; Queiroz, O.C.M.; Jiang, Y.; Drouin, P.; Wu, F.; Vyas, D.; Adesogan, A.T. Silage Review: Mycotoxins in Silage: Occurrence, Effects, Prevention, and Mitigation. *J. Dairy Sci.* **2018**, *101*, 4034–4059. [CrossRef] [PubMed]
6. Bervis, N.; Lorán, S.; Juan, T.; Carramiñana, J.J.; Herrera, A.; Ariño, A.; Herrera, M. Field Monitoring of Aflatoxins in Feed and Milk of High-Yielding Dairy Cows under Two Feeding Systems. *Toxins* **2021**, *13*, 201. [CrossRef] [PubMed]
7. Waqas, M.; Pervaiz, W.; Zia, K.M.; Iqbal, S.Z. Assessment of Aflatoxin B1 in Animal Feed and Aflatoxin M1 in Raw Milk Samples of Different Species of Milking Animals from Punjab, Pakistan. *J. Food Saf.* **2021**, *41*, e12893. [CrossRef]
8. Tarja, L. Russia's War on Ukraine: EU Food Policy Implications. Available online: https://policycommons.net/artifacts/2325126/russias-war-on-ukraine/3085659/ (accessed on 16 June 2022).
9. Min, L.; Fink-Gremmels, J.; Li, D.; Tong, X.; Tang, J.; Nan, X.; Yu, Z.; Chen, W.; Wang, G. An Overview of Aflatoxin B1 Biotransformation and Aflatoxin M1 Secretion in Lactating Dairy Cows. *Anim. Nutr.* **2021**, *7*, 42–48. [CrossRef]
10. Wang, Q.; Zhang, Y.; Zheng, N.; Guo, L.; Song, X.; Zhao, S.; Wang, J. Biological System Responses of Dairy Cows to Aflatoxin B1 Exposure Revealed with Metabolomic Changes in Multiple Biofluids. *Toxins* **2019**, *11*, 77. [CrossRef]
11. Mavrommatis, A.; Giamouri, E.; Tavrizelou, S.; Zacharioudaki, M.; Danezis, G.; Simitzis, P.E.; Zoidis, E.; Tsiplakou, E.; Pappas, A.C.; Georgiou, C.A.; et al. Impact of Mycotoxins on Animals' Oxidative Status. *Antioxidants* **2021**, *10*, 214. [CrossRef] [PubMed]
12. EFSA (EFSA Panel on Contaminants in the Food Chain). Scientific Opinion—Risk assessment of aflatoxins in food. *EFSA J.* **2020**, *18*, e06040. [CrossRef]
13. Nidhina, N.; Bhavya, M.L.; Bhaskar, N.; Muthukumar, S.P.; Murthy, P.S. Aflatoxin Production by Aspergillus Flavus in Rumen Liquor and Its Implications. *Food Control* **2017**, *71*, 26–31. [CrossRef]
14. Battacone, G.; Nudda, A.; Cannas, A.; Borlino, A.C.; Bomboi, G.; Pulina, G. Excretion of Aflatoxin M1 in Milk of Dairy Ewes Treated with Different Doses of Aflatoxin B1. *J. Dairy Sci.* **2003**, *86*, 2667–2675. [CrossRef] [PubMed]
15. Battacone, G.; Nudda, A.; Palomba, M.; Pascale, M.; Nicolussi, P.; Pulina, G. Transfer of Aflatoxin B1 from Feed to Milk and from Milk to Curd and Whey in Dairy Sheep Fed Artificially Contaminated Concentrates. *J. Dairy Sci.* **2005**, *88*, 3063–3069. [CrossRef] [PubMed]
16. Firmin, S.; Morgavi, D.P.; Yiannikouris, A.; Boudra, H. Effectiveness of Modified Yeast Cell Wall Extracts to Reduce Aflatoxin B1 Absorption in Dairy Ewes. *J. Dairy Sci.* **2011**, *94*, 5611–5619. [CrossRef] [PubMed]
17. MAPA (Ministerio de Agricultura, Pesca y Alimentación). El Sector Ovino y Caprino de Leche En Cifras: Principales Indicadores Económicos. Subdirección General de Producciones Ganaderas y Cinegéticas, Dirección General de Producciones y Mercados Agrarios. Available online: https://www.mapa.gob.es/es/ganaderia/estadisticas/indicadoreseconomicosdelsectorovinoycaprinodeleche2022_tcm30-553590.pdf (accessed on 28 November 2022).
18. Milán, M.J.; Caja, G.; González-González, R.; Fernández-Pérez, A.M.; Such, X. Structure and Performance of Awassi and Assaf Dairy Sheep Farms in Northwestern Spain. *J. Dairy Sci.* **2011**, *94*, 771–784. [CrossRef]
19. Legaz, E.A. Caracterización de la Raza Assaf en España. Ph.D. Thesis, Universidad Complutense de Madrid, Madrid, Spain, 2016.
20. *Standard 6496:1999*; ISO Animal Feeding Stuffs—Determination of Moisture Adn Other Volatile Matter Content. International Organization for Standardization: Geneva, Switzerland, 1999.
21. *Standard 5984:2002*; ISO Animal Feeding Stuffs—Determination of Crude Ash. International Organization for Standardization: Geneva, Switzerland, 2002.
22. *Standard 5983-2:2005*; ISO Animal Feeding Stuffs—Determination of Nitrogen Content and Calculation of Crude Protein Content—Part 2: Block Digestion and Steam Distillation Method. International Organization for Standardization: Geneva, Switzerland, 2005.
23. *Ankom Technology Method 8*; Ankom Technology Acid Detergent Fiber in Feeds. Filter Bag Technique (For A2000, A2000I). Ankom Technology: Macedon, NY, USA, 2006.
24. *Ankom Technology Method 9*; Ankom Technology Neutral Detergent Fiber in Feeds. Filter Bag Technique (For A2000, A2000I). Ankom Technology: Macedon, NY, USA, 2006.
25. American Oil Chemists' Society (AOCS). *Official Methods and Recommended Practices*, 5th ed.; American Oil Chemists' Society: Champaign, IL, USA, 2008.
26. *Standard 9622:1999*; ISO Whole Milk—Determination of Milkfat, Protein and Lactose Content—Guidance on the Operation of Mid-Infrared Instruments. International Organization for Standardization: Geneva, Switzerland, 1999.
27. Pulina, G.; Macciotta, N.; Nudda, A. Milk Composition and Feeding in the Italian Dairy Sheep. *Ital. J. Anim. Sci.* **2005**, *4*, 5–14. [CrossRef]

28. Kuznetsova, A.; Brockhoff, P.B.; Christensen, R.H.B. LmerTest Package: Tests in Linear Mixed Effects Models. *J. Stat. Softw.* **2017**, *82*, 1–26. [CrossRef]
29. R Core Team. *R: A Language and Environment for Statistical Computing*; R Foundation for Statistical Computing: Vienna, Austria, 2022.
30. Pulido, E.; Giráldez, F.J.; Bodas, R.; Andrés, S.; Prieto, N. Effect of Reduction of Milking Frequency and Supplementation of Vitamin E and Selenium above Requirements on Milk Yield and Composition in Assaf Ewes. *J. Dairy Sci.* **2012**, *95*, 3527–3535. [CrossRef]
31. Battacone, G.; Nudda, A.; Palomba, M.; Mazzette, A.; Pulina, G. The Transfer of Aflatoxin M1 in Milk of Ewes Fed Diet Naturally Contaminated by Aflatoxins and Effect of Inclusion of Dried Yeast Culture in the Diet. *J. Dairy Sci.* **2009**, *92*, 4997–5004. [CrossRef]
32. Huang, S.; Zheng, N.; Fan, C.; Cheng, M.; Wang, S.; Jabar, A.; Wang, J.; Cheng, J. Effects of Aflatoxin B1 Combined with Ochratoxin A and/or Zearalenone on Metabolism, Immune Function, and Antioxidant Status in Lactating Dairy Goats. *Asian-Australas. J. Anim. Sci.* **2018**, *31*, 505–513. [CrossRef] [PubMed]
33. Rodrigues, R.O.; Rodrigues, R.O.; Ledoux, D.R.; Rottinghaus, G.E.; Borutova, R.; Averkieva, O.; McFadden, T.B. Feed Additives Containing Sequestrant Clay Minerals and Inactivated Yeast Reduce Aflatoxin Excretion in Milk of Dairy Cows. *J. Dairy Sci.* **2019**, *102*, 6614–6623. [CrossRef] [PubMed]
34. David, C.M.G.; Costa, R.L.D.; Parren, G.A.E.; Rua, M.A.S.; Nordi, E.C.P.; Paz, C.C.P.; Quirino, C.R.; Figueiredo, R.S.; Bohland, E.; David, C.M.G.; et al. Hematological, Parasitological and Biochemical Parameters in Sheep during the Peripartum Period. *Rev. Colomb. Cienc. Pecu* **2020**, *33*, 81–95. [CrossRef]
35. The Merck Veterinary Manual. Available online: https://search.library.wisc.edu/catalog/9911027735002121 (accessed on 30 June 2022).
36. Nedeva, I.; Slavov, T.; Varlyakov, I.; Radev, V.; Panayotov, D. Haematological and Blood Biochemical Parameters in Lacaune Dairy Sheep. *Bulg. J. Agric. Sci.* **2019**, *25*, 91–95.
37. Ogunade, I.M.; Arriola, K.G.; Jiang, Y.; Driver, J.P.; Staples, C.R.; Adesogan, A.T. Effects of 3 Sequestering Agents on Milk Aflatoxin M1 Concentration and the Performance and Immune Status of Dairy Cows Fed Diets Artificially Contaminated with Aflatoxin B1. *J. Dairy Sci.* **2016**, *99*, 6263–6273. [CrossRef] [PubMed]
38. Sulzberger, S.A.; Melnichenko, S.; Cardoso, F.C. Effects of Clay after an Aflatoxin Challenge on Aflatoxin Clearance, Milk Production, and Metabolism of Holstein Cows. *J. Dairy Sci.* **2017**, *100*, 1856–1869. [CrossRef] [PubMed]
39. Wang, Q.; Zhang, Y.; Zheng, N.; Zhao, S.; Li, S.; Wang, J. The Biochemical and Metabolic Profiles of Dairy Cows with Mycotoxins-Contaminated Diets. *PeerJ* **2020**, *8*, e8742. [CrossRef]
40. Zhang, Y.; Zhang, N.; Chen, D.; Huang, G.; Cao, H. Investigation of the Transport of Aflatoxin M1 by the Transporter ABCG2 in Bovine Mammary Epithelial Cells. *Med. Weter.* **2020**, *76*, 646–651. [CrossRef]
41. Queiroz, O.C.M.; Han, J.H.; Staples, C.R.; Adesogan, A.T. Effect of Adding a Mycotoxin-Sequestering Agent on Milk Aflatoxin M1 Concentration and the Performance and Immune Response of Dairy Cattle Fed an Aflatoxin B1-Contaminated Diet. *J. Dairy Sci.* **2012**, *95*, 5901–5908. [CrossRef]

animals

MDPI

Article

Zinc Oxide Nanoparticles (ZnO-NPs) Induce Cytotoxicity in the Zebrafish Olfactory Organs via Activating Oxidative Stress and Apoptosis at the Ultrastructure and Genetic Levels

Sheren A. Al-Zahaby [1], Mayada R. Farag [2], Mahmoud Alagawany [3,*], Heba S. A. Taha [4], Maria Vittoria Varoni [5,*], Giuseppe Crescenzo [6,†] and Suzan Attia Mawed [1,†]

1 Zoology Department, Faculty of Science, Zagazig University, Zagazig 44519, Egypt; sherin@zu.edu.eg (S.A.A.-Z.); samoawad@zu.edu.eg (S.A.M.)
2 Forensic Medicine and Toxicology Department, Faculty of Veterinary Medicine, Zagazig University, Zagazig 44519, Egypt; dr.mayadarf@gmail.com
3 Poultry Department, Faculty of Agriculture, Zagazig University, Zagazig 44519, Egypt
4 Genetics Department, Faculty of Agriculture, Zagazig University, Zagazig 44519, Egypt; hebasayedtaha@gmail.com
5 Department of Veterinary Medicine, University of Sassari, 07100 Sassari, Italy
6 Department of Veterinary Medicine, University of Bari, 70010 Valenzano, Italy; giuseppe.crescenzo@uniba.it
* Correspondence: dr.mahmoud.alagwany@gmail.com (M.A.); varoni@uniss.it (M.V.V.)
† These authors contributed equally to this work.

Simple Summary: Zinc oxide nanoparticles (ZnO-NPs) can exert toxic effects on living organisms. The fish olfactory epithelium is considered the first organ affected by ZnO-NPs, and we demonstrated that a 60-day exposure to ZnO-NPs induced significant malformations of the olfactory rosettes at histological, ultrastructural, and genetic levels in zebrafish, affecting the cellular repairing mechanisms. The present study shows that ZnO-NPs can mediate the cellular oxidative stress and arrest cell growth that induces apoptosis without the ability of cellular regeneration, damaging the olfactory epithelium and affecting fish smell and appetite.

Abstract: Nanotechnology has gained tremendous attention because of its crucial characteristics and wide biomedical applications. Although zinc oxide nanoparticles (ZnO-NPs) are involved in many industrial applications, researchers pay more attention to their toxic effects on living organisms. Since the olfactory epithelium is exposed to the external environment, it is considered the first organ affected by ZnO-NPs. Herein, we demonstrated the cytotoxic effect of ZnO-NPs on the olfactory organ of adult zebrafish after 60 days post-treatment. We opted for this period when fishes stop eating their diet from the aquarium, appear feeble, and cannot swim freely. Our study demonstrated that ZnO-NPs induced significant malformations of the olfactory rosettes at histological, ultrastructural, and genetic levels. At the ultrastructure level, the olfactory lamellae appeared collapsed, malformed, and twisted with signs of degeneration and loss of intercellular connections. In addition, ZnO-NPs harmed sensory receptor and ciliated cells, microvilli, rodlet, crypt, and Kappe cells, with hyperactivity of mucous secretion from goblet cells. At the genetic level, ZnO-NPs could activate the reactive oxygen species (ROS) synthesis expected by the down-regulation of mRNA expression for the antioxidant-related genes and up-regulation of DNA damage, cell growth arrest, and apoptosis. Interestingly, ZnO-NPs affected the odor sensation at 60 days post-treatment (60-dpt) more than at 30-dpt, severely damaging the olfactory epithelium and irreparably affecting the cellular repairing mechanisms. This induced a dramatically adverse effect on the cellular endoplasmic reticulum (ER), revealed by higher CHOP protein expression, that suppresses the antioxidant effect of Nrf2 and is followed by the induction of apoptosis via the up-regulation of Bax expression and down-regulation of Bcl-2 protein.

Keywords: zebrafish; zinc oxide nanoparticles (ZnO-NPs); olfactory epithelium; oxidative stress; apoptosis

1. Introduction

The future insight into nanomaterials utilization has grown considerably. Along with silicon dioxide nanoparticles, zinc oxide nanoparticles (ZnO-NPs) are considered one of the most applied nanomaterials in biomedical industries [1–6]. The bio-safety of ZnO-NPs is still a controversial issue since increasing studies assumed that they are biocompatible and could be applied to biomedical materials [7–10]; at the same time, others indicated the toxicological influences of ZnO-NPs on living species from bacteria to humans [11–20].

Zebrafish have gained great importance in developmental genetics, aquatic toxicology, and neuroscience research [21,22] due to their unique physiological aspects, such as external fertilization, rapid development, and rapid recovery rate from damage [23]. Although extensive research has been conducted on the zebrafish at the embryonic and larval stages [24,25], studies of ZnO-NPs' influence on the adult stage are still limited.

For most living creatures, olfaction is one of the most important ways of interacting with the environment. It is one of the oldest senses, permitting organisms with receptors for the odorant to identify the surrounding environment and territory [26,27], contributing to food finding, predator escaping, and mating in wildlife [27]. The olfactory system is known for its role in associative behaviors mediated by odorants sensed in the olfactory mucosa and olfactory receptors in the olfactory epithelium of the nasal cavity, so it plays a fundamental role in the daily life of all animal species [26].

Olfactory dysfunction has received increased attention recently because it is a common age-related disease associated with some pathologies [1,2,28]. These pathologies include viral infection and the intake of toxic substances related to the progress of olfactory dysfunction [29]. Other studies have also demonstrated that olfactory dysfunction is an independent risk factor, even in mortality [30,31]. This is because the peripheral olfactory organs are open to the environment; therefore, they are always at risk of being injured by extrinsic pathogens and chemicals, unlike the peripheral structures of most other sensory systems [27].

Indeed, few studies referred to the toxic effects of nanoparticles on the olfactory bulb and sensory epithelium, especially in teleost. Exposure to copper nanoparticles in rainbow trout led to detrimental effects, including oxidative stress and immune suppression [32], silver nanoparticles induced a toxic effect on the olfaction of Crucian carp [33], and ZnO-NPs exhibited a toxic effect on the rat olfactory system [34].

Therefore, the main goal of the present work was to study the hazardous effect of ZnO-NPs on the olfactory sensory cells in the zebrafish model via investigating the histological and ultrastructural alterations but also the changes in the mRNA expressions of antioxidant-, stress-, and apoptotic-related genes to clarify the mechanisms of ZnO-NPs toxicity.

2. Materials and Methods

2.1. Zebrafish Husbandry and ZnO-NPs Exposure

Adult zebrafish (*Danio rerio*) were bought from a local fish supplier (Cairo, Egypt). The fish supplier reared only wild-type zebrafish in large glass tanks (1270 mm × 610 mm × 457 mm) with known reared dates. Adult males (n = 90; average weight 0.62 ± 0.21 g, 6 months old) were acclimatized for two weeks before the experiment. During the acclimatization and throughout the investigation, fishes were kept in aerated de-chlorinated tap water at 27.5 ± 1 °C in glass aquaria (80 × 40 × 30 cm, water capacity 60 L) 14 h light:10 h dark, pH 6.7 ± 0.2 and dissolved oxygen 6.3 ± 0.5 mg/L. The fish were fed twice daily on *Artemia nauplii* (hatched shrimp eggs) according to well-established protocols [35]. Acclimatized fishes were randomly divided into two experimental groups (n = 45/group), each in triplicate (15 fish in each replication in separate tanks). The first group served received no treatment (control group), while the second group was exposed to 1/5th of the estimated LC_{50} of ZnO-NPs (0.69 mg/L) in the water daily for 60 days (treated). All the animal procedures used in this study were approved by the Institutional Animal Care and Use Committee of the Zagazig University, Zagazig, Egypt (Approval number: ZU-IACUC/1/F/213/2023).

The synthesis and characterization of ZnO-NPs were previously described in Mawed et al. (2022), where the UV-VIS spectroscopy results of the characterization of ZnO-NPs show the maximum peak at 340 nm [36]. TEM analysis reveals a spherical shape with an average size of 108 nm. The net surface charge is −33 mV based on the data from the zeta potential analysis. The hydrodynamic size is 89 nm based on the DLS analysis. The LC_{50} of ZnO-NPs was estimated in our laboratory and found to be 3.48 mg/L.

2.2. Scanning Electron Microscopy (SEM) Preparations

The sacrificed adult zebrafish heads were dissected under a stereoscopic binocular microscope (ZEISS LuMAR.V12, Oberkochen, Germany) to expose olfactory rosettes in the bottom of the olfactory chamber; then, they were quickly fixed in vivo by perfusion with a mixture solution (2% formaldehyde, 1.25% glutaraldehyde in 0.1 M sodium cacodylate buffer, pH 7.2) for about 24 h at 4 °C. After fixation, the rosettes, which were lifted in their natural position, were rinsed in the same buffer for about 10 min and subjected to post-fixation in 1% osmium tetroxide in 0.1 M cacodylate buffer (pH 7.2) for 2 h. The setting rosettes were washed with the same buffer and dehydrated through a graded acetone series, which was followed by amyl acetate. The dehydrated rosettes were then dried using a Critical Point Dryer (Hitachi Ltd., Tokyo, Japan) [37]. The dried specimens were then fixed to stubs with the colloidal carbon and coated by gold–palladium in a sputtering device. Then, they were examined and photographed by a JEOL SEM device (Faculty of Science, Alexandria, Egypt) at an accelerating voltage of 15 kV, a working distance of 5.6–6.6 mm, and a standard acquisition resolution of 1536 × 1024.

2.3. Transmission Electron Microscopy (TEM) and Semi-Thin Sections Preparations

The fixed olfactory rosettes were cut into small pieces and then post-fixed for 2 h at room temperature in the same glutaraldehyde solution and 1% osmium tetroxide. Rosette pieces were then dehydrated in a graded ethanol series and embedded in an Epon–Araldite mixture. Then, using a Reichert ultra-microtome, ultrathin sections of 1.5 mm were cut and stained with toluidine blue contrasted in a 50% alcohol–uranyl acetate solution and lead citrate with a transmission Philips EM 400 electron microscope (Philips, INCAEDX, Oxford, UK) [30]. The semi-thin sections after toluidine staining were examined and photographed (Faculty of Science, Alexandria, Egypt).

2.4. Histological Assessments by Light Microscope

The newly separated olfactory rosettes were fixed in 10% formalin. After 24 h, rosettes were appropriately dehydrated through an ascending series of ethyl alcohols, cleared with xylene, and embedded in paraffin wax. Tissue sections at 5 μm were prepared using a microtome (Leica Model, RM2125 Biosystems, Deer Park, NY, USA) and stained with hematoxylin and eosin (H&E) to be examined and photographed by light with a PANNORAMIC MIDI I (Digital Slide Scanners MIDI, 3D HISTECH Company, Budapest, Hungary) [38].

2.5. Total RNA Extraction and Quantitative Real-Time PCR (qRT-PCR)

Total RNA was isolated from the control and treated olfactory rosettes (n = 10/group) using TRIzol reagent according to the manufacturer's instructions (Life Technologies, Carlsbad, CA, USA). RNA purity and concentration were evaluated using gel electrophoresis and the spectrophotometer (METTLER, TOLEDO, Mississauga, ON, Canada). First, 1 μg from the isolated RNA was reverse transcribed into cDNAs by PrimeScript TM RT reagent Kit with gDNA Eraser (Stratagene, Takara, Shiga, Japan). Quantitative real-time PCR was performed on the MSLPCR30 Thermal Cycler system (Biobase Biozone Co., Ltd., Shaanxi, Guangdong, China) with thermal cycling conditions comprised denaturation at 95 °C for 1 min followed by 40 cycles of 95 °C for 10 s and then 60 °C for 20 s and 72 °C for 30 s. The mRNA expressions of the studied genes were normalized to β-actin, and the primers used in the study are listed in Table 1.

Table 1. Primer sequences (forward and reverse) used for real-time qPCR analysis.

Gene	Name	Primers	Accession (Gene ID)
sod1	Superoxide dismutase1	F: 5′ CGCACTTCAACCCTCATGAC 3′ R: 5′ TGAATCACCATGGTCCTCCC 3′	NM_131294
sod2	Superoxide dismutase2	F:5′ CCTCCAGACAGAAGCA 3′ R:5′ CTGAAATGAGCCAAAGT 3′	NM_199976
gpx1a	glutathione peroxidase 1a	F:5′ GCACAACAGTCAGGGAT 3′ R:5′ TCAGGAACGCAAACAG 3′	NM_001007281
gstp1.2	glutathione S-transferase pi 1.2	F: 5′ CCAACCACCTCAAATGCT 3′ R: 5′ ACGGGAAAGAGTCCAGACAG 3′	NM_131734
cat	Catalase	F: 5′ TGTGGAAGGAGGGTCG 3′ R: 5′ CTTTGGCTTTGGAGTAG 3′	NM_130912
p21	cyclin-dependent kinase inhibitor 1A (cdkn1a)	F: 5′ CCTACGTTCACTCGGTAATGGG 3′ R: 5′ CACTAGACGCTTCTTGGCTTGG 3′	NM_001128420
p53	Tumor protein p53 (tp53), transcript variant 2	F: 5′ GCAGTCTGGCACAGCAAAATCTGT 3′ R: 5′ TCAGCCACATGCTCGGACTTCTTA 3′	NM_131327
gadd45aa	Growth arrest and DNA-damage-inducible, alpha, a	F: 5′ GCTGCGAGAACGACATCAACA 3′ R: 5′ GGGCACCCACTGATCCATACA 3′	NM_200576
siva1	Apoptosis-inducing factor	F: 5′ CCGCTACCGACAGGAGATCTACGA 3′ R: 5′ GGTGTGGAGCGCGCTCTGTGCAGT 3′	NM_001327928
baxa	BCL2 associated X, apoptosis regulator	F: 5 GACAGGGATGCTGAAGTGA 3′ R: 5′ TGAGTCGGCTGAAGATTAGA 3′	NM_131562
caspa	caspase a (caspa)	F: 5′ GACGGTGAGCCTGATGAGCCAA 3′ R: 5′ CCTGAACAGTTCCTCGATGTGA 3′	NM_131505
Actin b1	actin, beta 1 (actb1)	F: 5′ ATGGATGAGGAAATCGCTGC 3′ R:5′ CTTTCTGTCCCATGCCAACC 3′	NM_131031

2.6. Protein Extraction and Western Blot Analysis

Total protein was extracted from homogenates of 8 frozen olfactory organs (stored at −80 °C) for each experimental group, including control and ZnO-NPs treated for 30 and 60 days. Western blot was performed according to a previous report [36]. After the processes of electrophoresis and electro-transferase, Nylon Fluoride membranes (Millipore, Burlington, MA, USA) were cut at the desired band of protein marker and then washed by Tris-Buffered Saline Tween (TBST) for 15 min; then, they were blocked against 5% BSA (Bovine Serum Albumin, AUG pharma, Giza, Egypt) for 1 h in room temperature. Nylon membranes were blotted with primary antibodies overnight at 4 °C. Primary antibodies were kindly provided from the National Research Central (El-Dokii, Giza, Egypt), and procedures were performed according to the manufacturer's instructions: Nrf2 antibody (N2C2) (1:500 dilution, Internal Cat. No. GTX103322, Gene Tex, Alton, IL, USA), rabbit anti-Chop protein (GADD153) (1:400, G6916, Sigma Aldrich, Taufkirchen, Germany), Bax polyclonal antibody (1:5000 dilution, 50599-2-lg, proteintech, Manchester, UK), Becl-2 antibody N1N2 (1:1000, GTx100064, GeneTex, Alton, IL, USA) and rabbit anti-β-actin was used for normalization (1:1000 dilution, Cell signaling, 4967S, Inc., Global Headquarters, USA), respectively. The next day, blots were probed with a secondary antibody (HRP-conjugated, Abcam, Cambridge, UK) and then visualized by ECL Western blot detection reagents. Band scanning and protein area quantifications were detected by NIH software Image J. 1.51 k; Java 1.6.0_24.

2.7. Statistical Analysis and Graphs Preparation

Statistical analysis was performed using SPSS. Data were analyzed by Student's *t*-test when comparing two groups and one-way ANOVA when comparing more than two groups. All data are presented as the means ± standard error of the mean and were first checked for normality using the D'Agostino–Pearson normality test. Histological image quantification and analysis were calculated by the 3D Histech Quant Center (3DHISTECH Budapest, Hungary). For protein band quantification, images were analyzed using Image J software (1.51k, Java1.6.0., National Institutes of Health, Bethesda, Maryland, USA). All plots and graphs were designed using Graph Pad Prism 8 package (GraphPad Inc., La Jolla, CA, USA). The significance was given as (* $p < 0.05$; ** $p < 0.01$; *** $p < 0.001$) [39–45].

3. Results

3.1. Macrostructure of Zebrafish Olfactory Organ

Anatomically, zebrafish have two nasal cavities (olfactory chamber) anterodorsally positioned and slightly close to the orbits and mouth; in a parasagittal section at the orbital level, each nasal cavity is covered by a boat sail-shaped skin flap that outlines the funnel-shaped inlet and outlet. Through these openings, water conveying odorants circulates via the olfactory chamber to submerge the sensory structure (olfactory rosette) sitting on the bottom. Longitudinal sections show normal olfactory rosette organization in the control fish (Figure 1A–C). On the other hand, the ZnO-NPs treated group showed a malformed olfactory rosette with stacked lamellae (Figure 1D–F).

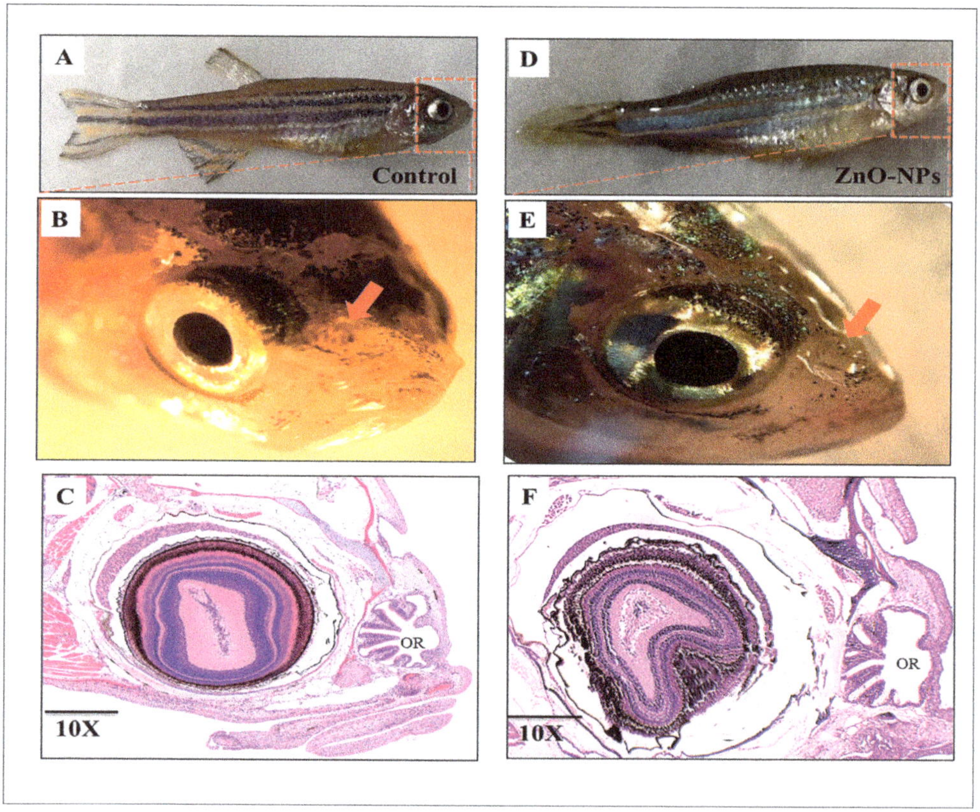

Figure 1. Gross morphology of the adult zebrafish (*Danio rerio*) olfactory rosette and main olfactory system structures: (**A**) Control zebrafish, (**B**) Lateral view of a dissected olfactory rosette (OR) of control fish (red arrow), (**C**) H&E histological assay of a longitudinal section of the whole control OR showing some lamellae; (**D**) ZnO-NPs treated zebrafish, (**E**) Lateral view of a dissected OR of treated fish (red arrow), and (**F**) H&E histological assay of a longitudinal section of the whole treated OR showing some lamellae.

3.2. ZnO-NPs Alter the Histological Architecture of the Olfactory Rosette

Light microscope observations for the control group revealed the normal histological architecture of the olfactory rosette. In Figure 2A, the arranged olfactory lamellae radiating from the midline raphe are represented. Each olfactory lamella appears to be covered on both sides by a pseudostratified columnar epithelium that encloses a central lamellar stromal sheet, the central core. This central core comprises loose connective tissues of collagenous fibers comprising a network of blood capillaries and nerve fibers which run from the olfactory epithelium to the olfactory bulb. The olfactory epithelia on both sides of the central core are of unequal thickness (Figure 2A(b–d)). The sensory epithelium comprises spindle-shaped (bipolar neuron) ciliated receptor cells with oval nuclei and cylindrical non-sensory supporting cells arranged in alternate rows besides rounded basal cells and goblet mucous cells. However, besides the last two types of cells, basal and mucous goblet cells, the non-sensory epithelium embraces round to cubical indifferent epidermal cells and some cylindrical supporting cells, as shown in Figure 2A(c,d). The basal cells are relatively small and spherical, with rounded nuclei scattered in the whole epithelium's deeper part just above the basal lamina. They are a reservoir for forming receptors and supporting cells as they migrate toward the upper part of the olfactory epithelium. The goblet mucous cells are scattered all over the superficial layer of the olfactory epithelium, particularly in the non-sensory area (Figure 2A(c,d,f)). They vary in size and shape according to the activity; most are oval with basal nuclei.

On the other hand, the ZnO-NPs treated group showed an obvious disorganization of the lamellar arrangement of the treated fish. Olfactory lamellae appeared collapsed, malformed, and twisted with signs of degeneration and loss of intercellular connections (Figure 2B(a,b)). The olfactory epithelium appeared swollen with many holes between the central core and detached from the basal lamina (Figure 2B(c,d)). It was also evident that the cilia of different olfactory sensory and non-sensory were decreased in number, adherent, and stuck together. Also, goblet mucous cells were hyperactivated (Figure 2B(d,f)) with a higher precipitation of ZnO-NPs in the central core of the olfactory lamellae and appeared as large black accumulations (Figure 2B(c,e,f)). Statistical analysis of histopathological alterations in the olfactory rosette for both control and ZnO-NPs treated zebrafish indicated high ZnO-NPs precipitation in the treated fishes, lamellar adhesion, epithelial separation, and goblet cells were also well distributed. At the same time, the percentages of ciliated receptor cells, supporting cells, and distributed cilia were scarcely observed (Figure 2C).

3.3. ZnO-NPs-Treated Rosette Exhibited Lamellar Sensory Area Destruction at the Scanning Electron Microscope (SEM) Level

On the bottom of each nasal cavity of the control group, the olfactory rosette appears as an oval-shaped multi-lamellar sensory structure. Its olfactory lamellae are lined up on a wide midline raphe to support the lamellae, which radiate outward and extend toward the periphery of the nasal cavity, increasing in size as it goes from the rostral to caudal direction. The young lamellae are rostral built at both sides of the midline raphe; these olfactory lamellae range from 12 up to 15 (Figure 3A(a–c)). On higher magnification, the olfactory epithelia covering each olfactory lamella are separated into non-sensory and sensory epithelia (Figure 3A(d,e)). The edge of each lamella is covered with the ciliated non-sensory epithelium of ciliated non-sensory cells organized in a valleys-like system that extends to the upper edges of the lamellae as well as indifferent epithelium with apparent micro-ridges and goblet mucous cells observed in between (Figure 3A(f)). However, the medial part of each side of the lamellae encloses the olfactory sensory epithelium continuously planned with its receptor cells. It also covers the intervening areas between every two successive lamellae at the midline raphe.

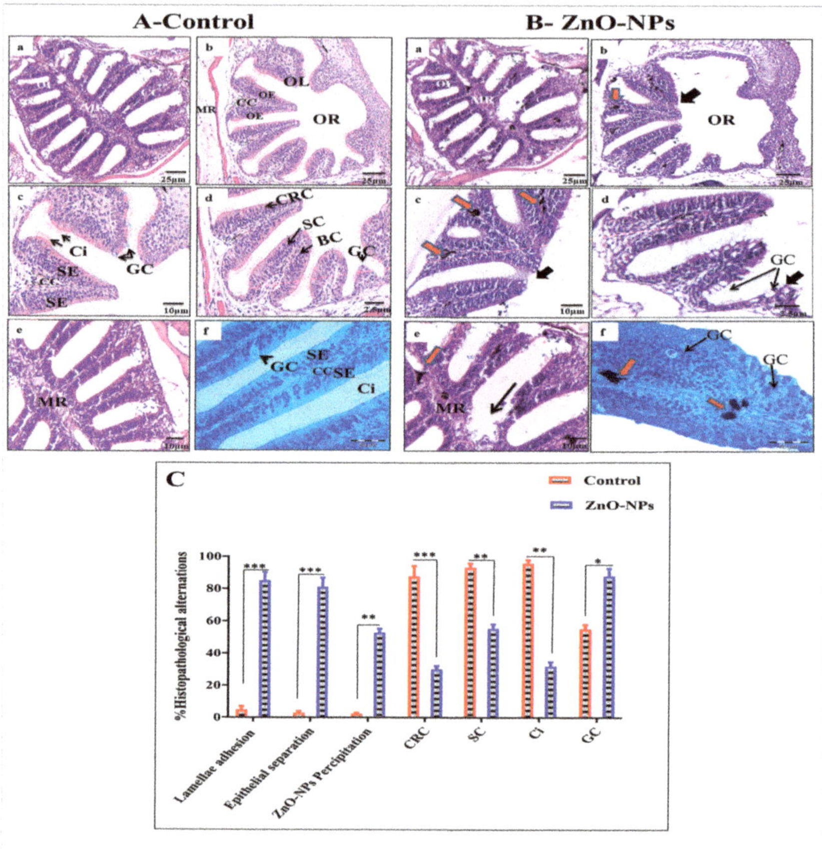

Figure 2. H&E histological assay of (**A**) the control and (**B**) ZnO-NPs-treated zebrafish olfactory rosettes: (**A**(**a**)) horizontal section of the whole control olfactory rosette (OR), olfactory lamellae (OL), median raphe (MR); (**A**(**b**)) transverse section of the whole control OR, OL, MR, and central core (CC); (**A**(**c**)) magnified part of the OR showing CC, sensory epithelium (SE), ciliated receptor cells have darken spindle shape (CRC), cilia of the ciliated non-sensory cell (Ci), and goblet cell (GC); (**A**(**d**)) magnified part of the olfactory rosette showing supporting cell (SC) and basal cell (BC); (**A**(**e**)) magnified portion of the olfactory rosette showing CC; (**A**(**f**)) photomicrographs of the semi-thin section stained with toluidine blue of the olfactory lamella showing CC, SE, Ci, and GC (black arrow); (**B**(**a**)) horizontal section of the whole treated OR, collapsed OL, necrosis in MR; (**B**(**b**,**c**)) transverse section of the whole treated olfactory rosette showing swollen and detached olfactory epithelium (black arrow) and precipitation of ZnO-NPs in the olfactory epithelium and the central core (red arrow); (**B**(**d**)) magnified part of the olfactory rosette showing a large number of GC (black arrow); (**B**(**e**)) magnified portion of the olfactory rosette showing lamellar destruction (black arrow) and precipitation of ZnO-NPs (red arrow); (**B**(**f**)) photomicrographs of the semi-thin section of the olfactory lamella showing a large number of GC (black arrow) and precipitation of ZnO-NPs (red arrow). (**C**) Statistical analysis for three different sections from the OR of the control and treated group showing histopathological alterations after ZnO-NPs treatment. The results are the mean ± SEM.* $p < 0.05$, ** $p < 0.01$, *** $p < 0.001$.

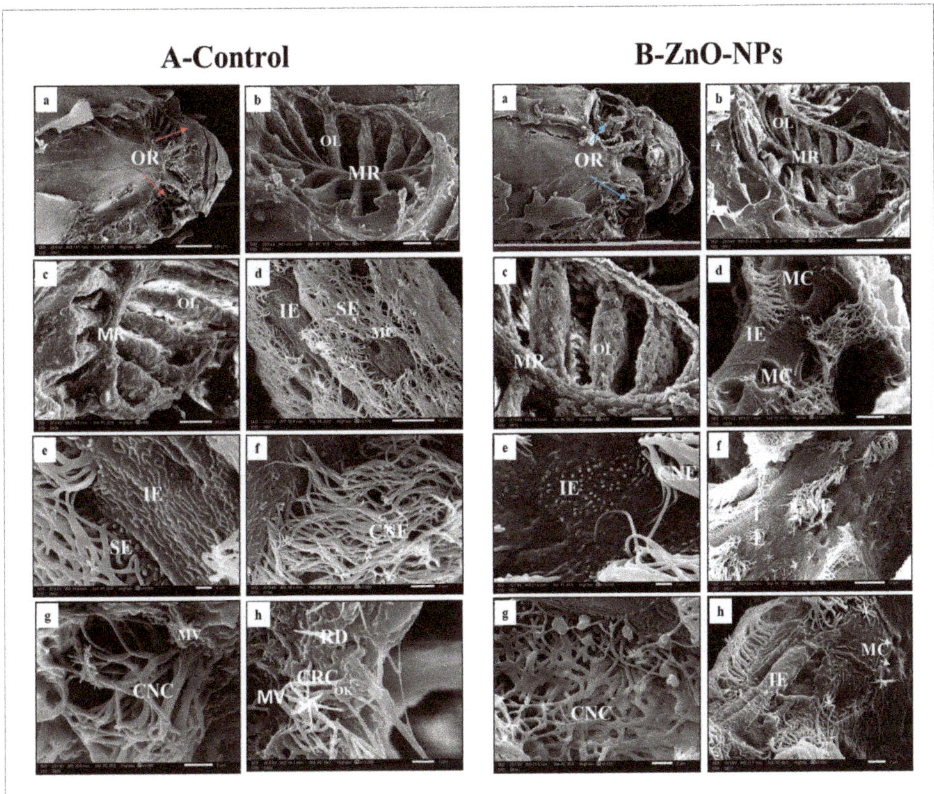

Figure 3. Scanning electron microscopy observations of the epithelial surface of (**A**) the control and (**B**) ZnO-NPs zebrafish olfactory rosette: (**A**(**a**)) scanning electron micrograph of the head of an adult zebrafish with two olfactory rosettes (ORs) (red arrows); (**A**(**b**)) olfactory rosette located in the nasal cavity, with olfactory lamellae (OL) arranged on both sides of the midline raphe (MR); (**A**(**c**)) higher magnification of the OL and the MR; (**A**(**d**,**e**)) sensory epithelium (SE) and indifferent epithelium (IE) are strictly separated; (**A**(**f**)) lamella is covered with ciliated non-sensory epithelium (CNE); (**A**(**g**)) cilia of the ciliated non-sensory cell (CNC); (**A**(**h**)) the surface of the sensory epithelium shows ciliated receptor cells (CRC) with olfactory knobs (OK), microvillous receptor cells (MV), and rod cells (RD); (**B**(**a**)) scanning electron micrograph of the head of an adult zebrafish with two treated OR (blue arrows); (**B**(**b**,**c**)) the olfactory rosette stunted appearance with preserved OL and the MR; (**B**(**d**)) numerous pores of mucous cells (MC), the IE without micro ridges; (**B**(**e**)) IE without micro-ridges; (**B**(**f–h**)) cilia of CNC fused with a decreased number.

On SEM, we could detect three receptor cell types based on the structure and shape of their apical dendrites, whether ciliated, microvillar, or rod-shaped (Figure 3A(g,h)). The sensory cells can be organized by scanning microscopy into:

i. Ciliated receptor cells, their dendritic part protrudes slightly beyond the supporting cells' boundary, forming a small terminal swelling hillock-like apex, the olfactory knob. From this knob, six to eight long cilia or flagella arise radially projecting into the lumen of the olfactory cavity (Figure 3A(h)).
ii. Microvillous receptor cells with apical surfaces full of numerous shorter microvilli protruding into the olfactory space (Figure 3A (g,h)).
iii. Rod cell shows rod-like projection and protrudes from its free surface by an olfactory knob. Rod neurons can be observed randomly between the ciliated sensory cells (Figure 3A(h)).

Contrarily, the olfactory rosette of the zebrafish treated with ZnO-NPs showed a stunted appearance with preserved olfactory lamellae and degenerated olfactory rosette (Figure 3B(a–c)). The long cilia of ciliated non-sensory cells were decreased in number, thinned out, curled, and fused. This was observed mainly in the outer distal region of the lamella with massive mucus secretion given by the activated mucous cells with wider pores compared to the normal non-treated fish (Figure 3B(d)). The micro-ridges of the indifferent epithelium lost their linear appearance and sometimes disappeared entirely in some areas (Figure 3B (e,f)).

Concerning the sensory epithelia, they were extensively damaged, with almost complete loss of cilia and microvilli of all receptor cells to the extent that some of their knobs appeared utterly naked, and some with a rod-like extension, the ciliated and microvillous neurons had been hardly detected (Figure 3B(f–h)).

3.4. ZnO-NPs Induce Sensory Cell Apoptosis and Cytoplasmic Organelles Destruction at the Transmission Electron Microscope (TEM) Level

TEM observations highlighted the olfactory epithelium of the control group into ciliated non-sensory cells and seven distinct types of olfactory sensory receptor cells. All these cells are closely crowded, including ciliated receptor cells, microvillous receptor cells, rod cells, rodlet cells, crypt cells, Kappe cells, and pear-shaped cells in addition to the supporting cells, the small rounded basal cells, and the mucous goblet.

i. Ciliated non-sensory cells are club-shaped with a narrow, deep surface and a relatively flat, broad, free surface. They do not have dendrites and axons but have numerous long rootlet cilia arising as a tuft oriented in the same direction from the cell's surface (Figure 4A(a)). At the most apical cytoplasmic region, plentiful oval or rounded mitochondria are found without preferential orientation (Figure 4A(a,b)). Each cilium's basal structure comprises a pair of centrioles and one rootlet (Figure 4A(c)). These cilia are kino-cilia, showing a typical axonemal pattern (9 + 2) of microtubules (mi) (Figure 4A(c,d)).
ii. Ciliated receptor cells are long, slender-shaped bipolar sensory cells (neurons). Their most basally located somata are highly granulated cytoplasm packed with elongated or rounded mitochondria. A basal axonal process penetrates the basal lamina, and apical long dendritic processes extend toward the surface of the olfactory epithelium. These processes (cilia) randomly arise from an olfactory knob. Each cilium has a basal body without any rootlets but is associated with centrioles with several neuro-filaments present just beneath the plasma membrane of the olfactory knob (Figure 4A(e)).
iii. Microvillous receptor cells are also elongated bipolar cells (neurons), their bodies featuring short dendrites and visible nuclei located at intermediate depths of the olfactory epithelium. Their apical surface is provided with a tuft of shorter dendrites, microvilli, which project radially outwards in the olfactory lumen from a concave olfactory knob under the surface level of the adjacent supporting cells. Some basal bodies are arranged in two rows at the microvilli's base. Numerous elongated or rounded mitochondria are scattered in the cell cytoplasm (Figure 4A(f)).
iv. Rod receptor cells are elongated bipolar cells (neurons) but differ from the other receptor cells in having a single thick cilium, rod-like projection, so they are known as rod receptor cells. This rod-like projection extends from a knob-like apex and has a pair of basal bodies at the base of its axonemal microtubules. As in all receptor cells, the cell body of a rod cell is fully packed with mitochondria scattered within its granulated cytoplasm (Figure 4A(g)).
v. Rodlet cells are ovoid-shaped cells enclosed by a distinctive thick cuticula-like wall, found against the inner aspect of the cell plasma membrane, with a narrow apex pore. So, there is not any junction with neighboring cells. These cells have a typical animal cell structure with a basally located nucleus of various forms and shapes. Their cytoplasm is crowded with rounded to elongated vesicular mitochondria as well as few vesicular vacuoles and free ribosomes in addition to clusters of its most striking club or rod-shaped electron-opaque vesicles, rodlets (Figure 4A(h)).

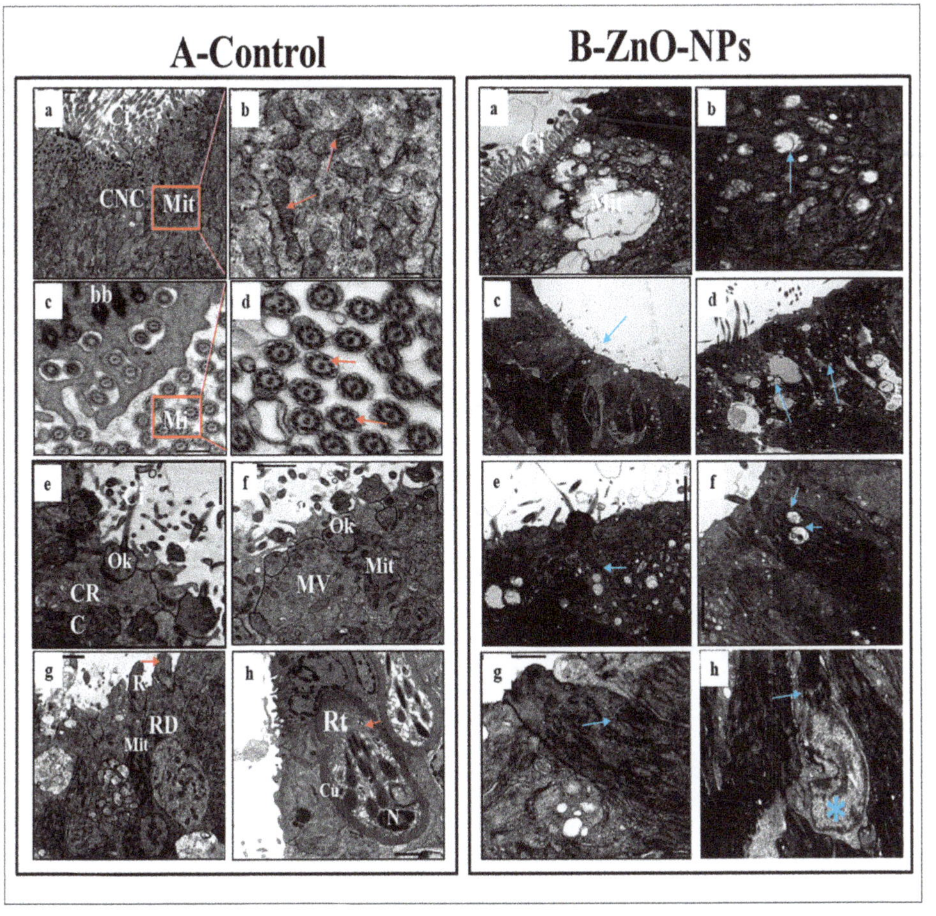

Figure 4. Transmission electron micrographs of (**A**) the control and (**B**) ZnO-NPs-treated zebrafish olfactory epithelium: (**A**(**a**)) olfactory epithelium consisting of ciliated non-sensory cells (CNC) with cilia (Ci) and mitochondria (Mit); (**A**(**b**)) magnified part of ciliated non-sensory cells showing Mit; (**A**(**c**,**d**)) cross-section of cilia exhibits nine pairs of outer microtubules (Mi) and two central ones (red arrow), basal body (bb); (**A**(**e**)) magnified view of ciliated receptor cells (CRC) showed an olfactory knob (Ok) bearing cilia (Ci). (**A**(**f**)) magnified view of microvillous receptor cell (MV), which showed an Ok bearing short microvillar processes (Mi) on its apical surface and Mit; (**A**(**g**)) magnified view of rod cell (RD) shows parallel oriented microtubules (red arrows) in rod-like cilia (R) and Mit. (**A**(**h**)) the rodlet cell (Rt) is identified by the thick cuticle (cu) and its typical rodlets (red arrows) and nucleus (N); (**B**(**a–d**)) olfactory epithelium consisting of ciliated non-sensory cells with decreased number of Ci and Mit swelling and vacuolation (blue arrow); (**B**(**e–g**)) the cilia, microvilli, and rods of all olfactory neurons injured mitochondria swollen and vacuolated (blue arrow); (**B**(**h**)) rodlet cell with hypertrophy nucleus (blue star) and detached apical rodlets (blue arrow).

vi. Crypt cells are olfactory sensory neurons (OSNs) with elongated pear-shaped somata found near the apical surface of the sensory epithelium of examined zebrafish.

Although crypt cells occur regularly in all lamellae, their absolute number is low and not as high as that of ciliated and microvillous OSNs. They bear cilia and submerged microvilli (Figure 5A(a,b)). These cilia, as those of ciliated OSNs, show the typical (9 + 2) axonemal pattern of microtubules (Figure 5A(b)); the cytoplasm of these crypt cells is electron-dense, packed with elongated or rounded mitochondria and free, abundant ribosomes, but its nucleus fills about one-third of the cell body (Figure 5A(a)). These crypt cells are surrounded by one or two specialized electron-lucent supporting cells bearing micro-ridges but do not have cilia.

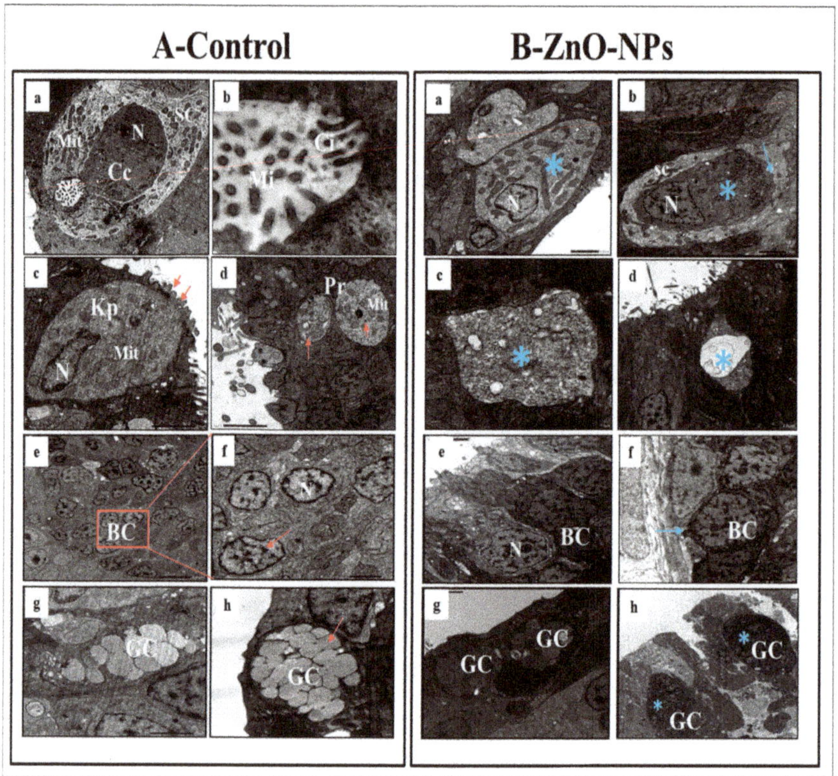

Figure 5. Transmission electron micrographs of the degenerated sensory cells of (**A**) the control and (**B**) ZnO-NPs-treated zebrafish olfactory epithelium: (**A**(**a**)) crypt cell (Cc) with in-sunk cilia, the nucleus (N) in the lower portion of the cell, supporting cell (SC) surrounding the crypt cell and mitochondria (Mit); (**A**(**b**)) higher magnification of the upper portion of a crypt cell, (Cc) showing cilia (Ci) and microtubules (Mi). (**A**(**c**)) the Kappe cells (KP), the nucleus (N) in the basal part of the cell, micro-ridges upper part (red arrows), and mitochondria (Mit); (**A**(**d**)) pear-shaped cell (Pr), the cytoplasm with mitochondria (Mit) and ribosomes (red arrows); (**A**(**e**,**f**)) basal cells (BC, red arrow) with N; (**A**(**g**,**h**)) goblet cells (GC); (**B**(**a**,**b**)) crypt cell (Cc) showing the disappearance of cilia, elongated mitochondria (blue star), and the surrounding supporting cells (SC) thinned out; (**B**(**c**,**d**)) the Kappe and pear-shaped cells that have lost their distinct shape (blue star); (**B**(**e**,**f**)) basal cells (BC) increased in size, and with the nucleus (N) enlarged; (**B**(**g**,**h**)) hyper-activated goblet cells (GC) with retention of a large amount of ZnO-NPs (blue star).

vii. Kappe cells are found in the most apical epithelial positions close to the olfactory lumen. Their cell bodies are elongated pear-shaped, similar to crypt cells, but their inward superficial cap apical end is fortified with few cilia and microvilli. Their less flattened nuclei are positioned in the basal part of the cell body and swim in the ground cytoplasm with fully packed rounded mitochondria (Figure 5A(c)).

viii. Morphologically, a pear-shaped cell is similar to Kappe cells but rounded and variable in size. It is located in the apical part of the epithelium, and its cytoplasm has numerous rounded mitochondria-free ribosomes (Figure 5A(d)).

ix. Basal cells are intermingled with the basal portion of the other cell types in the olfactory epithelium. They are small polyhedral cells having a distinct globular shape and darkly stained centrally located nuclei. Basal cells are grouped and interposed by the bases of the sensory and non-sensory supporting cells, forming a discontinuous layer in the deeper part of the epithelium just above the basal lamina and did not reach the free surface of the epithelium (Figure 5A(e,f)).

x. Goblet mucous cells are restricted to the non-sensory epithelium. They are oval-shaped, having basally located nuclei, and about two-thirds of the cell body is filled with large mucous granules. They are surrounded by ciliated non-sensory or epidermal cells bearing micro-ridges. Mature goblet cells secrete their mucous granules into the lumen of the olfactory cavity over the non-sensory epidermal cell surface (Figure 5A(g,h)).

Conversely, in ZnO-NPs-treated fishes, the cilia emitted from the ciliated non-sensory cells appeared shrunken and decreased in number. The mitochondria showed signs of partial or complete degeneration through swelling and vacuolation; tight junctions between different cells were diminished and rarely noticed (Figure 4B(a–d)).

Cilia, microvilli, and rods of all olfactory ciliated microvillus and rod cells (neurons) were significantly injured with large cytoplasmic empty vacuoles (Figure 4B(e–g)), respectively. The mitochondria in all these sensory cells (neurons) were swollen and vacuolated compared with the control siblings. They had a clear matrix and lost their electron-dense deposits with destructive changes in their cristae (Figure 4B(d–f)). Furthermore, the appearance of swollen or filamentous mitochondria in the rod cells was evident (Figure 4B(g)).

Moreover, the rodlet cell lost its thick cuticle-like characterized by degenerated rodlets and hypertrophy nucleus with an irregular crescent shape containing detached chromatin as a sign of oncocytic changes (Figure 4B(h)).

Alongside, the crypt cells lost their distinctive shape. The nucleus appeared irregular and highly condensed; dark chromatin masses were observed but with a continuous nuclear envelope. Their mitochondria were swollen and vacuolated with stacked cilia and microvilli, and the surrounding supporting cells were squeezed and decreased in size (Figure 5B(a,b)).

The Kappe cells and pear-shaped cells appeared empty and lost their distinct shape. The nucleus seemed shrunken with decreased chromatin without a nuclear envelope; the mitochondria were swollen and vacuolated (Figure 5B(c,d)). Basal cells showed a compensatory increase in size; the nucleus was enlarged with condensed chromatin surrounded by a distinct nuclear membrane (Figure 5B(e,f)). The goblet mucous cells+ showed an increased number and became hyper-activated. Their secretions covered the olfactory epithelium's surface with many ZnO-NPs retaining the black stain on the goblet granules (Figure 5B(g,h)).

3.5. ZnO-NPs Induce Apoptosis in the Olfactory Epithelium via Mediating Oxidative Stress and DNA Damage

To detect the underlying mechanisms of ZnO-NPs cytotoxicity effect on the zebrafish olfactory organs, the mRNA expression of antioxidant, DNA damage, and apoptosis-related genes was evaluated by qRT-PCR [44] to support our TEM observations between the control and ZnO-NPs treated groups. It has been observed that ZnO-NPs alter mitochondrial structure and function, resulting in the generation of excessive reactive oxygen species (ROS) that weaken the antioxidant enzyme activity, altogether placing the olfactory cells at oxidative stress risk [46–49]. Accordingly, the mRNA expression of antioxidant-related genes, including *sod1*, *sod2*, *gpx1a*, *gstp1.2*, and *cat*, was down-regulated in the treated olfactory rosette compared with the control one (Figure 6A). In addition, the ROS mediate genotoxicity, which results in chromosomal alteration and DNA damage [50,51], and this is revealed by the up-regulation of cyclin-dependent kinase inhibitor (CDKN1A) or *p21*, tumor suppressor protein *p53*, and growth arrest and DNA damage-inducible alpha a *gadd45aa*, all of which play an essential role in inhibiting DNA replication and subsequently induce cell cycle arrest, apoptosis, and senescence (Figure 6B). In the present study, cellular apoptosis was revealed in the TEM of the treated rosette by destroying the sensory and supporting cells' cytoplasmic components. The latter observations were confirmed by the mRNA up-regulation of pro-apoptotic related genes, including *siva1*, *baxa*, and *caspa*, in the treated group compared with the control group (Figure 6C).

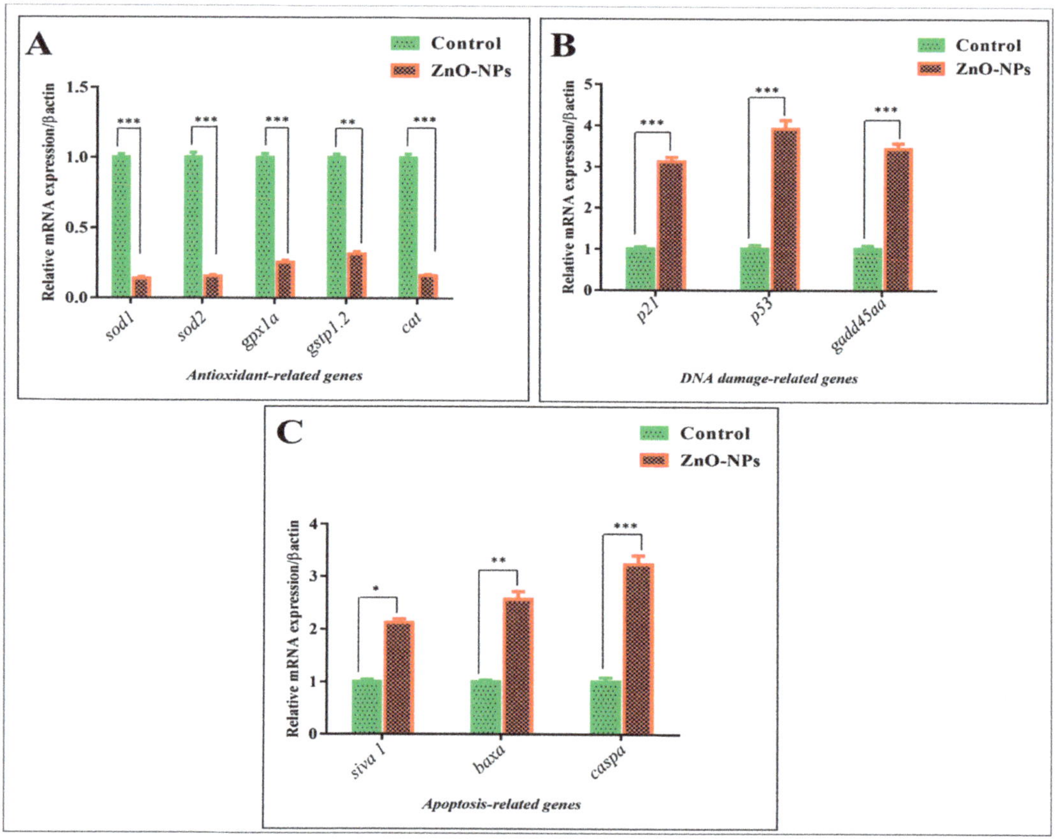

Figure 6. ZnO-NPs-induced cellular apoptosis via oxidative stress and DNA damage at the genetic level: (**A**) mRNA expression evaluated by qRT-PCR for antioxidant-related genes; (**B**) mRNA expression evaluated by qRT-PCR for DNA damage-related genes; (**C**) mRNA expression evaluated by qRT-PCR for apoptosis-related genes. The results are the mean ± SEM.* $p < 0.05$, ** $p < 0.01$, *** $p < 0.001$.

Western blot analysis was conducted on the control, (30-dpt), and (60-dpt) groups to reveal the dramatic changes in the protein expression for the previously mentioned pathways. Herein, nuclear factor erythroid 2-related factor 2 (Nrf2), a crucial regulator in the cellular defense against oxidative stress, was slightly up-regulated after 30-dpt, indicating the cytoprotective effect and antioxidative response of Nrf2 against ZnO-NPs toxicity. Nrf2 was suddenly down-regulated after 60-dpt, indicating its suppression due to high ROS accumulation (Figure 7A,B). At the same time, CHOP, which is involved in apoptosis via DNA damage and growth arrest [52], exhibited higher expression at 60-dpt (Figure 7A–C). In addition, Bax, a core regulator of the cellular pathway of apoptosis, was highly up-regulated in the 60-dpt group compared with the control or 30-dpt groups (Figure 7A–D). Contrarily, the anti-apoptotic protein, BecL-2, exhibited a lower expression in the 60-dpt group compared with the control or the 30-dpt groups (Figure 7A–E). Altogether, these results ensure the highly oxidative damage in the olfactory epithelium after 60-dpt of ZnO-NPs, leading to DNA damage and cellular apoptosis.

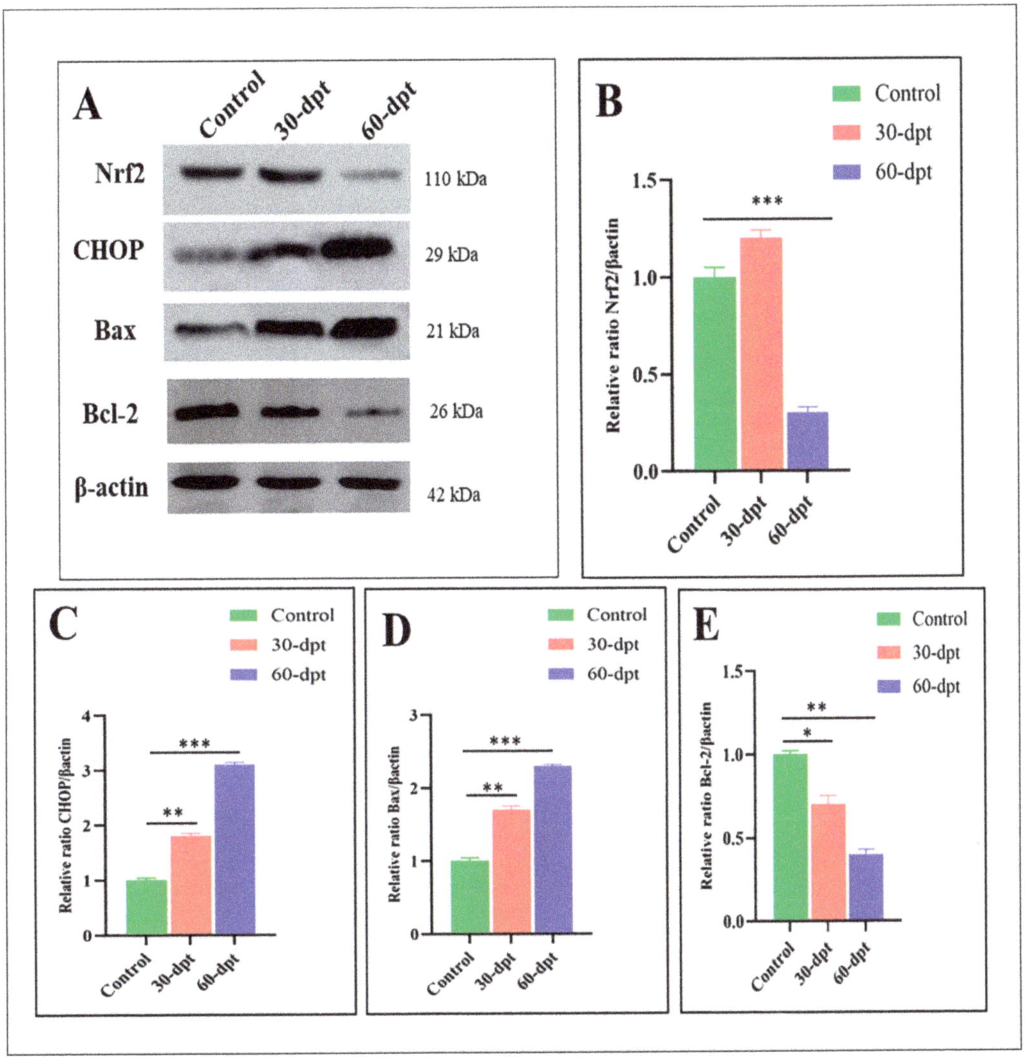

Figure 7. Apoptotic pathway induction by ZnO-NPs via oxidative stress induction: (**A**) immunoblots showing Nrf2, CHOP, Bax, and Bcl-2 proteins of control, 30-dpt, and 60-dpt (β-actin was used for normalization and relative protein levels were quantified using NIH software Image J), (**B–E**) protein expression revealing the ratio analysis of Nrf2/βactin, CHOP/βactin, BAX/β actin, Bcl-2/βactin quantified by the Image J 1.51k; Java 1.6.0_24 (64-Bit). The results are the mean ± SEM. * $p < 0.05$, ** $p < 0.01$, *** $p < 0.001$.

4. Discussion

Unlike most other sensory systems, the olfactory organs are externally open to the surrounding environment, allowing exposure to various toxicants [53]. Although the cytotoxicity of ZnO-NPs has been widely studied, the underlying mechanisms are still unclear [24,54–60]. Olfaction is a critical sense for detecting and discriminating the surrounding environment of all vertebrates, finding food, and recognizing adverse conditions [61]. Generally, the environmental chemical information is transmitted from the olfactory organ to the brain via the olfactory nerve, causing alarm response, predator avoidance, food search, social communication, reproductive activity, and migration [62–64].

Zebrafish, as with other animals [65,66], possess a well-developed sense of smell, responsible for various behaviors involved in reproduction, appetite, and fear. Moreover, the functional properties within its sensory epithelium and the olfactory bulb are comparable to those of mammals [67].

Despite the morphological variations and anatomy of the olfactory system within different vertebrates, the neural basis of odor detection is well maintained since the sense of smell is necessary to perform key functions, mainly securing survival [68,69]. Teleost, such as zebrafish, have a sole olfactory epithelium located on the floor of the nasal cavity and lack the separate vomeronasal organs of higher vertebrates [70]. This olfactory epithelium is organized in lamellae, which radiate from a central ridge or raphe and give rise to an olfactory rosette set on the bottom surface of the nasal cavity on each side of the skull [9,71]. From each olfactory sensory cell, outspread axonal projection forms a fasciculate olfactory nerve [72] and a well-organized neuronal circuitry [73]. So, zebrafish is a key model organism for studying the olfactory system [74].

In all teleosts, there are two main types of OSNs: ciliated and microvillous OSNs. These two morphologically distinct receptor cell types have been distributed in differential patterns within the olfactory epithelium since they are the foremost OSNs in the zebrafish [73]. Nonetheless, teleost, in addition to these two major types of OSN, have two more minor OSN types: crypt OSNs, which express only a single olfactory receptor [75], and the recently identified Kappe neurons [76] that are believed to be absent in tetrapods [77].

All four OSN types are recognized by their morphological features like the cell shape and position within the olfactory epithelium, axons, and dendritic features and preferential response to different stimuli [78]. Ciliated OSNs tend to have a very slender pattern and instead basally situated cell bodies with long apical dendrite-bearing cilia usually radiating from an olfactory knob at its distal ends and extending to the surface of the lamellae, as also shown in channel catfish [10,78] and zebrafish [79,80]. On the other side, the microvillous OSNs are located at the intermediate depths of the epithelium. They have short apical microvilli stemming from a thick dendrite. These microvillous neurons are responded to by amino acids, as mentioned in Salmonids [81], Rainbow trout [82], channel catfish [78], and zebrafish [79,83]. In other words, the ciliated OSNs serve as generalists, whereas microvillous are specialists. Salmonids and cyprinids have shown that both ciliated and microvillous OSNs generally respond to amino acid odorants, but bile acids stimulate ciliated OSNs, and nucleotides activate microvillous OSNs [71]. Earlier, Cancalon (1982) clarified that zinc could induce an extensive degeneration of the olfactory sensory cells and result in severe damage [84].

Exposure to mercury, a toxic and harmful metal for the olfactory organs, reacted differently with the three main types of OSNs. Bazáes and Schmachtenberg (2012) recently showed that microvillous OSNs are more susceptible to mercury exposure than ciliated OSNs, and crypt cell density decreases [85].

Crypt neurons constitute an exciting cell population comprising the third type of olfactory receptor neurons. They appeared early in vertebrate evolution since they are common in almost all marine and freshwater actinopterygian fish, even in cartilaginous fish, but not sarcopterygian lungfishes [77,86]. Such cells are observed by TEM only at the olfactory lamellar surface, which was probably due to their positioning and enwrapping between other closely adjacent receptors and supporting cells [63]. Crypt neurons are located close to the epithelial surface in addition to relatively short microvilli and submerged cilia without olfactory knobs [74,85]. Many attempts have been made to clarify the function of the crypt cell during spawning, indicating its significant relation to the reproductive status and sex pheromone detectors [87].

Conversely, Kappe neurons are a limited cell population exhibiting conspicuous short globular shape somata equipped with a few cilia and microvilli. They are positioned superficially within the olfactory epithelium close to the lumen and far away from the basal lamina [75]. Ahuja et al. (2015) suggested that they are new types of OSNs characterized by their cap apical end [76].

Their absolute existence in the olfactory epithelium shows an astonishing complexity of odor signs already in the periphery of the olfactory system. In addition, the present study described the pear-shaped cell, which is located in the apical part of the epithelium, with numerous mitochondria, ribosomes, and extremely short dendrites, and this is in agreement with other authors, who declared that these cells are present in a very small number in the most superficial layer of the olfactory epithelium and serving for detection of adenosine [73,88].

Cheung et al. (2021) later confirmed the presence of a rare rod cell in the olfactory epithelium of zebrafish, especially in the early stages [89]. They are morphologically distinguishing from the other well-known sensory cells as they possess a conspicuous single compound cilium-like-rod extending from the center of a knob-like apex without a detectable axon. So, they do not belong to the two broad classes of sensory receptors, ciliated and microvillous, but have been identified based on morphology, receptor expression, and projection pattern [90]. Olfactory rod cells have been previously described in many other teleost fish species, including several eel species [91], goldfish [92], rainbow trout [93], common bleak [94], catfish [95], *Mugil cephalus,* and *Malapterurus electricus* [96] cave loach species [97,98]. However, some authors presumed that the existence of receptor cells bearing rod cilium or microvilli represented intermediate stages of the ciliated one [99,100].

Interestingly, rod cells are more distinctive from rodlet cells, described in many different epithelial tissues of all fish, including zebrafish [101,102]. The rodlet cells appeared in the olfactory epithelia of the presently studied zebrafish, often among sensory and non-sensory epithelia. These are ovoid-shaped cells enclosed by a distinctive thick cuticula-like wall and have been reported as being immature stages of goblet cells [103].

Nonetheless, these cells, initially supposed to be protozoan parasites, are prevalent in fish organ tissue and are not parasitic [104–106]. These confusing rodlet cells are often associated with fish viscera and epithelium such as skin, intestine, kidney tubules, and biliary duct [105,107–110]. These rodlet cells represent inflammatory cells closely related to other innate immune cells and potential biomarkers for stressors and chemical agents [111].

Among other nanoparticles, zinc oxide might enhance the odorant responses of OSNs [112]. However, in the present investigation, the cilia, microvilli, and rod of all olfactory ciliated microvilli and rod cells were adversely affected by ZnO-NPs. These dendritic projections were atrophied, minimized in number, and significantly injured. The mitochondria in all these sensory neurons swelled or became filamentous and showed distinctive signs of degeneration compared to the normal, non-treated fish, particularly in the rod cells. Nonetheless, although the crypt cells have both cilia and microvilli not directly immersed in the water flow in the olfactory chamber [113], these were less affected by zinc nanoparticles. Crypt cells' density dropped and lost their distinctive shape, nuclei shrunk, and their mitochondria were elongated, becoming filamentous, according to other literature reports [114,115]. Alongside, the cilia and micro-ridges of ciliated non-sensory cells were shortened, minimized, or erased.

Furthermore, their surrounding supporting cells were also squeezed and decreased in size [116]. Nonetheless, the goblet mucous cells increased in number and became hyper-activated. Their mucous secretions covered the surface of all the olfactory epithelium with retention of large amounts of ZnO-NPs, as reported by Ghosh et al. (2014), who observed the same effect upon mercury exposure and interpreted it as a type of protection [117]. When the mucous layer becomes excessive, it can prevent pollutants from directly contacting the epithelial surface and decrease toxicity effects [118].

Accordingly, ZnO-NPs in the present study induced mitochondrial damage and impaired the genetic antioxidant enzymes synthesized at the genetic level, releasing ROS that modulate oxidative stress, which agrees with previous studies [27,59,119,120]. The super oxidase dismutase (sod1) and (sod2), catalase (cat), and glutathione peroxidase (gpx) are important markers in defending cells against oxidative stress by catalyzing the conversion of superoxide free radicals ($O2^-$) into hydrogen peroxide then reduced to water [121–123]. Earlier, it was found that ROS can cause severe damage to DNA molecules [124–128], and this was ensured by the up-regulation of cyclin-dependent kinase inhibitor p21, tumor protein p53, and growth arrest gadd45aa expressions indicating the cell cycle arrest after DNA damage [56,129–133]. As a result, damaged DNA activates apoptosis via the loss of membrane integrity, cytoplasmic content fragmentation, and chromatin condensation, as demonstrated earlier [134–136].

Nrf2 is a transcription factor activated in response to stress. It significantly enhances the antioxidant defense of stressed cells and helps detoxify and eliminate exogenous chemicals and their toxic metabolites [137]. Herein, Nrf2 was down-regulated after 60-dpt, which might be a defense mechanism against ROS accumulation. Moreover, in the 60-dpt group, there was an up-regulation of the apoptotic CHOP and Bax expression and a down-regulation of the anti-apoptotic protein BcL-2 expression, confirming the apoptotic effect of ZnO-NPs. Similar to these findings, in zebrafish embryos exposed to ZnO-NPs, the gene expression analysis of several genes of antioxidant proteins (Bcl-2, Nqo1, and Gstp2) revealed an important down-regulation [54].

Furthermore, the production of ROS, which is the basis of oxidative stress, was confirmed by an altered expression of anti-apoptotic genes (Bcl-2, B-cell lymphoma2) and pro-apoptotic (bax, puma, and apaf-1) genes in zebrafish exposed to ZnO-NPs, where the expression of BCL2-associated X apoptosis regulator (Bax) was significantly up-regulated, while Bcl-2 was down-regulated [138]. The overexpression of CHOP and microinjection of CHOP protein have been reported to lead to cell cycle arrest and/or apoptosis [139]. Moreover, the overexpression of CHOP leads to decreased Bcl-2 protein and translocation of Bax protein from the cytosol to the mitochondria [140].

5. Conclusions

The present study shows that ZnO-NPs can mediate the cellular oxidative stress and arrest cell growth that induces apoptosis without the ability of cellular regeneration, hence leading to sensory toxicity that directly damages the olfactory epithelium and affects fish smell.

Author Contributions: Conceptualization, S.A.A.-Z. and M.A.; methodology, M.R.F., H.S.A.T. and M.A.; software, H.S.A.T. and S.A.M.; validation, M.R.F., M.A. and G.C.; formal analysis, S.A.M., S.A.A.-Z. and M.R.F.; investigation, M.R.F. and M.A.; resources, M.R.F. and M.V.V.; data curation, M.R.F.; writing—original draft preparation, H.S.A.T., M.A., S.A.M., S.A.A.-Z. and G.C.; writing—review and editing, M.A., M.R.F., M.V.V. and G.C.; visualization, M.A., M.R.F., H.S.A.T. and G.C.; project administration, S.A.M., M.A., M.V.V. and M.R.F. All authors have read and agreed to the published version of the manuscript.

Funding: The research project was partially founded by the University of Sassari (Fondo di Ateneo per la Ricerca 2020), www.uniss.it.

Institutional Review Board Statement: This study conformed to the guidance of ethical animal treatment for the care and use of experimental animals and was approved by the Institutional Animal Care and Use Committee of the Zagazig University, Zagazig, Egypt (Approval number: ZU-IACUC/1/F/213/2023, approved on 22 June 2023).

Informed Consent Statement: Not applicable.

Data Availability Statement: The data presented in this study are available on request from the corresponding authors.

Conflicts of Interest: The authors declare no conflict of interest.

References

1. Keller, A.A.; McFerran, S.; Lazareva, A.; Suh, S. Global life cycle releases of engineered nanomaterials. *J. Nanoparticle Res.* **2013**, *15*, 1692. [CrossRef]
2. Piccinno, F.; Gottschalk, F.; Seeger, S.; Nowack, B. Industrial production quantities and uses of ten engineered nanomaterials in Europe and the world. *J. Nanoparticle Res.* **2012**, *14*, 1109. [CrossRef]
3. Di Cerbo, A.; Pezzuto, F.; Scarano, A. Cytotoxic and Bacteriostatic Activity of Nanostructured TiO_2 Coatings. *Pol. J. Microbiol.* **2016**, *65*, 225–229. [CrossRef]
4. Di Cerbo, A.; Mescola, A.; Iseppi, R.; Canton, R.; Rossi, G.; Stocchi, R.; Loschi, A.R.; Alessandrini, A.; Rea, S.; Sabia, C. Antibacterial Effect of Aluminum Surfaces Untreated and Treated with a Special Anodizing Based on Titanium Oxide Approved for Food Contact. *Biology* **2020**, *9*, 456. [CrossRef]
5. Di Cerbo, A.; Rosace, G.; Rea, S.; Stocchi, R.; Morales-Medina, J.C.; Canton, R.; Mescola, A.; Condo, C.; Loschi, A.R.; Sabia, C. Time-Course Study of the Antibacterial Activity of an Amorphous $SiO_{(x)}C_{(y)}H_{(z)}$ Coating Certified for Food Contact. *Antibiotics* **2021**, *10*, 901. [CrossRef]
6. Di Cerbo, A.; Mescola, A.; Rosace, G.; Stocchi, R.; Rossi, G.; Alessandrini, A.; Preziuso, S.; Scarano, A.; Rea, S.; Loschi, A.R.; et al. Antibacterial Effect of Stainless Steel Surfaces Treated with a Nanotechnological Coating Approved for Food Contact. *Microorganisms* **2021**, *9*, 248. [CrossRef] [PubMed]
7. Berube, D.M. Rhetorical gamesmanship in the nano debates over sunscreens and nanoparticles. *J. Nanoparticle Res.* **2008**, *10*, 23–37. [CrossRef]
8. Jiang, J.; Pi, J.; Cai, J. The Advancing of Zinc Oxide Nanoparticles for Biomedical Applications. *Bioinorg. Chem. Appl.* **2018**, *2018*, 1062562. [CrossRef] [PubMed]
9. Wiesmann, N.; Mendler, S.; Buhr, C.R.; Ritz, U.; Kammerer, P.W.; Brieger, J. Zinc Oxide Nanoparticles Exhibit Favorable Properties to Promote Tissue Integration of Biomaterials. *Biomedicines* **2021**, *9*, 1462. [CrossRef] [PubMed]
10. Zhang, Y.; Nayak, T.R.; Hong, H.; Cai, W. Biomedical applications of zinc oxide nanomaterials. *Curr. Mol. Med.* **2013**, *13*, 1633–1645. [CrossRef]
11. Ahamed, M.; Khan, M.A.M.; Akhtar, M.J.; Alhadlaq, H.A.; Alshamsan, A. Role of Zn doping in oxidative stress mediated cytotoxicity of TiO_2 nanoparticles in human breast cancer MCF-7 cells. *Sci. Rep.* **2016**, *6*, 30196. [CrossRef] [PubMed]
12. Franklin, N.M.; Rogers, N.J.; Apte, S.C.; Batley, G.E.; Gadd, G.E.; Casey, P.S. Comparative Toxicity of Nanoparticulate ZnO, Bulk ZnO, and $ZnCl_2$ to a Freshwater Microalga (*Pseudokirchneriella subcapitata*): The Importance of Particle Solubility. *Environ. Sci. Technol.* **2007**, *41*, 8484–8490. [CrossRef] [PubMed]
13. Kumar, N.; Chandan, N.K.; Wakchaure, G.C.; Singh, N.P. Synergistic effect of zinc nanoparticles and temperature on acute toxicity with response to biochemical markers and histopathological attributes in fish. *Comp. Biochem. Physiol. C Toxicol. Pharmacol.* **2020**, *229*, 108678. [CrossRef]
14. Lin, D.; Xing, B. Phytotoxicity of nanoparticles: Inhibition of seed germination and root growth. *Environ. Pollut.* **2007**, *150*, 243–250. [CrossRef]
15. Park, S.; Lee, Y.K.; Jung, M.; Kim, K.H.; Chung, N.; Ahn, E.K.; Lim, Y.; Lee, K.H. Cellular toxicity of various inhalable metal nanoparticles on human alveolar epithelial cells. *Inhal. Toxicol.* **2007**, *19* (Suppl. 1), 59–65. [CrossRef]
16. Sardoiwala, M.N.; Kaundal, B.; Choudhury, S.R. Toxic impact of nanomaterials on microbes, plants and animals. *Environ. Chem. Lett.* **2018**, *16*, 147–160. [CrossRef]
17. Zhang, L.; Jiang, Y.; Ding, Y.; Povey, M.; York, D. Investigation into the antibacterial behaviour of suspensions of ZnO nanoparticles (ZnO nanofluids). *J. Nanoparticle Res.* **2007**, *9*, 479–489. [CrossRef]
18. Khalil, S.R.; Zheng, C.; Abou-Zeid, S.M.; Farag, M.R.; Elsabbagh, H.S.; Siddique, M.S.; Azzam, M.M.; Di Cerbo, A.; Elkhadrawey, B.A. Modulatory effect of thymol on the immune response and susceptibility to *Aeromonas hydrophila* infection in Nile tilapia fish exposed to zinc oxide nanoparticles. *Aquat. Toxicol.* **2023**, *259*, 106523. [CrossRef]
19. Mawed, S.A.; Centoducati, G.; Farag, M.R.; Alagawany, M.; Abou-Zeid, S.M.; Elhady, W.M.; El-Saadony, M.T.; Di Cerbo, A.; Al-Zahaby, S.A. *Dunaliella salina* Microalga Restores the Metabolic Equilibrium and Ameliorates the Hepatic Inflammatory Response Induced by Zinc Oxide Nanoparticles (ZnO-NPs) in Male Zebrafish. *Biology* **2022**, *11*, 1447. [CrossRef] [PubMed]
20. Di Cerbo, A.; Canello, S.; Guidetti, G.; Fiore, F.; Corsi, L.; Rubattu, N.; Testa, C.; Cocco, R. Adverse food reactions in dogs due to antibiotic residues in pet food: A preliminary study. *Vet. Ital.* **2018**, *54*, 137–146. [CrossRef]
21. Arunachalam, M.; Raja, M.; Vijayakumar, C.; Malaiammal, P.; Mayden, R.L. Natural history of zebrafish (*Danio rerio*) in India. *Zebrafish* **2013**, *10*, 1–14. [CrossRef]
22. Schilling, T.F.; Webb, J. Considering the zebrafish in a comparative context. *J. Exp. Zool. B Mol. Dev. Evol.* **2007**, *308*, 515–522. [CrossRef]
23. Becker, C.G.; Becker, T. Adult zebrafish as a model for successful central nervous system regeneration. *Restor. Neurol. Neurosci.* **2008**, *26*, 71–80. [PubMed]
24. Choi, J.S.; Kim, R.O.; Yoon, S.; Kim, W.K. Developmental Toxicity of Zinc Oxide Nanoparticles to Zebrafish (*Danio rerio*): A Transcriptomic Analysis. *PLoS ONE* **2016**, *11*, e0160763. [CrossRef]
25. Kteeba, S.M.; El-Ghobashy, A.E.; El-Adawi, H.I.; El-Rayis, O.A.; Sreevidya, V.S.; Guo, L.; Svoboda, K.R. Exposure to ZnO nanoparticles alters neuronal and vascular development in zebrafish: Acute and transgenerational effects mitigated with dissolved organic matter. *Environ. Pollut.* **2018**, *242*, 433–448. [CrossRef] [PubMed]

26. Brooker, R.M.; Dixson, D.L. Assessing the Role of Olfactory Cues in the Early Life History of Coral Reef Fish: Current Methods and Future Directions. In *Chemical Signals in Vertebrates 13*; Springer: Cham, Switzerland, 2016; pp. 17–31.
27. Kondo, K.; Kikuta, S.; Ueha, R.; Suzukawa, K.; Yamasoba, T. Age-Related Olfactory Dysfunction: Epidemiology, Pathophysiology, and Clinical Management. *Front. Aging Neurosci.* **2020**, *12*, 208. [CrossRef]
28. Attems, J.; Walker, L.; Jellinger, K.A. Olfaction and Aging: A Mini-Review. *Gerontology* **2015**, *61*, 485–490. [CrossRef]
29. Hummel, T.; Whitcroft, K.L.; Andrews, P.; Altundag, A.; Cinghi, C.; Costanzo, R.M.; Damm, M.; Frasnelli, J.; Gudziol, H.; Gupta, N.; et al. Position paper on olfactory dysfunction. *Rhinology* **2016**, *56*, 1–30. [CrossRef]
30. Liu, B.; Luo, Z.; Pinto, J.M.; Shiroma, E.J.; Tranah, G.J.; Wirdefeldt, K.; Fang, F.; Harris, T.B.; Chen, H. Relationship Between Poor Olfaction and Mortality among Community-Dwelling Older Adults: A Cohort Study. *Ann. Intern. Med.* **2019**, *170*, 673–681. [CrossRef]
31. Schubert, C.R.; Fischer, M.E.; Pinto, A.A.; Klein, B.E.K.; Klein, R.; Tweed, T.S.; Cruickshanks, K.J. Sensory Impairments and Risk of Mortality in Older Adults. *J. Gerontol. Ser. A Biomed. Sci. Med. Sci.* **2017**, *72*, 710–715. [CrossRef] [PubMed]
32. Razmara, P.; Lari, E.; Mohaddes, E.; Zhang, Y.; Goss, G.G.; Pyle, G.G. The effect of copper nanoparticles on olfaction in rainbow trout (*Oncorhynchus mykiss*). *Environ. Sci. Nano* **2019**, *6*, 2094–2104. [CrossRef]
33. Bilberg, K.; Døving, K.B.; Beedholm, K.; Baatrup, E. Silver nanoparticles disrupt olfaction in Crucian carp (*Carassius carassius*) and Eurasian perch (*Perca fluviatilis*). *Aquat. Toxicol.* **2011**, *104*, 145–152. [CrossRef]
34. Gao, L.; Yang, S.T.; Li, S.; Meng, Y.; Wang, H.; Lei, H. Acute toxicity of zinc oxide nanoparticles to the rat olfactory system after intranasal instillation. *J. Appl. Toxicol.* **2013**, *33*, 1079–1088. [CrossRef]
35. Westerfield, M. *The Zebrafish Book: A Guide for the Laboratory Use of Zebrafish (Danio rerio)*; University of Oregon Press: Eugene, OR, USA, 2000.
36. Mawed, S.A.; Marini, C.; Alagawany, M.; Farag, M.R.; Reda, R.M.; El-Saadony, M.T.; Elhady, W.M.; Magi, G.E.; Di Cerbo, A.; El-Nagar, W.G. Zinc Oxide Nanoparticles (ZnO-NPs) Suppress Fertility by Activating Autophagy, Apoptosis, and Oxidative Stress in the Developing Oocytes of Female Zebrafish. *Antioxidants* **2022**, *11*, 1567. [CrossRef] [PubMed]
37. Ruzhinskaya, N.N.; Gdovskii, P.A.; Devitsina, G.V. Chloride Cells, A Constituent of the Fish Olfactory Epithelium. *J. Evol. Biochem. Physiol.* **2001**, *37*, 89–94. [CrossRef]
38. Slaoui, M.; Fiette, L. Histopathology procedures: From tissue sampling to histopathological evaluation. *Drug Saf. Eval. Methods Protoc.* **2011**, *691*, 69–82. [CrossRef]
39. Di Cerbo, A.; Canello, S.; Guidetti, G.; Laurino, C.; Palmieri, B. Unusual antibiotic presence in gym trained subjects with food intolerance; a case report. *Nutr. Hosp.* **2014**, *30*, 395–398. [CrossRef]
40. Di Cerbo, A.; Palmieri, B. Review: The market of probiotics. *Pak. J. Pharm. Sci.* **2015**, *28*, 2199–2206.
41. Mazzeranghi, F.; Zanotti, C.; Di Cerbo, A.; Verstegen, J.P.; Cocco, R.; Guidetti, G.; Canello, S. Clinical efficacy of nutraceutical diet for cats with clinical signs of cutaneus adverse food reaction (CAFR). *Pol. J. Vet. Sci.* **2017**, *20*, 269–276. [CrossRef]
42. Di Cerbo, A.; Rubino, V.; Morelli, F.; Ruggiero, G.; Landi, R.; Guidetti, G.; Canello, S.; Terrazzano, G.; Alessandrini, A. Mechanical phenotyping of K562 cells by the Micropipette Aspiration Technique allows identifying mechanical changes induced by drugs. *Sci. Rep.* **2018**, *8*, 1219. [CrossRef]
43. Di Cerbo, A.; Palmieri, B. The economic impact of second opinion in pathology. *Saudi Med. J.* **2012**, *33*, 1051–1052.
44. Iannitti, T.; Palmieri, B.; Aspiro, A.; Di Cerbo, A. A preliminary study of painless and effective transdermal botulinum toxin A delivery by jet nebulization for treatment of primary hyperhidrosis. *Drug Des. Dev. Ther.* **2014**, *8*, 931–935. [CrossRef]
45. Destefanis, S.; Giretto, D.; Muscolo, M.C.; Di Cerbo, A.; Guidetti, G.; Canello, S.; Giovazzino, A.; Centenaro, S.; Terrazzano, G. Clinical evaluation of a nutraceutical diet as an adjuvant to pharmacological treatment in dogs affected by Keratoconjunctivitis sicca. *BMC Vet. Res.* **2016**, *12*, 214. [CrossRef]
46. Farag, M.R.; Zizzadoro, C.; Alagawany, M.; Abou-Zeid, S.M.; Mawed, S.A.; El Kholy, M.S.; Di Cerbo, A.; Azzam, M.M.; Mahdy, E.A.A.; Khedr, M.H.E.; et al. In ovo protective effects of chicoric and rosmarinic acids against Thiacloprid-induced cytotoxicity, oxidative stress, and growth retardation on newly hatched chicks. *Poult. Sci.* **2023**, *102*, 102487. [CrossRef] [PubMed]
47. Farag, M.R.; Abo-Al-Ela, H.G.; Alagawany, M.; Azzam, M.M.; El-Saadony, M.T.; Rea, S.; Di Cerbo, A.; Nouh, D.S. Effect of Quercetin Nanoparticles on Hepatic and Intestinal Enzymes and Stress-Related Genes in Nile Tilapia Fish Exposed to Silver Nanoparticles. *Biomedicines* **2023**, *11*, 663. [CrossRef]
48. Farag, M.R.; Moselhy, A.A.A.; El-Mleeh, A.; Aljuaydi, S.H.; Ismail, T.A.; Di Cerbo, A.; Crescenzo, G.; Abou-Zeid, S.M. Quercetin Alleviates the Immunotoxic Impact Mediated by Oxidative Stress and Inflammation Induced by Doxorubicin Exposure in Rats. *Antioxidants* **2021**, *10*, 1906. [CrossRef]
49. Farag, M.R.; Khalil, S.R.; Zaglool, A.W.; Hendam, B.M.; Moustafa, A.A.; Cocco, R.; Di Cerbo, A.; Alagawany, M. Thiacloprid Induced Developmental Neurotoxicity via ROS-Oxidative Injury and Inflammation in Chicken Embryo: The Possible Attenuating Role of Chicoric and Rosmarinic Acids. *Biology* **2021**, *10*, 1100. [CrossRef] [PubMed]
50. Gallo, A.; Landi, R.; Rubino, V.; Di Cerbo, A.; Giovazzino, A.; Palatucci, A.T.; Centenaro, S.; Guidetti, G.; Canello, S.; Cortese, L.; et al. Oxytetracycline induces DNA damage and epigenetic changes: A possible risk for human and animal health? *PeerJ* **2017**, *5*, e3236. [CrossRef]
51. Guildford, A.L.; Poletti, T.; Osbourne, L.H.; Di Cerbo, A.; Gatti, A.M.; Santin, M. Nanoparticles of a different source induce different patterns of activation in key biochemical and cellular components of the host response. *J. R. Soc. Interface* **2009**, *6*, 1213–1221. [CrossRef] [PubMed]

52. Lebeaupin, C.; Vallee, D.; Hazari, Y.; Hetz, C.; Chevet, E.; Bailly-Maitre, B. Endoplasmic reticulum stress signalling and the pathogenesis of non-alcoholic fatty liver disease. *J. Hepatol.* **2018**, *69*, 927–947. [CrossRef]
53. Hentig, J.T.; Byrd-Jacobs, C.A. Exposure to Zinc Sulfate Results in Differential Effects on Olfactory Sensory Neuron Subtypes in Adult Zebrafish. *Int. J. Mol. Sci.* **2016**, *17*, 1445. [CrossRef]
54. Bai, W.; Zhang, Z.; Tian, W.; He, X.; Ma, Y.; Zhao, Y.; Chai, Z. Toxicity of zinc oxide nanoparticles to zebrafish embryo: A physicochemical study of toxicity mechanism. *J. Nanoparticle Res.* **2010**, *12*, 1645–1654. [CrossRef]
55. Du, J.; Wang, S.; You, H.; Jiang, R.; Zhuang, C.; Zhang, X. Developmental toxicity and DNA damage to zebrafish induced by perfluorooctane sulfonate in the presence of ZnO nanoparticles. *Environ. Toxicol.* **2016**, *31*, 360–371. [CrossRef] [PubMed]
56. Hou, J.; Liu, H.; Zhang, S.; Liu, X.; Hayat, T.; Alsaedi, A.; Wang, X. Mechanism of toxic effects of Nano-ZnO on cell cycle of zebrafish (*Danio rerio*). *Chemosphere* **2019**, *229*, 206–213. [CrossRef] [PubMed]
57. Kteeba, S.M.; El-Adawi, H.I.; El-Rayis, O.A.; El-Ghobashy, A.E.; Schuld, J.L.; Svoboda, K.R.; Guo, L. Zinc oxide nanoparticle toxicity in embryonic zebrafish: Mitigation with different natural organic matter. *Environ. Pollut.* **2017**, *230*, 1125–1140. [CrossRef] [PubMed]
58. Lee, G.; Lee, B.; Kim, K.-T. Mechanisms and effects of zinc oxide nanoparticle transformations on toxicity to zebrafish embryos. *Environ. Sci. Nano* **2021**, *8*, 1690–1700. [CrossRef]
59. Zhao, X.; Wang, S.; Wu, Y.; You, H.; Lv, L. Acute ZnO nanoparticles exposure induces developmental toxicity, oxidative stress and DNA damage in embryo-larval zebrafish. *Aquat. Toxicol.* **2013**, *136–137*, 49–59. [CrossRef]
60. Zhu, X.; Wang, J.; Zhang, X.; Chang, Y.; Chen, Y. The impact of ZnO nanoparticle aggregates on the embryonic development of zebrafish (*Danio rerio*). *Nanotechnology* **2009**, *20*, 195103. [CrossRef]
61. Wyatt, T.D. Pheromones and signature mixtures: Defining species-wide signals and variable cues for identity in both invertebrates and vertebrates. *J. Comp. Physiol. A Neuroethol. Sens. Neural. Behav. Physiol.* **2010**, *196*, 685–700. [CrossRef]
62. Eisthen, H.L. Evolution of vertebrate olfactory systems. *Brain Behav. Evol.* **1997**, *50*, 222–233. [CrossRef]
63. Hamdani, E.H.; Doving, K.B. Specific projection of the sensory crypt cells in the olfactory system in crucian carp, *Carassius carassius*. *Chem. Senses* **2006**, *31*, 63–67. [CrossRef]
64. Døving, K.; Kasumyan, A. Chemoreception. In *Fish Larval Physiology*; CRC Press: Boca Raton, FL, USA, 2008; pp. 331–394. [CrossRef]
65. Di Cerbo, A.; Sechi, S.; Canello, S.; Guidetti, G.; Fiore, F.; Cocco, R. Behavioral Disturbances: An Innovative Approach to Monitor the Modulatory Effects of a Nutraceutical Diet. *J. Vis. Exp.* **2017**, *119*, e54878. [CrossRef]
66. Sechi, S.; Di Cerbo, A.; Canello, S.; Guidetti, G.; Chiavolelli, F.; Fiore, F.; Cocco, R. Effects in dogs with behavioural disorders of a commercial nutraceutical diet on stress and neuroendocrine parameters. *Vet. Rec.* **2017**, *180*, 18. [CrossRef] [PubMed]
67. Kermen, F.; Franco, L.; Wyatt, C.; Yaksi, E. Neural circuits mediating olfactory-driven behavior in fish. *Front. Neural Circuits* **2013**, *7*, 62. [CrossRef]
68. Biechl, D.; Tietje, K.; Gerlach, G.; Wullimann, M.F. Crypt cells are involved in kin recognition in larval zebrafish. *Sci. Rep.* **2016**, *6*, 24590. [CrossRef] [PubMed]
69. Lazzari, M.; Bettini, S.; Milani, L.; Maurizii, M.G.; Franceschini, V. Differential response of olfactory sensory neuron populations to copper ion exposure in zebrafish. *Aquat. Toxicol.* **2017**, *183*, 54–62. [CrossRef]
70. Hansen, A.; Zeiske, E. The peripheral olfactory organ of the zebrafish, *Danio rerio*: An ultrastructural study. *Chem. Senses* **1998**, *23*, 39–48. [CrossRef]
71. Hansen, A.; Zielinski, B.S. Diversity in the olfactory epithelium of bony fishes: Development, lamellar arrangement, sensory neuron cell types and transduction components. *J. Neurocytol.* **2005**, *34*, 183–208. [CrossRef]
72. Miyasaka, N.; Wanner, A.A.; Li, J.; Mack-Bucher, J.; Genoud, C.; Yoshihara, Y.; Friedrich, R.W. Functional development of the olfactory system in zebrafish. *Mech. Dev.* **2013**, *130*, 336–346. [CrossRef]
73. Olivares, J.; Schmachtenberg, O. An update on anatomy and function of the teleost olfactory system. *PeerJ* **2019**, *7*, e7808. [CrossRef]
74. Calvo-Ochoa, E.; Byrd-Jacobs, C.A. The Olfactory System of Zebrafish as a Model for the Study of Neurotoxicity and Injury: Implications for Neuroplasticity and Disease. *Int. J. Mol. Sci.* **2019**, *20*, 1639. [CrossRef] [PubMed]
75. Gayoso, J.; Castro, A.; Anadon, R.; Manso, M.J. Crypt cells of the zebrafish *Danio rerio* mainly project to the dorsomedial glomerular field of the olfactory bulb. *Chem. Senses* **2012**, *37*, 357–369. [CrossRef]
76. Ahuja, G.; Nia, S.B.; Zapilko, V.; Shiriagin, V.; Kowatschew, D.; Oka, Y.; Korsching, S.I. Kappe neurons, a novel population of olfactory sensory neurons. *Sci. Rep.* **2014**, *4*, 4037. [CrossRef]
77. Hansen, A.; Finger, T.E. Phyletic distribution of crypt-type olfactory receptor neurons in fishes. *Brain Behav Evol* **2000**, *55*, 100–110. [CrossRef] [PubMed]
78. Hansen, A.; Rolen, S.H.; Anderson, K.; Morita, Y.; Caprio, J.; Finger, T.E. Correlation between olfactory receptor cell type and function in the channel catfish. *J. Neurosci.* **2003**, *23*, 9328–9339. [CrossRef]
79. Lipschitz, D.L.; Michel, W.C. Amino acid odorants stimulate microvillar sensory neurons. *Chem. Senses* **2002**, *27*, 277–286. [CrossRef] [PubMed]
80. Sato, Y.; Miyasaka, N.; Yoshihara, Y. Mutually exclusive glomerular innervation by two distinct types of olfactory sensory neurons revealed in transgenic zebrafish. *J. Neurosci.* **2005**, *25*, 4889–4897. [CrossRef]

81. Hara, T.J.; Zhang, C. Topographic bulbar projections and dual neural pathways of the primary olfactory neurons in salmonid fishes. *Neuroscience* **1998**, *82*, 301–313. [CrossRef] [PubMed]
82. Sato, K.; Suzuki, N. Whole-cell response characteristics of ciliated and microvillous olfactory receptor neurons to amino acids, pheromone candidates and urine in rainbow trout. *Chem. Senses* **2001**, *26*, 1145–1156. [CrossRef]
83. Oka, Y.; Korsching, S.I. Shared and unique G alpha proteins in the zebrafish versus mammalian senses of taste and smell. *Chem. Senses* **2011**, *36*, 357–365. [CrossRef]
84. Cancalon, P. Degeneration and regeneration of olfactory cells induced by $ZnSO_4$ and other chemicals. *Tissue Cell* **1982**, *14*, 717–733. [CrossRef]
85. Bazaes, A.; Schmachtenberg, O. Odorant tuning of olfactory crypt cells from juvenile and adult rainbow trout. *J. Exp. Biol.* **2012**, *215*, 1740–1748. [CrossRef] [PubMed]
86. Ferrando, S.; Bottaro, M.; Gallus, L.; Girosi, L.; Vacchi, M.; Tagliafierro, G. Observations of crypt neuron-like cells in the olfactory epithelium of a cartilaginous fish. *Neurosci. Lett.* **2006**, *403*, 280–282. [CrossRef] [PubMed]
87. Hamdani, E.H.; Lastein, S.; Gregersen, F.; Doving, K.B. Seasonal variations in olfactory sensory neurons—Fish sensitivity to sex pheromones explained? *Chem. Senses* **2008**, *33*, 119–123. [CrossRef]
88. Wakisaka, N.; Miyasaka, N.; Koide, T.; Masuda, M.; Hiraki-Kajiyama, T.; Yoshihara, Y. An Adenosine Receptor for Olfaction in Fish. *Curr. Biol.* **2017**, *27*, 1437–1447.E4. [CrossRef] [PubMed]
89. Cheung, K.Y.; Jesuthasan, S.J.; Baxendale, S.; van Hateren, N.J.; Marzo, M.; Hill, C.J.; Whitfield, T.T. Olfactory Rod Cells: A Rare Cell Type in the Larval Zebrafish Olfactory Epithelium with a Large Actin-Rich Apical Projection. *Front. Physiol.* **2021**, *12*, 626080. [CrossRef]
90. Elsaesser, R.; Paysan, J. The sense of smell, its signalling pathways, and the dichotomy of cilia and microvilli in olfactory sensory cells. *BMC Neurosci.* **2007**, *8*, S1. [CrossRef]
91. Yamamoto, M. Comparative Morphology of the Peripheral Olfactory Organ in Teleosts. In *Chemoreception in Fishes*; Hara, T.J., Ed.; Elsevier: New York, NY, USA, 1982; pp. 39–59.
92. Ichikawa, M.; Ueda, K. Fine structure of the olfactory epithelium in the goldfish, Carassius auratus. *Cell Tissue Res.* **1977**, *183*, 445–455. [CrossRef]
93. Rhein, L.D.; Cagan, R.H.; Orkand, P.M.; Dolack, M.K. Surface specializations of the olfactory epithelium of rainbow trout, Salmo gairdneri. *Tissue Cell* **1981**, *13*, 577–587. [CrossRef]
94. Hernadi, L. Fine structural characterization of the olfactory epithelium and its response to divalent cations Cd^{2+} in the fish Alburnus alburnus (Teleostei, Cyprinidae): A scanning and transmission electron microscopic study. *Neurobiology* **1993**, *1*, 11–31.
95. Datta, N.C.; Bandopadhyay, S. Ultrastructure of cell types of the olfactory epithelium in a catfish, *Heteropneustesfossilis* (Bloch). *J. Biosci.* **1997**, *22*, 233–245. [CrossRef]
96. Ismail, M.H.; Salem, M.A.; Nassar, S.A.; Mawed, S.A. Comparative morphological and histological studies on the olfactory organ in two models of bony fishes (*Mugil cephalus* and *Malapterurus electricus*): Light and electron microscopic studies. *Egypt. J. Zool.* **2013**, *60*, 223–244. [CrossRef]
97. Waryani, B.; Zhao, Y.; Zhang, C.; Abbasi, A.R.; Ferrando, S.; Dai, R.; Soomro, A.N.; Baloch, W.A.; Abbas, G. Surface architecture of the olfactory epithelium of two Chinese cave loaches (Cypriniformes: Nemacheilidae: *Oreonectes*). *Ital. J. Zool.* **2015**, *82*, 179–185. [CrossRef]
98. Zhang, X.Y.; Huang, Z.Q.; Ning, T.; Xiang, X.H.; Li, C.Q.; Chen, S.Y.; Xiao, H. Microscopic and Submicroscopic Gradient Variation of Olfactory Systems among Six *Sinocyclocheilus* Species Living in Different Environments. *Zool. Sci.* **2018**, *35*, 411–420. [CrossRef]
99. Zielinski, B.S.; Hara, T.J. Ciliated and microvillar receptor cells degenerate and then differentiate in the olfactory epithelium of rainbow trout following olfactory nerve section. *Microsc. Res. Tech.* **1992**, *23*, 22–27. [CrossRef]
100. Pashchenko, N.I.; Kasumyan, A.O. Scanning electron microscopy of development of the olfactory organ in ontogeny of grass carp *Ctenopharyngodon idella*. *J. Ichthyol.* **2015**, *55*, 880–899. [CrossRef]
101. DePasquale, J.A. Tropomyosin and alpha-actinin in teleost rodlet cells. *Acta Zool.* **2021**, *102*, 323–332. [CrossRef]
102. Dezfuli, B.S.; Capuano, S.; Simoni, E.; Previati, M.; Giari, L. Rodlet cells and the sensory systems in zebrafish (*Danio rerio*). *Anat. Rec.* **2007**, *290*, 367–374. [CrossRef]
103. Al-Hussaini, A.H. On the Nature of Certain Pear-Shaped Cells in the Intestinal Epithelium of Fish. *Bull. Inst. Egypte* **1964**, *40*, 23–31.
104. Grunberg, W.; Hager, G. Ultrastructural and histochemical aspects of the rodlet cells from the bulbus arteriosus of *Cyprinus carpio* L. (Pisces: Cyprinidae) (author's transl). *Anat. Anzeiger.* **1978**, *143*, 277–290.
105. Dezfuli, B.S.; Simoni, E.; Rossi, R.; Manera, M. Rodlet cells and other inflammatory cells of *Phoxinus phoxinus* infected with *Raphidascaris acus* (Nematoda). *Dis. Aquat. Org.* **2000**, *43*, 61–69. [CrossRef]
106. Blaiotta, G.; Murru, N.; Di Cerbo, A.; Succi, M.; Coppola, R.; Aponte, M. Commercially standardized process for probiotic "Italico" cheese production. *LWT-Food Sci. Technol.* **2017**, *79*, 601–608. [CrossRef]
107. Dezfuli, B.S.; Capuano, S.; Manera, M. A description of rodlet cells from the alimentary canal of *Anguilla anguilla* and their relationship with parasitic helminths. *J. Fish Biol.* **1998**, *53*, 1084–1095. [CrossRef]
108. Fishelson, L.; Becker, K. Rodlet cells in the head and trunk kidney of the domestic carp (*Cyprinus carpio*): Enigmatic gland cells or coccidian parasites? *Naturwissenschaften* **1999**, *86*, 400–403. [CrossRef] [PubMed]
109. Iger, Y.; Abraham, M. Rodlet cells in the epidermis of fish exposed to stressors. *Tissue Cell* **1997**, *29*, 431–438. [CrossRef]

110. Scarano, A.; Murmura, G.; Vantaggiato, G.; Lauritano, D.; Silvestre-Rangil, J.; Di Cerbo, A.; Lorusso, F. Delayed expansion of atrophic mandible (deam): A case report. *Oral Implant.* **2017**, *10*, 190–196. [CrossRef] [PubMed]
111. Dezfuli, B.S.; Pironi, F.; Maynard, B.; Simoni, E.; Bosi, G. Rodlet cells, fish immune cells and a sentinel of parasitic harm in teleost organs. *Fish Shellfish Immunol.* **2022**, *121*, 516–534. [CrossRef] [PubMed]
112. Viswaprakash, N.; Dennis, J.C.; Globa, L.; Pustovyy, O.; Josephson, E.M.; Kanju, P.; Morrison, E.E.; Vodyanoy, V.J. Enhancement of odorant-induced responses in olfactory receptor neurons by zinc nanoparticles. *Chem. Senses* **2009**, *34*, 547–557. [CrossRef]
113. Lazzari, M.; Bettini, S.; Ciani, F.; Franceschini, V. Light and transmission electron microscopy study of the peripheral olfactory organ of the guppy, *Poecilia reticulata* (Teleostei, Poecilidae). *Microsc. Res. Tech.* **2007**, *70*, 782–789. [CrossRef]
114. Lazzari, M.; Bettini, S.; Milani, L.; Maurizii, M.G.; Franceschini, V. Differential nickel-induced responses of olfactory sensory neuron populations in zebrafish. *Aquat. Toxicol.* **2019**, *206*, 14–23. [CrossRef]
115. Lazzari, M.; Bettini, S.; Milani, L.; Maurizii, M.G.; Franceschini, V. Response of Olfactory Sensory Neurons to Mercury Ions in Zebrafish: An Immunohistochemical Study. *Microsc. Microanal.* **2022**, *28*, 227–242. [CrossRef] [PubMed]
116. Razmara, P.; Pyle, G.G. Recovery of rainbow trout olfactory function following exposure to copper nanoparticles and copper ions. *Aquat. Toxicol.* **2022**, *245*, 106109. [CrossRef]
117. Ghosh, D.; Mandal, D.K. Mercuric chloride induced toxicity responses in the olfactory epithelium of *Labeo rohita* (Hamilton): A light and electron microscopy study. *Fish Physiol. Biochem.* **2014**, *40*, 83–92. [CrossRef] [PubMed]
118. Roy, D.; Ghosh, D.; Mandal, D.K. Induction of Metallothionein in the Olfactory Epithelium of *Channa punctatus* (Bloch) in Response to Cadmium Exposure: An Immunohistochemical Study. *Proc. Zool. Soc.* **2012**, *65*, 40–44. [CrossRef]
119. Saliani, M.; Jalal, R.; Goharshadi, E. Mechanism of oxidative stress involved in the toxicity of ZnO nanoparticles against eukaryotic cells. *Nanomed. J.* **2016**, *3*, 1–14. Available online: https://profdoc.um.ac.ir/paper-abstract-1053987.html (accessed on 29 August 2023).
120. Verma, S.K.; Panda, P.K.; Jha, E.; Suar, M.; Parashar, S.K.S. Altered physiochemical properties in industrially synthesized ZnO nanoparticles regulate oxidative stress; induce in vivo cytotoxicity in embryonic zebrafish by apoptosis. *Sci. Rep.* **2017**, *7*, 13909. [CrossRef]
121. Wang, Y.; Branicky, R.; Noe, A.; Hekimi, S. Superoxide dismutases: Dual roles in controlling ROS damage and regulating ROS signaling. *J. Cell Biol.* **2018**, *217*, 1915–1928. [CrossRef]
122. Hwang, J.; Jin, J.; Jeon, S.; Moon, S.H.; Park, M.Y.; Yum, D.Y.; Kim, J.H.; Kang, J.E.; Park, M.H.; Kim, E.J.; et al. SOD1 suppresses pro-inflammatory immune responses by protecting against oxidative stress in colitis. *Redox Biol.* **2020**, *37*, 101760. [CrossRef]
123. Ighodaro, O.M.; Akinloye, O.A. First line defence antioxidants-superoxide dismutase (SOD), catalase (CAT) and glutathione peroxidase (GPX): Their fundamental role in the entire antioxidant defence grid. *Alex. J. Med.* **2018**, *54*, 287–293. [CrossRef]
124. Preedia Babu, E.; Subastri, A.; Suyavaran, A.; Lokeshwara Rao, P.; Suresh Kumar, M.; Jeevaratnam, K.; Thirunavukkarasu, C. Extracellularly synthesized ZnO nanoparticles interact with DNA and augment gamma radiation induced DNA damage through reactive oxygen species. *RSC Adv.* **2015**, *5*, 62067–62077. [CrossRef]
125. Barzilai, A.; Yamamoto, K. DNA damage responses to oxidative stress. *DNA Repair* **2004**, *3*, 1109–1115. [CrossRef]
126. Panda, K.K.; Golari, D.; Venugopal, A.; Achary, V.M.M.; Phaomei, G.; Parinandi, N.L.; Sahu, H.K.; Panda, B.B. Green Synthesized Zinc Oxide (ZnO) Nanoparticles Induce Oxidative Stress and DNA Damage in *Lathyrus sativus* L. Root Bioassay System. *Antioxidants* **2017**, *6*, 35. [CrossRef]
127. Payne, C.M.; Bernstein, C.; Bernstein, H. Apoptosis overview emphasizing the role of oxidative stress, DNA damage and signal-transduction pathways. *Leuk. Lymphoma* **1995**, *19*, 43–93. [CrossRef]
128. Di Cerbo, A.; Pezzuto, F.; Guidetti, G.; Canello, S.; Corsi, L. Tetracyclines: Insights and updates of their use in human and animal pathology and their potential toxicity. *Open Biochem. J.* **2019**, *13*, 1–12. [CrossRef]
129. Chen, Z.; Wan, X.; Hou, Q.; Shi, S.; Wang, L.; Chen, P.; Zhu, X.; Zeng, C.; Qin, W.; Zhou, W.; et al. GADD45B mediates podocyte injury in zebrafish by activating the ROS-GADD45B-p38 pathway. *Cell Death Dis.* **2016**, *7*, e2068. [CrossRef] [PubMed]
130. Kumar, A.; Najafzadeh, M.; Jacob, B.K.; Dhawan, A.; Anderson, D. Zinc oxide nanoparticles affect the expression of p53, Ras p21 and JNKs: An ex vivo/in vitro exposure study in respiratory disease patients. *Mutagenesis* **2015**, *30*, 237–245. [CrossRef]
131. Macleod, K.F.; Sherry, N.; Hannon, G.; Beach, D.; Tokino, T.; Kinzler, K.; Vogelstein, B.; Jacks, T. p53-dependent and independent expression of p21 during cell growth, differentiation, and DNA damage. *Genes Dev.* **1995**, *9*, 935–944. [CrossRef]
132. Setyawati, M.I.; Tay, C.Y.; Leong, D.T. Effect of zinc oxide nanomaterials-induced oxidative stress on the p53 pathway. *Biomaterials* **2013**, *34*, 10133–10142. [CrossRef]
133. Ng, K.W.; Khoo, S.P.; Heng, B.C.; Setyawati, M.I.; Tan, E.C.; Zhao, X.; Xiong, S.; Fang, W.; Leong, D.T.; Loo, J.S. The role of the tumor suppressor p53 pathway in the cellular DNA damage response to zinc oxide nanoparticles. *Biomaterials* **2011**, *32*, 8218–8225. [CrossRef] [PubMed]
134. Norbury, C.J.; Zhivotovsky, B. DNA damage-induced apoptosis. *Oncogene* **2004**, *23*, 2797–2808. [CrossRef]
135. Roos, W.P.; Kaina, B. DNA damage-induced cell death by apoptosis. *Trends Mol. Med.* **2006**, *12*, 440–450. [CrossRef] [PubMed]
136. Wang, C.; Hu, X.; Gao, Y.; Ji, Y. ZnO Nanoparticles Treatment Induces Apoptosis by Increasing Intracellular ROS Levels in LTEP-a-2 Cells. *BioMed Res. Int.* **2015**, *2015*, 423287. [CrossRef] [PubMed]
137. Lu, H.; Lei, X.; Zhang, Q. Moderate activation of IKK2-NF-kB in unstressed adult mouse liver induces cytoprotective genes and lipogenesis without apparent signs of inflammation or fibrosis. *BMC Gastroenterol.* **2015**, *15*, 94. [CrossRef]

138. Du, J.; Cai, J.; Wang, S.; You, H. Oxidative stress and apoptosis to zebrafish (*Danio rerio*) embryos exposed to perfluorooctane sulfonate (PFOS) and ZnO nanoparticles. *Int. J. Occup. Med. Environ. Health* **2017**, *30*, 213–229. [CrossRef]
139. Gotoh, T.; Oyadomari, S.; Mori, K.; Mori, M. Nitric oxide-induced apoptosis in RAW 264.7 macrophages is mediated by endoplasmic reticulum stress pathway involving ATF6 and CHOP. *J. Biol. Chem.* **2002**, *277*, 12343–12350. [CrossRef]
140. McCullough, K.D.; Martindale, J.L.; Klotz, L.O.; Aw, T.Y.; Holbrook, N.J. Gadd153 sensitizes cells to endoplasmic reticulum stress by down-regulating Bcl2 and perturbing the cellular redox state. *Mol. Cell. Biol.* **2001**, *21*, 1249–1259. [CrossRef]

animals

Article

Do Organochlorine Contaminants Modulate the Parasitic Infection Degree in Mediterranean Trout (*Salmo trutta*)?

Anna Monnolo [1,†], Maria Teresa Clausi [2,†], Filomena Del Piano [1], Mario Santoro [3], Maria Lorena Fiorentino [4], Lorella Barca [5], Giovanna Fusco [6], Barbara Degli Uberti [6], Luigia Ferrante [7], Raffaelina Mercogliano [1,‡] and Maria Carmela Ferrante [1,*,‡]

1 Department of Veterinary Medicine and Animal Productions, University of Naples Federico II, Via Federico Delpino 1, 80137 Naples, Italy; anna.monnolo@unina.it (A.M.); filomena.delpiano@unina.it (F.D.P.); raffaelina.mercogliano@unina.it (R.M.)
2 Experimental Zooprophylactic Institute of Southern Italy, Calabria Section, 88100 Catanzaro, Italy; mariateresa.clausi@izsmportici.it
3 Department of Integrative Marine Ecology, Stazione Zoologica Anton Dohrn, 80121 Naples, Italy; mario.santoro@szn.it
4 Environmental Research Center, Istituti Clinici Scientifici Maugeri IRCCS, 27100 Pavia, Italy; marialorena.fiorentino@icsmaugeri.it
5 Experimental Zooprophylactic Institute of Southern Italy, Calabria Section, 87100 Cosenza, Italy; lorella.barca@izsmportici.it
6 Experimental Zooprophylactic Institute of Southern Italy, 80055 Portici, Italy; giovanna.fusco@izsmportici.it (G.F.); barbara.degliuberti@izsmportici.it (B.D.U.)
7 Department of Biomedical Sciences, Humanitas University, 20072 Milan, Italy; luigia.ferrante@st.hunimed.eu
* Correspondence: ferrante@unina.it
† These authors contributed equally to this work.
‡ These authors equally contributed as senior authors.

Simple Summary: Living organisms may be simultaneously exposed to several stressors. Trout are a clear example of this scenario, being usually exposed to chemical contaminants and parasites. Moreover, it is also an intensely farmed fish, often caught for human consumption. Thus, trout may be considered a sentinel species, and the related evidence is a matter of importance. We looked at a sample of wild brown trout from a protected area of Southern Italy. Different numbers of gastro-intestinal helminths and concentrations of organochlorine pollutants were detected among sample units. In particular, a negative correlation between the presence of parasites and the concentration of polychlorinated biphenyls was assessed, suggesting that these organochlorine pollutants can affect parasite survival. Our results provide a contribution to the advancement of the knowledge of the interplay among environment, parasites, and host.

Abstract: We investigated the occurrence of organochlorine pollutants (OCs) in the muscle of brown trout and evaluated their potential modulation of parasite infection. The toxicological risk for consumer health was assessed, too. Trout were collected from the Sila National Park (Calabria region, South of Italy). The highest concentrations emerged for the sum of the 6 non-dioxin-like (ndl) indicator polychlorinated biphenyls (Σ6ndl-PCBs), followed by the 1,1,1-trichloro-2,2-di(4-chlorophenyl)-ethane (DDT), dioxin-like PCBs, hexachlorobenzene (HCB), and dieldrin. Measured on lipid weight (LW), the mean value of Σ6ndl-PCBs amounted to 201.9 ng g^{-1}, that of ΣDDTs (the sum of DDT-related compounds) to 100.2 ng g^{-1}, with the major contribution of the DDT-metabolite *p,p'*-DDE which was detected in all sample units (97.6 ng g^{-1} on average). Among dioxin-like congeners, PCB 118 showed the highest mean concentration (21.96 ng g^{-1} LW) and was detected in all sample units. Regression analysis of intestinal parasites on OC concentration was performed, controlling for two potential confounding factors, namely sex and sexual stage. The results evidenced the existence of interactions between the dual stressors in the host-parasite system in the wild. A negative and statistically significant correlation was estimated, suggesting that OCs may decrease parasite infection degree. Regarding the toxicological risk evaluation, OC concentrations were consistently below the current European Maximum Residue Limits.

Keywords: organochlorine contaminants; parasite infection; brown trout; risk evaluation

1. Introduction

Polychlorinated biphenyls (PCBs) and organochlorine pesticides (OCPs) are organochlorine compounds (OCs) widely used in the past that still persist in the environment due to their high chemical stability and lipophilicity. Aquatic organisms living in a contaminated ecosystem undergo OC biomagnification processes [1], resulting in high OC concentrations in the case of predatory species [2].

OCs are endocrine disruptors that induce a wide range of adverse effects, including alterations of reproductive, nervous, and immune systems, in both humans and wild animals, especially aquatic species [3]. In general, exposure to OCs leads to a suppression of the immune system's capability in fish [4–9]; in some cases, it leads to stimulation [10,11] or lack of adverse effects [12]. The extent of stimulus or suppression may be influenced by the exposure level and physiological factors, including sex and age [13,14]. For instance, Duffy and coauthors observed that the immunodepression increased in young Japanese medaka (*Oryzias latipes*) exposed to PCB 126, whereas it was unaffected in mature fish [15].

Digenean trematodes are the most common eukaryotic parasites in the aquatic environment with roughly 25,000 species identified and widely distributed in European ecosystems [16,17]. In particular, the intestine of freshwater teleost commonly harbors trematodes of the genus *Crepidostomum* [18]. Some authors suggest that these parasites do not cause relevant damage to fish [19], just exploiting the intestinal fluids [20].

Chemical xenobiotics and parasites may co-contaminate living beings [21], determining a host response that may depend on their interaction [22]. Recent research based on donkey milk [23] provided evidence of a positive correlation between intestinal parasitic infection and OC contamination, the latter being probably responsible for weakened immune system defense. Henríquez-Hernández et al. [24] hypothesized that intestinal parasites in dogs might reduce OCs bioavailability and their body burden in the host by bioaccumulating OCs introduced through food intake by the host itself. OCs may impair parasite success in reaching the host [25] and decrease the population density of those parasites with complex life cycles [22] and free-life stages [26].

The main goal of the present study was to investigate the potential interaction between OCs and parasites in freshwater fish. We analyzed wild brown trout (*Salmo trutta*) from a protected area of Southern Italy for the presence of parasites and OCs contamination of the fillet. We looked at brown trout because it is a predatory species, common in freshwaters and coastal marine fish faunas, endemic in Europe [27]. Trout are frequently exposed to OCs [28–30] and gastro-intestinal (GI) helminths [31,32]. In rainbow trout, these parasites may induce moderate pathogenicity, such as gut inflammation and malabsorption as well as decreased hemoglobin level and hematocrit [33].

Since trout are intensely farmed and often caught for human consumption [34], their contamination by several PCBs and OCPs could be a cause of concern for human health. We thus also evaluated the ensuing risk to human health due to the consumption of contaminated fillets.

2. Materials and Methods

2.1. Study Area and Fish Collection

Fish were collected in the Trionto River, in the municipality of Longobucco (Cosenza province of Calabria region in Southern Italy) (Figure 1). The Trionto River with a length of about 40 km arises in the province of Cosenza, from the mountains of the Sila National Park, and flows east, entering the Ionian Sea. This site has long suffered from inadequate urban waste disposal (including illegal dumps or not compliant landfills located very close to riverbeds), inefficient wastewater treatment plants, and the presence of some areas of concern for environmental remediation, including a National Interest Site (Rapporti ISTISAN 16/9).

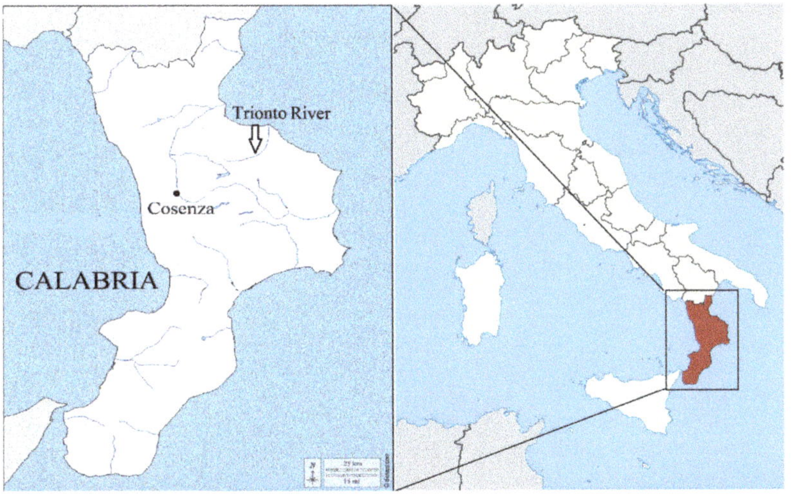

Figure 1. Italy and sampling area in Calabria Region.

A total of 87 brown trout were collected by electrofishing with an IG600 Scubla & C. Snc equipment in the daytime in June and July 2013. Electrofishing permits (n. 2283, 4 April 2013) were issued by the Parco Nazionale della Sila on request by the Istituto Zooprofilattico Sperimentale del Mezzogiorno (n. 0001933, 13 February 2013). Immediately after being caught, fish were euthanized by gills cutting to ensure death while still unconscious according to the recommendations by the European Directive 2010/63 and Jung-Schroers et al. [35]. Specimens were transported to the laboratory under refrigerated conditions (4–8 °C) and then stored at −20 °C until the analyses were performed. Soon after thawing, biometrical data, length (cm), and weight (g) of trout were recorded. Fish were weighed using an electronic balance to the nearest 0.1 g. The length was measured considering the fork length (FL), that is, from the tip of the snout to the fork of the tail to the nearest 0.1 cm, with the help of a digital caliper. The gonads of examined fish were fixed in 10% formalin, embedded in paraffin wax, sectioned at 6 μm thick, and stained with hematoxylin and eosin. Then, slices were microscopically examined to evaluate sex and gonadal maturity stage (mature and immature trout), on the basis of criteria by Hajirezaee et al. [36]. Prevalence, abundance, and mean abundance of infection were according to Bush et al. [37].

2.2. Analytical Sample Preparation

We started with 87 pieces of the dorsal muscle of as many trout. However, since each piece of trout was too small to be analyzed individually, we formed 22 statistical units, each one consisting of 3–5 trout pieces obtained from trout as homogenous as possible in terms of weight, sex, sexual developmental stage, and presence or absence of GI parasites. The length of each sample unit is the average fork length of the trout corresponding to these pieces.

2.3. Analytical Procedure

Each sample unit was examined for the presence of 5 OCPs, 15 non-dioxin-like (ndl)-PCBs, and 8 dioxin-like (dl)-PCBs. As regards OCPs, the concentrations of *p,p′*-DDT (1,1,1-trichloro-2,2-di(4-chlorophenyl)-ethane) and its main metabolites *p,p′*-DDE (1,1-dichloro-2,2-bis(4-chlorophenyl)-ethylene) and *p,p′*-DDD (1,1-dichloro-2,2-bis-(4-chlorophenyl)-ethane) as far as HCB (hexachlorobenzene) and dieldrin were determined. In the following, we reported as ΣDDTs the sum of DDT-related compounds. As regards ndl-PCBs, we measured the six indicator congeners (IUPAC nos. 28, 52, 101, 138, 153, and 180) and the other nine non-indicator ndl-PCBs (namely, IUPAC nos. 66, 74, 128, 146, 170, 183, 187, 194, and 196). The sum of the indicator PCBs was reported as Σ6ndl-PCBs, while Σ15ndl-PCBs denotes the sum of all ndl-congeners. Σ6ndl-PCBs is indicative overall of ndl-PCBs pollution and has been adopted since 2011 by EU legislation to set tolerance limits in several foodstuffs (EU Reg. no. 1259/2011). The other non-indicator ndl-PCBs were examined because previously detected in foods of animal origin and other biotic matrices [38,39]. Finally, among the dl-PCBs we measured 3 non-ortho congeners (IUPAC nos. 77, 126, 169) and 5 mono-ortho congeners (IUPAC nos. 105, 118, 156, 157, 167), selected because of their overall high toxic equivalency factors (TEFs). Their concentrations were summed up and reported as Σ3dl-PCBs and Σ5dl-PCBs, respectively.

2.3.1. Chemical Analysis

Regarding the OCs analysis, for the extraction procedure, including the separation of the analytes from the lipid fraction and the purification of the final extracts, we followed the method described by Ferrante et al. [40]. Briefly, each sample unit (roughly 3 g) was homogenized and manually cold-extracted using petroleum ether/acetone (1:1, *v*/*v*). After centrifugation, the extract was passed through a glass tube packed with anhydrous sodium sulfate. Extraction was repeated and additional extract was put into the column. The eluate was then evaporated to dryness by rotavapor, and the lipid content was gravimetrically determined. Separation of OCs from the lipid fraction was performed using a combined system of Extrelut-3/Extrelut-1 cartridges (Merck Kga A Darmstadt, Germany), previously modified by adding 0.36 g C-18 Isolute (40 to 60 mesh Merck Kga A Darmstadt, Germany). The analytes were eluted with acetonitrile and cleaned up on a glass column containing 2.5 g of heat-activated Florisil (60/100 mesh Supelco, Bellefonte, PA, USA) to separate OCs in three fractions. The column was eluted with 30 mL of n-hexane, 25 mL of n-hexane/toluene (80:20, *v*/*v*), and 30 mL of n-hexane/toluene/ethyl acetate (180:19:1, *v*/*v*/*v*) in subsequent order. The first fraction contained all PCBs, HCB, and *p,p′*-DDE, the second one contained *p,p′*-DDT and *p,p′*-DDD, while dieldrin was obtained with the third fraction. The three fractions were then concentrated to a small volume and PCB 209 was added as an internal standard (IS) for instrumental analysis. The choice of using PCB 209 as IS was due to its almost absence in the environment [41]; a more detailed explanation has been previously reported [38].

2.3.2. Instrumental Analysis

OCs analysis was carried out using an Agilent 7890A/7000A GC triple quadrupole mass spectrometer system (GC/QQQ), and the gas chromatograph was equipped with the Agilent 7693 autosampler. Data analysis and quantification of individual OCs were conducted using Agilent MassHunter Workstation software—Quantitative Analysis. The fractions were injected in the splitless mode and the injector was kept at 270 °C. A (35% Phenyl)-methylpolysiloxane DB 35 ms capillary column (30 m × 0.25 mm id, 0.25 mm film thickness) (J&W Scientific from Agilent, Santa Clara, CA, USA) was used for analytes separation and helium was employed as carrier gas. The oven temperature was programmed as follows: hold for 1 min at 120 °C, increase 15 °C min^{-1} to 160 °C, increase 3 °C min^{-1} to 220 °C, hold for 2 min at 220 °C, increase 8 °C min^{-1} to 280 °C, hold for 4 min at 280 °C. The GC/MS/MS operated in multiple reaction monitoring (MRM). The QQQ collision cell helium quench gas was set to 2.25 mL min^{-1} with N2 collision gas at 1.5 mL min^{-1}. Two MRM transitions were used for each OC to quantify and qualify the compounds. The calibration curves were linear with a R^2 coefficient greater than 0.998.

For quality assurance and quality control, we mainly followed the guidelines proposed by the European Commission Regulation No. 644/2017. To confirm method selectivity and to check for cross-contamination, matrix, and procedural blanks were extracted and analyzed. Pure reference standard solutions (Dr. Ehrenstorfer Laboratory) were used for instrument calibration and analytes quantification, as well as for precision and recovery tests. Recovery rates, calculated at 3 concentration levels, ranged from 81% to 105% depending on the compound. Analytical performances of the method were also assured by the analyses of reference materials: IAEA-406 for OCPs and ndl-PCBs and WMF-01 for dl-PCBs (International Atomic Energy Agency and Wellington Laboratories, respectively). Since the GC-MS/MS produces virtually no noise in the chromatogram, the standard deviation (SD) of the lowest reference standard solution in seven replicates was calculated and used to determine the limit of detection (LOD) and limit of quantification (LOQ) values (assumed as 3 × SD and 10 × SD, respectively). They ranged from 0.005 ng mL^{-1} to 0.03 ng mL^{-1} and from 0.02 ng mL^{-1} to 0.10 ng mL^{-1} (on solvent), respectively, for detection and quantification limits. Data, not corrected for recovery, were expressed as ng g^{-1} on lipid weight (LW), as well as on wet weight (WW). and they were reported as not detectable (ND) when below LOD. For the calculation of sum and mean values, we chose to assume a value of zero for concentrations lower than LOD.

2.4. Parasitological Examination

Skin, gills, mouth cavity, GI tract (stomach and intestine), liver, heart, gonads, visceral cavity, and mesenteries of each fish were dissected and studied for metazoan parasites using a Zeiss Axio Zoom V16 (Carl Zeiss, DE) dissecting microscope [42,43]. The musculature of each specimen was cut into thin slices (~0.5 cm) and examined under the same microscope for helminth parasites [44]. For each organ/tissue, ecto- and endo-parasites were studied, collected, counted, washed in physiological saline solution, and preserved in 70% ethanol. For morphological identification, trematodes and acanthocephalans were stained with Mayer's acid carmine dehydrated through a graded ethanol series, cleared in methyl salicylate, and mounted in Canada balsam; nematode larvae were clarified in Amman's lactophenol. All parasites were then studied by light microscope and identified to the lowest possible taxonomic level using the available literature. Parasites were found almost exclusively in the GI (mostly in the intestine). For this reason, we referred to GI parasites throughout the text.

2.5. Statistical Analysis

Statistical analysis was performed using STATA software. Data obtained from OC determinations and from parasite detection were preliminarily evaluated through summary statistics and presented as mean ± SD. To assess and quantify the relationship between parasitic infection and OC contamination levels, regression analysis was exploited. The outcome variable was either a dummy identifying sample units characterized by the presence of parasites or the variable measuring the (average) number of parasites; the right side of the regression contains a measure of OC compounds divided by the (average) length of the trout. In this latter case, since the outcome variable is a count variable that takes on nonnegative integer values, we considered a Poisson regression model, which is well suited for modeling count variables. Moreover, we also provided evidence by adding two control variables, that is sex and sexual stage, to check whether differences in these parameters can be responsible for a confounding effect on the results of the previous analysis.

Measures of OCs concentrations were the sum of OCs concentrations on LW, considering the following groups of compounds: Σ6ndl-PCBs, Σ15ndl-PCBs, Σ3dl-PCBs, Σ5dl-PCBs, ΣDDTs, HCB and dieldrin. The null hypothesis (absence of a relationship between the two variables of interest) was rejected in the case of a p-value lower than 0.05.

3. Results and Discussion

Fork length ranged from 10.65 to 20.1 cm (mean value: 14.18, SD: 2.49); the weight ranged from 18.9 to 151.3 g (mean value: 57.18, SD: 29). Among the 22 sample units assembled, 11 units consisted of only female trout and 11 of only male ones; 45% of female sample units and 27% of male sample units were sexually mature. The sample mean fat content was 0.033 g g^{-1} muscle (range 0.080–0.130 g). GI parasites infested 54% of sample units.

3.1. OCs in Trout Muscle

PCBs were the most plentiful OCs followed by DDTs, HCB, and dieldrin (Tables 1 and 2). Among PCBs, the mean concentration was highest for the Σ15ndl-PCBs group, followed by Σ6ndl-PCBs, Σ5dl-PCBs, and Σ3dl-PCBs (Table 1). The Σ6ndl-PCBs amounted to roughly 72% of Σ15ndl-PCBs.

Table 1. Summary statistics of ndl-PCB and dl-PCB concentrations (ng g^{-1}).

	Mean	SD	Min	Max
Panel A (LW)				
Σ6ndl-PCBs	201.99	80.69	97.82	408.04
Σ15ndl-PCBs	281.18	111.23	140.03	560.86
Σ3dl-PCBs	11.3	6.53	0.00	22.04
Σ5dl-PCBs	35.44	16.85	14.61	79.79
Panel B (WW)				
Σ6ndl-PCBs	6.58	2.55	3.61	13.60
Σ15ndl-PCBs	9.15	3.49	5.10	18.69
Σ3dl-PCBs	0.36	0.21	0.00	0.74
Σ5dl-PCBs	1.16	0.55	0.49	2.66

Notes: The table reports PCB concentrations expressed as ng g^{-1} on lipid weight basis (LW, Panel A) and wet weight basis (WW, Panel B). Σ6ndl-PCBs refers to the sum of the concentrations of six indicator PCBs; Σ15ndl-PCBs indicate the sum of indicator and non-indicator ndl- congeners.; Σ3dl-PCBs and Σ5dl-PCBs are the sums of concentrations of 3 non-ortho and 5 mono-ortho congeners, respectively.

Table 2. Summary statistics of OCP concentrations (ng g^{-1}).

	Mean	SD	Min	Max
Panel A (LW)				
HCB	8.09	3.11	2.63	13.97
Dieldrin	1.25	1.60	0.00	5.09
p,p'-DDT	0.79	1.78	0.00	7.51
p,p'-DDD	1.86	1.94	0.00	8.60
p,p'-DDE	97.57	43.45	38.33	228.42
ΣDDTs	100.23	43.69	42.72	228.42
Panel B (WW)				
HCB	0.27	0.11	0.10	0.49
Dieldrin	0.04	0.05	0.00	0.14
p,p'-DDT	0.02	0.05	0.00	0.20
p,p'-DDD	0.06	0.06	0.00	0.23
p,p'-DDE	3.19	1.46	1.42	7.61
ΣDDTs	3.28	1.45	1.43	7.61

Notes: The table reports OCP concentrations expressed as ng g^{-1} on lipid weight and wet weight basis (Panel A and Panel B, respectively). ΣDDTs refers to the sum of the three DDT-related compounds.

Each indicator ndl-PCB congener was detected in all sample units (Figure 2). The indicator hexa-chlorinated PCBs IUPAC Nos. 153 and 138 showed the highest mean concentrations among all OCs, with values of 63.25 and 49.74 ng g^{-1} LW, respectively. Adding up these two congeners, we accounted for 56% and about 40% of Σ6ndl-PCBs and Σ15ndl-PCBs, respectively. The tri-chlorinated PCB 28 followed with a mean concentration of 33.77 ng g^{-1} LW. The indicator tetra-chlorinated PCB 52 was detected at the lowest concentration, contributing to 7% of Σ6ndl-PCBs (Figure 2).

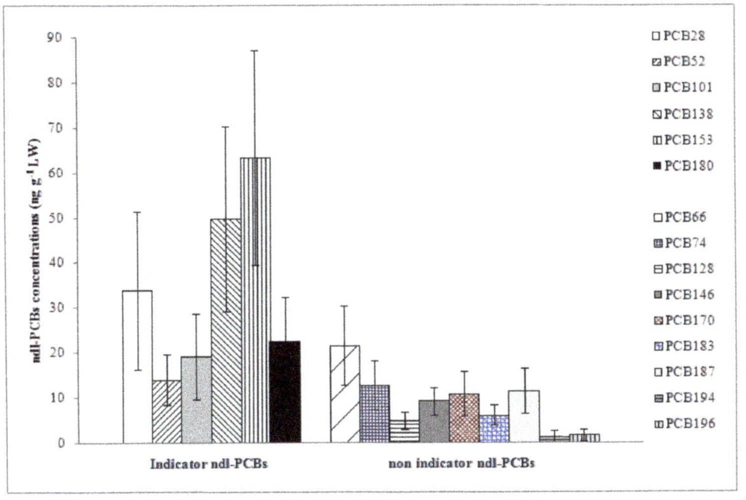

Figure 2. Mean concentrations and standard deviation of indicator and non-indicator ndl-PCBs expressed as ng g^{-1} on lipid weight basis (LW).

Regarding the non-indicator ndl-PCBs, the tetra-chlorinated PCB 66 was detected with the highest mean concentration (21.56 ng g^{-1} LW), accounting for 7.6% of Σ15ndl-PCBs, while the PCBs Nos. 194 and 196 were detected with the lowest ones (1.30 and 1.56 ng g^{-1} LW, respectively). The latter two congeners were found in 65% of sample units; other non-indicator ndl congeners were in all sample units.

Regarding dl-PCBs, Σ5dl-PCBs were higher than Σ3dl-PCBs (mean value of 35.44 ng g^{-1} LW vs. 11.30 ng g^{-1} LW) (Table 1). Among non-ortho congeners, PCBs Nos. 126 and 169 were never detected (Figure 3); therefore, the concentration of Σ3dl-PCBs is only due to PCB 77 (mean value of 11.28 ng g^{-1} LW and detection in 83% of sample units). Four out of five mono-ortho PCBs were detected; in particular, in all sample units, we found PCB 105 and PCB 118 (mean values 7.99 and 21.96 ng g^{-1} LW, respectively). The latter congener showed the highest concentration among dl-PCBs and contributed 62% to Σ5dl-PCBs. PCB 156 and PCB 167 had relatively low mean concentration levels (3.63 and 1.86 ng g^{-1} LW) (Figure 3); they were detected in 69% and 78% of the sample units, respectively. The congeners PCB 118, PCB 77, and PCB 105, recognized as more toxic and usually detected at lower concentrations than ndl ones [45], were instead found at mean concentrations roughly comparable to those of some indicator and non-indicator ndl-PCBs (i.e., PCB 52, 101, 180, 66, 74).

The finding of relatively high concentrations of PCBs fairly reflects our expectations. In fact, a National Interest Site and three sites contaminated with OCs undergoing remediation procedures are located in the same province of the study area.

Regarding OCPs, *p,p′*-DDE and HCB were found in all sample units with the highest mean concentrations (97.57 and 8.09 ng g^{-1} LW, respectively); *p,p′*-DDE was the dominant compound in terms of contribution to ΣDDTs (97%) (Table 2). *p,p′*-DDD, *p,p′*-DDT, and dieldrin were detected in 83%, 26%, and 43% of sample units, respectively, with quite low concentrations (Figure 4).

As it is well known, DDT is quickly metabolized to DDE that persists for a long time in the environment. Indeed, the relatively high *p,p′*-DDE concentration suggests that the parent compound was strongly used in the past. This hypothesis is supported by the value of the DDE/DDT ratio, based on the average concentration of the compounds, which is usually used to investigate the timing of DDT entering the environment [46]. In our case, the ratio is much higher than 1 (amounting to 123). The reasons behind the presence of

HCB can be identified both with its past use as a fungicide and because it is a by-product of several chlorine-containing chemicals [47].

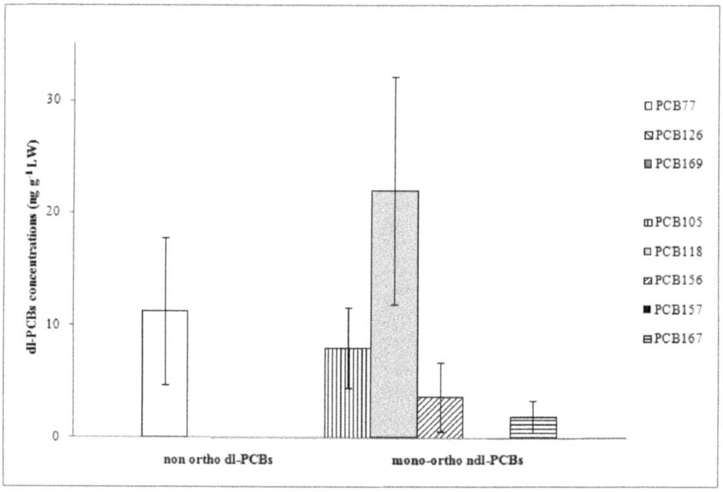

Figure 3. Mean concentrations and standard deviation of dl-PCBs expressed as ng g^{-1} on lipid weight basis (LW).

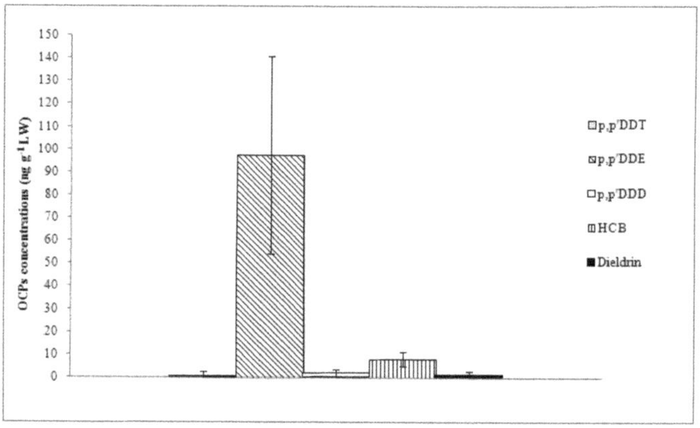

Figure 4. Mean concentrations and standard deviation of OCPs expressed as ng g^{-1} on lipid weight basis (LW).

Trout feeding could explain the presence of OCs. Crustaceans, insects, and small fish are the main components of trout's diet. These organisms live on the seabed in direct contact with sediments that accumulate OCs.

3.2. Regression Analysis of Parasites Infection and OCs

A total of 233 helminth parasites belonging to three taxa were found in the GI tract of 41 brown trout. The most prevalent (42.5%) and abundant taxon (mean abundance: 5.4 per specimen ranging from 1 to 35) was the trematode *Crepidostomum metoecus*, with the other trophically transmitted parasites found in 5.7% (the acanthocephalan *Echinorhynchus* sp.) and 2.3% (unidentified nematode larva) trout, respectively (Table 3). *Crepidostomum metoecus* has been previously reported as a common parasite of brown trout in European countries [31]. However, its presence has been rarely investigated in Italian rivers [48].

Table 3. Taxa and number of gastro-intestinal (GI) parasites found in the infected trout.

	Number of Parasites			Number of
	Total	Min	Max	Infected Trout
Crepidostomum metoecus	225	1	35	37
Echinorhynchus	4	1	1	4
Unidentified nematodes	2	1	1	2
Other unidentified parasites	2	1	1	2
All	233	1	35	41

Notes: some trout hosted more than one species of parasites.

The results of the regression analysis are shown in Tables 4–6. When the outcome variable identified the presence or not of parasite infection, that is, the outcome variable was a dummy, and OC concentration levels were expressed on LW basis, the relationship between OCs and parasite presence was (i) negative and statistically significant in the case of Σ6ndl-PCBs, Σ15ndl-PCBs, Σ5dl-PCBs, and ΣDDTs; and (ii) negative but insignificant in the case of Σ3dl-PCBs, HCB, and dieldrin (see Table 4). These results suggest that relatively high OC concentrations might reduce the probability of parasite infection.

Table 4. Regression analysis: presence of parasites and OCs.

	Presence of Parasites						
Σ6ndl-PCBs	−0.034 *** (−4.69)						
Σ15ndl-PCBs		−0.024 *** (−4.76)					
Σ3dl-PCBs			−0.350 (−2.03)				
Σ5dl-PCBs				−0.154 *** (−4.04)			
ΣDDTs					−0.055 ** (−3.54)		
HCB						−0.633 (−2.02)	
Dieldrin							−0.837 (−0.14)

Notes: The table reports results of the regression analysis of GI parasites on OC concentration levels (LW); t statistics in brackets. Number of observations: 22. Significance is denoted as follows: ** $p < 0.01$, *** $p < 0.001$.

The use of the two control variables enabled us to verify if previous results were biased by potential confounding factors. Table 5 shows that the negative and statistically significant relationship between parasite infection and OC concentration still emerged for Σ6ndl-PCBs, Σ15ndl-PCBs, and Σ5dl-PCBs. Moreover, we also notice that while the variable sex does not have any statistical impact, the coefficient attached to the stage of sexual development (immature versus mature) was estimated negative for all regressions, and statistically significant in several cases, consistent with the idea that immature younger fish had less time to accumulate parasite.

Our main evidence was also confirmed by exploiting the Poisson regression analysis where the outcome variable was the number of parasites (see Table 6). A negative and statistically significant relationship between parasite infection and OC concentration was estimated for Σ6ndl-PCBs, Σ15ndl-PCBs, and Σ5dl-PCBs.

Our evidence regarding the negative relationship between chemical pollutants and parasites accords with that of other authors. By relying on a meta-analysis of the effects of pollution on parasitism in aquatic animals, Blanar et al. [26] conclude with a strong, significant negative effect for Digenea and Monogenea, especially in response to metal pollution. For many other parasite/contaminant interactions, effect sizes were instead not significantly different from zero. However, few studies focus on OCs and do not reach a consensus [25,49].

Table 5. Regression analysis: presence of parasites and OCs, with control variables.

	Presence of Parasites						
Σ6ndl-PCBs	−0.024 * (−2.49)						
Σ15ndl-PCBs		−0.018 * (−2.49)					
Σ3dl-PCBs			−0.211 (−1.12)				
Σ5dl-PCBs				−0.115 * (−2.37)			
ΣDDT					−0.035 (−2.00)		
HCB						−0.175 (−0.51)	
Dieldrin							−5.771 (−1.50)
Immature	−0.395 (−1.91)	−0.395 (−1.90)	−0.463 * (−2.28)	−0.436 * (−2.21)	−0.422 (−1.98)	−0.494 * (−2.63)	−0.601 ** (−3.70)
Male	0.088 (0.48)	0.089 (0.48)	0.149 (0.79)	0.096 (0.52)	0.122 (0.64)	0.139 (0.70)	0.197 (1.03)

Notes: the table reports results of the regression analysis of GI parasites on OC concentration levels (LW) controlling for sex and sexual maturity; t statistics in brackets. Number of observations: 22. Significance is denoted as follows: * $p < 0.05$, ** $p < 0.01$.

Table 6. Poisson regression analysis.

	Number of Parasites						
Σ6ndl-PCBs	−0.079 ** (−2.59)						
Σ15ndl-PCBs		−0.056 * (−2.55)					
Σ3dl-PCBs			−0.464 (−1.06)				
Σ5dl-PCBs				−0.439 * (−2.09)			
ΣDDT					−0.104 (−1.43)		
HCB						−1.177 (−1.24)	
Dieldrin							−8.940 (−0.74)
Immature	−1.054 (−1.90)	−1.054 (−1.91)	−1.181 * (−2.30)	−1.160 * (−2.10)	−1.072 (−1.80)	−1.091 (−1.79)	−1.398 ** (−2.69)
Male	0.561 (1.39)	0.558 (1.39)	0.555 (1.35)	0.628 (1.40)	0.555 (1.28)	0.522 (1.27)	0.546 (1.21)

Notes: The table reports results of the Poisson regression analysis of the number of GI parasites on OC concentration levels (LW) controlling for sex and sexual maturity; t statistics in brackets. Number of observations: 22. Significance is denoted as follows: * $p < 0.05$, ** $p < 0.01$.

The digenetic class of trematodes, to which *Crepidostomum metoecus* belongs, has been reported as more vulnerable than other parasite species and a negative correlation with OCs has been noticed [26]; for freshwater taxa, the correlation was not determined due to lack of data relative to OC concentration levels. Vidal-Martinez et al. [50] evidenced a significant negative correlation between the degree of parasitism by larval trematode *Mesostephanus appendiculatoides* and DDT concentrations in the Mayan catfish collected in Chetumal Bay, Mexico. The authors reported that, although the catfish were highly contaminated, they seemed to be barely susceptible to the OCPs toxicity, which instead heavily affected parasites. A negative correlation was also documented with respect to the digenetic trematode *Steringophorus furciger* in the GI tract of flatfish species, which is a significantly greater presence of parasites in specimens poorly contaminated by PCBs [51]. Similar evidence was also reported by Carreras-Aubets et al. [25], who observed a lower abundance of adult digenean endoparasite *Opecoeloides furcatus* in *Mullus barbatus* fish related to higher concentrations of the sum of indicator PCBs plus PCB 118 in Western Mediterranean sediments. To the best of our knowledge, a positive relationship has never been recorded for the digenetic class of trematodes. With data from German Bight, Schmidt et al. [52] evidenced a negative relationship between the infection degree to some parasite species and OC concentrations measured in the muscle of European flounder, sediments, and blue mussels. In particular, they documented a lower abundance of parasites with higher concentrations of HCB, DDD, DDE, and the sum of indicator PCBs. In the liver and muscle of acanthocephalan-infected perch, Brázová and co-authors [53] detected PCB concentrations several times lower than in not parasitized perc. Similar findings, observed only for some PCB congeners, were recently reported by the same authors for another host-parasite system (GI cestode–freshwater bream) [54].

In addition to aquatic species, a negative correlation was also evidenced in dogs [55] and African immigrants [24]. The authors showed that serum concentration levels of some indicator PCBs (PCB 52, PCB 138, PCB 153) were significantly lower in subjects infected with GI parasites than in non-parasitized ones. The same results were found examining several OCs, including those that we analyzed in the present study, in dogs positive for earthworm *Dirofilaria immitis* [55]. Since OC serum concentrations remained low after antiparasitic treatment, the authors hypothesized that nematode parasites may metabolize OCs in addition to accumulating them.

Some other studies reported, instead, an increase in parasitism because of animal exposure to OCs. Parasitic infection prevalently by nematodes of the lung (but also intestine and uterus) was significantly and positively correlated to *p,p*′-DDT, *p,p*′-DDD, and *o,p*′-DDD concentrations measured in the blubber of finless porpoises (*Neophocaena phocaenoides*) [56]. In blubber of the same species, Isobe et al. [49] evidenced significantly higher concentrations of PCBs (expressed as the sum of 62 congeners including indicator congeners and dl-PCBs) in animals infected with liver trematodes, relative to non-infected ones. A similar correlation was also reported by Kannan and co-authors [57] for PCBs and infectious agents including intestinal acanthocephalans, protozoa, bacteria, and fungi in another marine mammal, the Southern Sea otter. Bamidele and co-authors [58,59] observed a significant positive correlation between the protozoa *Myxosoma sp* infection found in blackchin tilapia and silver catfish from Lagos lagoon (Nigeria) and *p,p*′-DDT concentrations in freshwaters; however, no correlation was determined between intestinal helminth parasites and OCP congeners [58].

Few potential explanations have been raised for the results obtained. Some authors related the findings of a positive relationship to the frequent immunosuppressive effect of the OCs reported in *in vivo* and *in vitro* studies [6,60–62]. Indeed, exposure to chemical xenobiotics can disrupt the host's immune response, so that adverse effects may depend on the indirect outcome of the pollutant on the host's capacity to cope with a pathogen [13], making the host itself more susceptible to parasitosis [63,64]. Instead, regarding the negative correlation, some authors suggest that high environmental OC concentrations may disrupt the parasite life cycle, impairing the ability of the free-life form to survive and reach the host [25,51,65]. To protect themselves from chemical contaminants, parasites may rely on their host for detoxification mechanisms, even though the parasitic infection itself could cause a decrease in host detoxification enzymes [65]. In the case of trematodes, which have a complex life cycle with a first intermediate host, usually a mollusk, several free-living forms, and, finally, one or multiple vertebrate hosts, the toxic effects of the pollutants may impair their ability to assimilate essential nutrients; as a consequence of this condition, also their reproductive potential results to be affected and some mutagenic damages could occur to developing embryos, leading to a reduced transmission [65].

The negative relationship has been also interpreted suggesting that parasites determine a decrease in OC concentrations. The explanation would be that, because of their lipid content, GI parasites, and thus also trematodes, are able to bioaccumulate OCs introduced by the animal host through contaminated feed consumption [21,53,54,66,67]. This makes OCs less bioavailable for the host and therefore may increase the tolerance of the host to contaminants-induced toxicity. For parasites other than helminths, another explanation may result from their metabolizing ability through cytochrome P-450 activity leading to the reduction of OCs body burden in the host [68]. Indeed, helminths perform limited OC detoxification because of the lack of cytochrome P450 mono-oxygenases [69,70]. Moreover, according to Brázová and co-authors [54], since a higher Fulton's condition factor was determined in infected breams, some parasites may even positively impact their hosts co-exposed to PCBs.

Overall, assessing the potential outcomes for parasites exploiting contaminated hosts is a crucial but neglected issue, since toxic effects on parasites may alter interspecific relationships. However, joint effects of parasites and chemical pollutants on host performance are extremely intricate depending on the level of parasitism, as well as the chemical pollutant, its mode of action, and the exposure levels. Contaminant accumulation by parasite results in positive effects among which is a reduction of both oxidative stress and histological modifications. This scenario indicates the possibility that a shift from parasitism to mutualism occurs. If concentration levels of the contaminant are high, they could induce damage to both host and parasites changing their relationships (see [71] and references therein).

3.3. Risk Assessment

Human exposure to OCs is due to a large extent to the consumption of foods of animal origin, mainly dairy and fishery products [72]. For consumer health risk assessment, the European Union (EU) established maximum residue limits (MRLs) for some OCs, namely dioxins, dl-PCBs, and six indicator ndl-PCBs in foodstuffs of animal origin (European Commission Regulation no. 1259/2011). The regulation fixed for "Muscle meat of wild caught freshwater fish, with the exception of diadromous fish species caught in freshwater, and products thereof" a MRL of 125 ng g^{-1} WW for ∑6ndl-PCBs. All the samples analyzed showed concentrations below this threshold.

For dioxins and dl-PCBs, MRLs are expressed as Toxic Equivalent Quantity (WHO-TEQ). To evaluate the compliance of any sample units with the thresholds set by the EU, we summed up the concentration of each congener of interest multiplied by the respective Toxic Equivalency Factor adopted by the World Health Organization (WHO-TEFs) and then compared the sum with the corresponding MRL. TEFs are the results of the comparison of the relative different toxicity of individual dioxins/furans and dl-PCBs congeners to that of 2,3,7,8-TCDD [73]. Since there is no specific limit for dl-PCBs, we considered a value of 3 pg g^{-1} fat arising from the difference between the MRL referred to as the sum of all dioxin-related compounds (PCDDs/Fs and dl-PCBs) and the value referred to PCDDs/Fs alone. Also, in this case, the measured concentrations were lower than the above-extrapolated value.

With respect to the considered pesticides, the EU has not set a specific MRL for fish and fish products to date. As far as concern Italian national legislation, tolerance limits for residues of chloro-organic substances in products of animal origin have been established by Decreto Ministeriale on 13 May 2005 (annex 4), which states limits differentiated according to the different fat content. All sample units in the present study showed a lipid percentage below 5%, thus falling into the so-called group 1, with tolerance limits for ∑DDTs, HCB, and Dieldrin, respectively, of 0.050, 0.010, and 0.005 μg g^{-1} WW. No sample units exceeded the limits of the above-mentioned pesticides established by the Italian legislation.

4. Conclusions

We investigated the potential existence of a relationship between parasitic infection degree and OC concentration levels found in brown trout specimens from the Calabria region. The regression analysis revealed the possibility that relatively high PCB concentrations lead to lower parasite infection degree. Results supporting this conjecture are summarized as follows: (i) there is a strongly significant negative relationship between parasites and PCB concentrations; (ii) such relationship is robust to the inclusion of two regressors in the empirical model that controls for sex and sexual maturity of trout, although the magnitude of the significance reduces due to the relatively low number of observations; (iii) the negative relationship is confirmed by results of the Poisson regression model for counting data; and (iv) among all considered OCs, concentrations of PCBs, that is, Σ15ndl-PCBs, Σ6ndl-PCBs and Σ5dl-PCBs, are the highest ones.

However, we are aware that the sample size may be an issue in our analysis and that the reverse causal direction cannot be dismissed. Therefore, more studies about the relationship between chemical pollutants and parasites in host–parasite systems, assessing whether a concern would arise for the host, the parasite, or the final consumers would be beneficial.

While OC concentration levels detected do not pose a risk to consumer health, being always below the threshold levels set by the EU, they signal non-negligible background pollution by PCBs and OCPs, although the monitored area is a protected one.

Author Contributions: Conceptualization, R.M. and M.C.F.; methodology, A.M., M.L.F., M.S., M.T.C., F.D.P., B.D.U., L.B., R.M. and M.C.F.; software, A.M., M.T.C., M.L.F. and F.D.P.; validation, M.C.F., R.M., M.L.F. and M.S.; formal analysis, A.M., M.T.C., F.D.P., L.F., R.M. and M.C.F.; investigation, A.M., M.T.C., M.L.F., M.S., B.D.U., L.B., R.M. and M.C.F.; resources, M.S., B.D.U., L.B. and M.C.F.; data curation, M.T.C., F.D.P., R.M. and M.C.F.; writing—original draft preparation, A.M., M.T.C., F.D.P., L.F. and M.C.F.; writing—review and editing, R.M. and M.C.F.; visualization, M.S., G.F. and L.F.; supervision, R.M. and M.C.F.; project administration, M.C.F., L.B., M.S. and G.F.; funding acquisition, G.F., L.B., B.D.U., M.S. and M.C.F. All authors have read and agreed to the published version of the manuscript.

Funding: This research was funded by Italian Ministry of Health, grant number C78C12000180001 (Ricerca corrente IZS ME 05/12).

Institutional Review Board Statement: Not applicable. The approval of the Ethics Committee was not required. The Italian Legislative Decree on the protection of animals used for scientific purposes was issued in 2014 (Decree No. 26 of 4 March 2014.), that is after fish collection and analytical sample preparation.

Informed Consent Statement: Not applicable.

Data Availability Statement: The data supporting the findings of the present study are available from the corresponding author upon reasonable request.

Acknowledgments: We would like to thank the guest editors and the reviewers for their suggestions that have substantially improved this manuscript.

Conflicts of Interest: The authors declare no conflict of interest.

References

1. Schmidt, S.N.; Burgess, R.M. Evaluating Polymeric Sampling as a Tool for Predicting the Bioaccumulation of Polychlorinated Biphenyls by Fish and Shellfish. *Environ. Sci. Technol.* **2020**, *54*, 9729–9741. [CrossRef]
2. Masset, T.; Frossard, V.; Perga, M.E.; Cottin, N.; Piot, C.; Cachera, S.; Naffrechoux, E. Trophic position and individual feeding habits as drivers of differential PCB bioaccumulation in fish populations. *Sci. Total Environ.* **2019**, *674*, 472–481. [CrossRef]
3. Ngoubeyou, P.S.K.; Wolkersdorfer, C.; Ndibewu, P.P.; Augustyn, W. Toxicity of polychlorinated biphenyls in aquatic environments—A review. *Aquat. Toxicol.* **2022**, *251*, 106284. [CrossRef] [PubMed]
4. Iwanowicz, L.R.; Blazer, V.S.; McCormick, S.D.; Vanveld, P.A.; Ottinger, C.A. Aroclor 1248 exposure leads to immunomodulation, decreased disease resistance and endocrine disruption in the brown bullhead, *Ameiurus nebulosus*. *Aquat. Toxicol.* **2009**, *93*, 70–82. [CrossRef] [PubMed]

5. Segner, H.; Bailey, C.; Tafalla, C.; Bo, J. Immunotoxicity of Xenobiotics in Fish: A Role for the Aryl Hydrocarbon Receptor (AhR)? *Int. J. Mol. Sci.* **2021**, *22*, 9460. [CrossRef] [PubMed]
6. Misumi, I.; Vella, A.T.; Leong, J.A.; Nakanishi, T.; Schreck, C.B. p, p′-DDE depresses the immune competence of chinook salmon (*Oncorhynchus tshawytscha*) leukocytes. *Fish. Shellfish Immunol.* **2005**, *19*, 97–114. [CrossRef]
7. Arkoosh, M.R.; Clemons, E.; Myers, M.; Casillas, E. Suppression of B-cell mediated immunity in juvenile chinook salmon (*Oncorhynchus tshawytscha*) after exposure to either a polycyclic aromatic hydrocarbon or to polychlorinated biphenyls. *Immunopharmacol. Immunotoxicol.* **1994**, *16*, 293–314. [CrossRef]
8. Martyniuk, C.J.; Doperalski, N.J.; Feswick, A.; Prucha, M.S.; Kroll, K.J.; Barber, D.S.; Denslow, N.D. Transcriptional networks associated with the immune system are disrupted by organochlorine pesticides in largemouth bass (*Micropterus salmoides*) ovary. *Aquat. Toxicol.* **2016**, *177*, 405–416. [CrossRef]
9. Burgos-Aceves, M.A.; Migliaccio, V.; Di Gregorio, I.; Paolella, G.; Lepretti, M.; Faggio, C.; Lionetti, L. 1,1,1-trichloro-2,2-bis (p-chlorophenyl)-ethane (DDT) and 1,1-Dichloro-2,2-bis (p, p′-chlorophenyl) ethylene (DDE) as endocrine disruptors in human and wildlife: A possible implication of mitochondria. *Environ. Toxicol. Pharmacol.* **2021**, *87*, 103684. [CrossRef]
10. Sawyna, J.M.; Spivia, W.R.; Radecki, K.; Fraser, D.A.; Lowe, C.G. Association between chronic organochlorine exposure and immunotoxicity in the round stingray (*Urobatis halleri*). *Environ. Pollut.* **2017**, *223*, 42–50. [CrossRef]
11. Quabius, E.S.; Krupp, G.; Secombes, C.J. Polychlorinated biphenyl 126 affects expression of genes involved in stress-immune interaction in primary cultures of rainbow trout anterior kidney cells. *Environ. Toxicol. Chem.* **2005**, *24*, 3053–3060. [CrossRef] [PubMed]
12. Cuesta, A.; Meseguer, J.; Angeles Esteban, M. Effects of the organochlorines p, p′-DDE and lindane on gilthead seabream leucocyte immune parameters and gene expression. *Fish Shellfish Immunol.* **2008**, *25*, 682–688. [CrossRef] [PubMed]
13. Segner, H.; Wenger, M.; Moller, A.M.; Kollner, B.; Casanova-Nakayama, A. Immunotoxic effects of environmental toxicants in fish—How to assess them? *Environ. Sci. Pollut. Res. Int.* **2011**, *19*, 2465–2476. [CrossRef] [PubMed]
14. Ekman, E.; Akerman, G.; Balk, L.; Norrgren, L. Impact of PCB on resistance to Flavobacterium psychrophilum after experimental infection of rainbow trout Oncorhynchus mykiss eggs by nanoinjection. *Dis. Aquat. Organ.* **2004**, *60*, 31–39. [CrossRef]
15. Duffy, J.E.; Carlson, E.A.; Li, Y.; Prophete, C.; Zelikofft, J.T. Age-related differences in the sensitivity of the fish immune response to a coplanar PCB. *Ecotoxicology* **2003**, *12*, 251–259. [CrossRef]
16. Esch, G.W.; Barger, M.A.; Fellis, K.J. The transmission of digenetic trematodes: Style, elegance, complexity. *Integr. Comp. Biol.* **2002**, *42*, 304–312. [CrossRef]
17. Couso-Perez, S.; Ares-Mazas, E.; Gomez-Couso, H. Gastrointestinal helminths in brown trout (*Salmo trutta* Linnaeus, 1758) captured in Galician rivers (NW Spain). *Parasitol. Int.* **2023**, *92*, 102676. [CrossRef]
18. Borgstrøm, R.; Mestrand, Ø.H.; Brittain, J.E.; Lien, L. The helminth fauna of brown trout (*Salmo trutta*) from a sub-alpine lake revisited after 40 years with introduced European minnow (*Phoxinus phoxinus*). *Fauna Nor.* **2021**, *41*, 15–26. [CrossRef]
19. Bullard, S.A.; Overstreet, R.M. Digeneans as Enemies of Fishes. In *Fish Diseases*, 1st ed.; Jorge, E., Ed.; Science Publishers, Inc.: Enfield, CT, USA, 2008; Volume 2, pp. 817–996.
20. Bartoli, P.; Boudouresque, C.F. Effect of the digenean parasites of fish on the fauna of Mediterranean lagoons. *Parassitologia* **2007**, *49*, 111–117.
21. Oluoch-Otiego, J.; Oyoo-Okoth, E.; Kiptoo, K.K.; Chemoiwa, E.J.; Ngugi, C.C.; Simiyu, G.; Omutange, E.S.; Ngure, V.; Opiyo, M.A. PCBs in fish and their cestode parasites in Lake Victoria. *Environ. Monit. Assess.* **2016**, *188*, 483. [CrossRef]
22. Sures, B.; Nachev, M.; Selbach, C.; Marcogliese, D.J. Parasite responses to pollution: What we know and where we go in 'Environmental Parasitology'. *Parasit. Vectors* **2017**, *10*, 65. [CrossRef] [PubMed]
23. Monnolo, A.; Clausi, M.T.; Mercogliano, R.; Fusco, G.; Fiorentino, M.L.; Buono, F.; Lama, A.; Ferrante, M.C. Levels of polychlorinated biphenyls and organochlorine pesticides in donkey milk: Correlation with the infection level by intestinal strongyles. *Chemosphere* **2020**, *258*, 127287. [CrossRef] [PubMed]
24. Henriquez-Hernandez, L.A.; Boada, L.D.; Perez-Arellano, J.L.; Carranza, C.; Ruiz-Suarez, N.; Jaen Sanchez, N.; Valeron, P.F.; Zumbado, M.; Camacho, M.; Luzardo, O.P. Relationship of polychlorinated biphenyls (PCBs) with parasitism, iron homeostasis, and other health outcomes: Results from a cross-sectional study on recently arrived African immigrants. *Environ. Res.* **2016**, *150*, 549–556. [CrossRef] [PubMed]
25. Carreras-Aubets, M.; Montero, F.E.; Kostadinova, A.; Carrasson, M. Parasite communities in the red mullet, *Mullus barbatus* L., respond to small-scale variation in the levels of polychlorinated biphenyls in the Western Mediterranean. *Mar. Pollut. Bull.* **2012**, *64*, 1853–1860. [CrossRef]
26. Blanar, C.A.; Munkittrick, K.R.; Houlahan, J.; Maclatchy, D.L.; Marcogliese, D.J. Pollution and parasitism in aquatic animals: A meta-analysis of effect size. *Aquat. Toxicol.* **2009**, *93*, 18–28. [CrossRef] [PubMed]
27. Filipe, A.F.; Markovic, D.; Pletterbauer, F.; Tisseuil, C.; De Wever, A.; Schmutz, S.; Bonada, N.; Freyhof, J. Forecasting fish distribution along stream networks: Brown trout (*Salmo trutta*) in Europe. *Divers. Distrib.* **2013**, *19*, 1059–1071. [CrossRef]
28. Piersanti, A.; Amorena, M.; Manera, M.; Tavoloni, T.; Lestingi, C.; Perugini, M. PCB concentrations in freshwater wild brown trouts (*Salmo trutta* trutta L) from Marche rivers, Central Italy. *Ecotoxicol. Environ. Saf.* **2012**, *84*, 355–359. [CrossRef]
29. Jaffal, A.; Givaudan, N.; Betoulle, S.; Terreau, A.; Paris-Palacios, S.; Biagianti-Risbourg, S.; Beall, E.; Roche, H. Polychlorinated biphenyls in freshwater salmonids from the Kerguelen Islands in the Southern Ocean. *Environ. Pollut.* **2011**, *159*, 1381–1389. [CrossRef]

30. Ondarza, P.M.; Gonzalez, M.; Fillmann, G.; Miglioranza, K.S. Polybrominated diphenyl ethers and organochlorine compound levels in brown trout (*Salmo trutta*) from Andean Patagonia, Argentina. *Chemosphere* **2011**, *83*, 1597–1602. [CrossRef]
31. Quilichini, Y.; Foata, J.; Orsini, A.; Mattei, J.; Marchand, B. Parasitofauna study of the brown trout, *Salmo trutta* (Pisces, Teleostei) from Corsica (Mediterranean island) rivers. *Parasite* **2007**, *14*, 257–260. [CrossRef]
32. Hartvigsen, R.; Halvorsen, O. Common and rare trout parasites in a small landscape system. *Parasitology* **1993**, *106 Pt 1*, 101–105. [CrossRef] [PubMed]
33. Klein, W.; Olsen, O.; Bowden, D. Effects of intestinal fluke, Crepidostomum farionis, on rainbow trout, Salmo gairdnerii. *Trans. Am. Fish. Soc.* **1969**, *98*, 1–6. [CrossRef]
34. European Commission. Directorate–General for Maritime Affairs and Fisheries. In *The EU Fish Market: 2020 Edition*; EU Publications: Luxembourg, 2020.
35. Jung-Schroers, V.; Hildebrandt, U.; Retter, K.; Esser, K.-H.; Hellmann, J.; Kleingeld, D.W.; Rohn, K.; Steinhagen, D. Is humane slaughtering of rainbow trout achieved in conventional production chains in Germany? Results of a pilot field and laboratory study. *BMC Vet. Res.* **2020**, *16*, 197. [CrossRef] [PubMed]
36. Hajirezaee, S.; Amiri, B.M.; Mehrpoosh, M.; Jafaryan, H.; Mirrasuli, E.; Golpour, A. Gonadal development and associated changes in gonadosomatic index and sex steroids during the reproductive cycle of cultured male and female Caspian brown trout, *Salmo trutta* caspius (Kessler, 1877). *J. Appl. Anim. Res.* **2012**, *40*, 154–162. [CrossRef]
37. Bush, A.O.; Lafferty, K.D.; Lotz, J.M.; Shostak, A.W. Parasitology meets ecology on its own terms: Margolis et al. revisited. *J. Parasitol.* **1997**, *83*, 575–583. [CrossRef]
38. Ferrante, M.C.; Fusco, G.; Monnolo, A.; Saggiomo, F.; Guccione, J.; Mercogliano, R.; Clausi, M.T. Food contamination by PCBs and waste disposal crisis: Evidence from goat milk in Campania (Italy). *Chemosphere* **2017**, *186*, 396–404. [CrossRef]
39. Ferrante, M.C.; Di Vaio, P.; Magli, E.; Frecentese, F.; Meli, R.; Caliendo, G.; Corvino, A.; Fiorino, F.; Giordano, F.; Monnolo, A.; et al. PCB levels in adipose tissue of dogs from illegal dumping sites in Campania region (Italy). *Chemosphere* **2020**, *244*, 125478. [CrossRef]
40. Ferrante, M.C.; Fusco, G.; Naccari, C.; Meli, R.; Clausi, M.T. Are Biometric Parameters Helpful to Assess the Health Risk of Consuming Organochlorine Compounds Contaminated Silver European Eel (*Anguilla anguilla*)? *J. Food Sci.* **2016**, *81*, T1024–T1030. [CrossRef]
41. Webster, L.; Roose, P.; Bersuder, P.; Kotterman, M.; Haarich, M.; Vorkamp, K. Determination of Polychlorinated Biphenyls (PCBs) in Sediment and Biota. In *ICES Techniques in Marine Environmental Sciences*; series number No. 53; International Council for the Exploration of the Sea (ICES) Publisher: Copenhagen, Denmark, 2013. [CrossRef]
42. Santoro, M.; Iaccarino, D.; Bellisario, B. Host biological factors and geographic locality influence predictors of parasite communities in sympatric sparid fishes off the southern Italian coast. *Sci. Rep.* **2020**, *10*, 13283. [CrossRef]
43. Santoro, M.; Bellisario, B.; Fernandez-Alvarez, F.A.; Crocetta, F.; Palomba, M. Parasites and prey of the nursehound shark Scyliorhinus stellaris (Linnaeus, 1758): Insights into hidden trophic web interactions in the Mediterranean Sea. *J. Fish. Biol.* **2023**, *102*, 271–280. [CrossRef]
44. Santoro, M.; Palomba, M.; Aco Alburqueque, R.; Mattiucci, S. Integrative Taxonomy Reveals Molicola uncinatus and *Gymnorhynchus gigas* (Cestoda: Trypanorhyncha) Coinfection in the Atlantic Pomfret Brama brama From the Mediterranean Sea, With Notes on the Phylogenetic Position of *G. gigas* within the Family Gymnorhynchidae. *Front. Vet. Sci.* **2022**, *9*, 909163. [CrossRef] [PubMed]
45. Giesy, J.P.; Kannan, K. Dioxin-like and non-dioxin-like toxic effects of polychlorinated biphenyls (PCBs): Implications for risk assessment. *Crit. Rev. Toxicol.* **1998**, *28*, 511–569. [CrossRef] [PubMed]
46. Bordajandi, L.R.; Gomez, G.; Fernandez, M.A.; Abad, E.; Rivera, J.; Gonzalez, M.J. Study on PCBs, PCDD/Fs, organochlorine pesticides, heavy metals and arsenic content in freshwater fish species from the River Turia (Spain). *Chemosphere* **2003**, *53*, 163–171. [CrossRef]
47. Bailey, R.E. Global hexachlorobenzene emissions. *Chemosphere* **2001**, *43*, 167–182. [CrossRef] [PubMed]
48. Paggi, L.; Orecchia, P.; Del Marro, M.; Iori, A.; Manilla, G. Parasites of *Salmo trutta* L. from the Tirino River. II. Host-parasite interactions of helminth species. *Parassitologia* **1978**, *20*, 161–168. [PubMed]
49. Isobe, T.; Oshihoi, T.; Hamada, H.; Nakayama, K.; Yamada, T.K.; Tajima, Y.; Amano, M.; Tanabe, S. Contamination status of POPs and BFRs and relationship with parasitic infection in finless porpoises (*Neophocaena phocaenoides*) from Seto Inland Sea and Omura Bay, Japan. *Mar. Pollut. Bull.* **2011**, *63*, 564–571. [CrossRef] [PubMed]
50. Vidal-Martínez, V.; Aguirre-Macedo, M.; Noreña-Barroso, E.; Gold-Bouchot, G.; Caballero-Pinzón, P. Potential interactions between metazoan parasites of the Mayan catfish Ariopsis assimilis and chemical pollution in Chetumal Bay, Mexico. *J. Helminthol.* **2003**, *77*, 173–184. [CrossRef]
51. Khan, M.A.; Hansen, L.G. Ortho-substituted polychlorinated biphenyl (PCB) congeners (95 or 101) decrease pituitary response to thyrotropin releasing hormone. *Toxicol. Lett.* **2003**, *144*, 173–182. [CrossRef]
52. Schmidt, V.; Zander, S.; Körting, W.; Broeg, K.; von Westernhagen, H.; Dizer, H.; Hansen, P.; Skouras, A.; Steinhagen, D. Parasites of flounder (*Platichthys flesus* L.) from the German Bight, North Sea, and their potential use in biological effects monitoring: C. Pollution effects on the parasite community and a comparison to biomarker responses. *Helgol. Mar. Res.* **2003**, *57*, 262–271. [CrossRef]

53. Brázová, T.; Hanzelová, V.; Miklisová, D. Bioaccumulation of six PCB indicator congeners in a heavily polluted water reservoir in Eastern Slovakia: Tissue-specific distribution in fish and their parasites. *Parasitol. Res.* **2012**, *111*, 779–786. [CrossRef]
54. Brázová, T.; Miklisová, D.; Barčák, D.; Uhrovič, D.; Šalamún, P.; Orosová, M.; Oros, M. Hazardous pollutants in the environment: Fish host-parasite interactions and bioaccumulation of polychlorinated biphenyls. *Environ. Pollut.* **2021**, *291*, 118175. [CrossRef]
55. Henriquez-Hernandez, L.A.; Carreton, E.; Camacho, M.; Montoya-Alonso, J.A.; Boada, L.D.; Valeron, P.F.; Falcon-Cordon, Y.; Falcon-Cordon, S.; Almeida-Gonzalez, M.; Zumbado, M.; et al. The heartworm (*Dirofilaria immitis*) seems to be able to metabolize organochlorine pesticides and polychlorinated biphenyls: A case-control study in dogs. *Sci. Total Environ.* **2017**, *575*, 1445–1452. [CrossRef]
56. Gui, D.; He, J.; Zhang, X.; Tu, Q.; Chen, L.; Feng, K.; Liu, W.; Mai, B.; Wu, Y. Potential association between exposure to legacy persistent organic pollutants and parasitic body burdens in Indo-Pacific finless porpoises from the Pearl River Estuary, China. *Sci. Total Environ.* **2018**, *643*, 785–792. [CrossRef] [PubMed]
57. Kannan, K.; Perrotta, E.; Thomas, N.J.; Aldous, K.M. A comparative analysis of polybrominated diphenyl ethers and polychlorinated biphenyls in Southern sea otters that died of infectious diseases and noninfectious causes. *Arch. Environ. Contam. Toxicol.* **2007**, *53*, 293–302. [CrossRef] [PubMed]
58. Bamidele, A.; Abiodun, K.T.; David, U.U.; Kayode, S.J. Gastrointestinal Parasites of *Sarotherodon melanotheron* (Ruppel, 1852) Histopathological Alterations and Organochlorine Pesticides Pollution from Lagos, Lagoon, Nigeria. *Egypt. Acad. J. Biol. Sci. E Med. Entomol. Parasitol.* **2018**, *10*, 15–29. [CrossRef]
59. Bamidele, A.; Abayomi, A.; Iyabo, A.; Giwa, M. Parasitic fauna, histopathological alterations, and organochlorine pesticides contamination in *Chrysichthys nigrodigitatus* (Lacepede, 1803) (Bagridae) from Lagos, Lagoon, Nigeria. *Sci. Afr.* **2019**, *5*, e00130. [CrossRef]
60. Ferrante, M.C.; Mattace Raso, G.; Esposito, E.; Bianco, G.; Iacono, A.; Clausi, M.T.; Amero, P.; Santoro, A.; Simeoli, R.; Autore, G.; et al. Effects of non-dioxin-like polychlorinated biphenyl congeners (PCB 101, PCB 153 and PCB 180) alone or mixed on J774A.1 macrophage cell line: Modification of apoptotic pathway. *Toxicol. Lett.* **2011**, *202*, 61–68. [CrossRef]
61. Santoro, A.; Ferrante, M.C.; Di Guida, F.; Pirozzi, C.; Lama, A.; Simeoli, R.; Clausi, M.T.; Monnolo, A.; Mollica, M.P.; Mattace Raso, G.; et al. Polychlorinated Biphenyls (PCB 101, 153, and 180) Impair Murine Macrophage Responsiveness to Lipopolysaccharide: Involvement of NF-kappaB Pathway. *Toxicol. Sci.* **2015**, *147*, 255–269. [CrossRef]
62. Sagerup, K.; Larsen, H.J.; Skaare, J.U.; Johansen, G.M.; Gabrielsen, G.W. The toxic effects of multiple persistent organic pollutant exposures on the post-hatch immunity maturation of glaucous gulls. *J. Toxicol. Environ. Health A* **2009**, *72*, 870–883. [CrossRef]
63. Luebke, R.W.; Copeland, C.B.; Diliberto, J.J.; Akubue, P.I.; Andrews, D.L.; Riddle, M.M.; Williams, W.C.; Birnbaum, L.S. Assessment of host resistance to Trichinella spiralis in mice following preinfection exposure to 2,3,7,8-TCDD. *Toxicol. Appl. Pharmacol.* **1994**, *125*, 7–16. [CrossRef]
64. Sures, B.; Knopf, K. Individual and combined effects of cadmium and 3,3′,4,4′,5-pentachlorobiphenyl (PCB 126) on the humoral immune response in European eel (*Anguilla anguilla*) experimentally infected with larvae of Anguillicola crassus (Nematoda). *Parasitology* **2004**, *128*, 445–454. [CrossRef] [PubMed]
65. Morley, N.J.; Lewis, J.W.; Hoole, D. Pollutant-induced effects on immunological and physiological interactions in aquatic host-trematode systems: Implications for parasite transmission. *J. Helminthol.* **2006**, *80*, 137–149. [CrossRef] [PubMed]
66. Yen Le, T.T.; Rijsdijk, L.; Sures, B.; Hendriks, A.J. Accumulation of persistent organic pollutants in parasites. *Chemosphere* **2014**, *108*, 145–151. [CrossRef] [PubMed]
67. Molbert, N.; Alliot, F.; Leroux-Coyau, M.; Medoc, V.; Biard, C.; Meylan, S.; Jacquin, L.; Santos, R.; Goutte, A. Potential Benefits of Acanthocephalan Parasites for Chub Hosts in Polluted Environments. *Environ. Sci. Technol.* **2020**, *54*, 5540–5549. [CrossRef]
68. Schafer, P.; Muller, M.; Kruger, A.; Steinberg, C.E.; Menzel, R. Cytochrome P450-dependent metabolism of PCB52 in the nematode Caenorhabditis elegans. *Arch. Biochem. Biophys.* **2009**, *488*, 60–68. [CrossRef]
69. Barrett, J. Helminth detoxification mechanisms. *J. Helminthol.* **1997**, *71*, 85–89. [CrossRef]
70. Barrett, J. Cytochrome P450 in parasitic protozoa and helminths. *Comp. Biochem. Physiol. C Pharmacol. Toxicol. Endocrinol.* **1998**, *121*, 181–183. [CrossRef]
71. Goutte, A.; Molbert, N. Benefits of Parasitism in Polluted Environments: A Review and Perspectives. *Front. Ecol. Evol.* **2022**, *97*, e34. [CrossRef]
72. Weber, R.; Herold, C.; Hollert, H.; Kamphues, J.; Blepp, M.; Ballschmiter, K. Reviewing the relevance of dioxin and PCB sources for food from animal origin and the need for their inventory, control and management. *Environ. Sci. Eur.* **2018**, *30*, 42. [CrossRef]
73. Van den Berg, M.; Birnbaum, L.S.; Denison, M.; De Vito, M.; Farland, W.; Feeley, M.; Fiedler, H.; Hakansson, H.; Hanberg, A.; Haws, L.; et al. The 2005 World Health Organization reevaluation of human and Mammalian toxic equivalency factors for dioxins and dioxin-like compounds. *Toxicol. Sci.* **2006**, *93*, 223–241. [CrossRef]

animals

Article

Dietary Curcumin Modulating Effect on Performance, Antioxidant Status, and Immune-Related Response of Broiler Chickens Exposed to Imidacloprid Insecticide

Naglaa Z. Eleiwa [1], Ahmed A. El-Shabrawi [1], Doaa Ibrahim [2,*], Abdelwahab A. Abdelwarith [3], Elsayed M. Younis [3], Simon J. Davies [4], Mohamed M. M. Metwally [5,6] and Ehsan H. Abu-Zeid [7,*]

[1] Department of Pharmacology, Faculty of Veterinary Medicine, Zagazig University, Zagazig 44519, Egypt; drnaglaa876@gmail.com (N.Z.E.); ahmedshabrawi@gmail.com (A.A.E.-S.)
[2] Department of Nutrition and Clinical Nutrition, Faculty of Veterinary Medicine, Zagazig University, Zagazig 44519, Egypt
[3] Department of Zoology, College of Science, King Saud University, P.O. Box 2455, Riyadh 11451, Saudi Arabia; awarith@ksu.edu.sa (A.A.A.); emyounis@ksu.edu.sa (E.M.Y.)
[4] Aquaculture Nutrition Research Unit ANRU, Carna Research Station, Ryan Institute, College of Science and Engineering, University of Galway, H91V8Y1 Galway, Ireland; sjdplymouth@live.co.uk
[5] Department of Pathology and Clinical Pathology, Faculty of Veterinary Medicine, King Salman International University, Ras Sudr 46612, Egypt; metywally@gmail.com
[6] Department of Pathology, Faculty of Veterinary Medicine, Zagazig University, Zagazig 44519, Egypt
[7] Department of Forensic Medicine and Toxicology, Faculty of Veterinary Medicine, Zagazig University, Zagazig 44519, Egypt
* Correspondence: ehelsharkawy@zu.edu.eg (E.H.A.); doibrahim@vet.zu.edu.eg (D.I.)

Simple Summary: This experiment was conducted to examine the protective role of curcumin (CUR) in mitigating imidacloprid (IMI)-induced toxic effects on broilers' growth performance, immune response, antioxidant status, and the expression of immune-associated genes. CUR significantly improved overall growth performance-related indices when compared to IMI-exposed birds. Additionally, CUR enhanced hematological indices, phagocytosis, and total protein, albumin, globulin, AST, ALT, lysozyme, and IgG levels when compared to the IMI-exposed birds. CUR supplementation significantly modulated oxidative stress-related indices, including TAC, SOD, CAT, and GPx, and decreased MDA levels when compared to IMI-exposed birds. The inflammatory response was modulated after CUR supplementation as supported by down-regulation of *IL-1β*, *TNF-α*, and *TLR4* mRNA expression levels and up-regulated the *IL-10* mRNA expression levels in the spleen when compared to IMI-exposed birds. These results collectively showed, for the first time, that CUR had an in vivo protective effect against IMI toxicity in broiler chickens.

Abstract: Birds appear to be especially vulnerable to adverse impacts from insecticides. This is especially true for imidacloprid (IMI), which is considered the most toxic to avian species. Recently, prospective studies aimed at including natural alternative products to alleviate the toxic impact that comes from insecticides have been increased. Focusing on herbal growth promoters and antioxidative medicament for the poultry industry, this ongoing experiment was conducted to examine the curcumin role (CUR) in mitigating IMI-prompted detrimental effects on broilers' performance, immunity, and antioxidant status. A total number of one hundred and fifty commercial meat-type Ross 308 broilers chicks (one-day-old) were randomly allocated into equal five groups (30 chicks/group and 10 birds/replicate). The first group (C) was the control; the second group (CUR) was fed a diet containing CUR at the level of 450 mg/kg; the third group (IMI) was fed control diet for 14 days and then was fed a diet containing IMI at the level of 50 mg/kg; the fourth group (CUR+IMI co-treated) was fed a diet containing CUR+IMI; and the fifth group (CUR+IMI pro/co-treated) was fed a diet containing CUR for 14 days as protective and then a diet containing CUR+IMI for the rest of the trial. CUR supplementation either in the (CUR pro/co-treated) or (CUR co-treated) groups significantly ($p < 0.05$) improved final body weight and total body weight gain while decreasing the total feed intake and feed conversion ratio when compared to the IMI-exposed and non-treated birds. CUR induced a significant ($p < 0.05$) enhancement in hematological indices, phagocytosis %, phagocytic index, intracellular killing capacity, total proteins, globulin, liver function enzymes, lysozyme activity, and immunoglobulin-G levels compared to IMI-exposed and non-treated birds. In addition, dietary supplementation of CUR significantly ($p < 0.05$) modulated oxidative stress-related biomarkers in splenic tissues (total antioxidant capacity, superoxide dismutase, catalase, and glutathione peroxidase) and decreased malondialdehyde levels ($p < 0.05$) when compared to IMI-exposed and non-treated birds. CUR significantly down-regulated mRNA levels expression of *IL-1β*, *TNF-α*, and *TLR4* and up-regulated *IL-10* mRNA expression levels in spleens of birds when compared to those exposed to IMI-and non-treated. Finally, our results provided new insight into IMI-induced immuno-toxicity in broiler chickens. Furthermore, for the first time, our study informed that CUR can cause an in vivo protective effect against IMI toxicity, principally as a protective and/or as concurrent supplementation during the exposure to IMI toxicity.

Keywords: curcumin; imidacloprid; immune-toxicity; hematological indices; phagocytosis; immune-related genes mRNA expression; oxidative stress; growth performance; 308 Ross Broiler

1. Introduction

Worldwide, poultry production has actively selected features that maximize birds' output as well as boost birds' immunity, thereby enhancing birds' productivity [1], feed profitability and utilization [2], and their performance [3,4]. In such a scenario, the poultry industry sector has seen a rise in the valuation of plant-based products and their bioactive components that are targeted to improve birds' health, productivity, and the products quality derived from them [5]. For broiler producers, boosting birds' immunity is a critical area [6,7]. Various approaches have been used, such as adding feed additives like natural extracts [8] with antioxidant potentials [9–12] and to modulate the metabolic homeostasis and immune status of birds [13]. To this end, turmeric, also known as *Curcuma longa* Linn (member of the *Zingiberaceae* family), is one of the most widely used nutritional supplements worldwide [14,15]. Turmeric is a potential medicinal herb used as a natural feed supplement in chickens' diets and has been used to replace dietary antibiotics with a beneficial impact on health [16]. According to Ashraf [17], CUR makes up the majority (80%) of the total amount of curcuminoids in turmeric powder. The hydrophobic phenolic compound gives turmeric its orange-yellow pigment [18]. It is mostly used to enhance food palatability, improve food appearance, preserve food, regulate aflatoxin-induced mutagenicity, and protect against hepatic carcinogenicity [19]. Owing to its capacity to affect a variety of signaling molecules, including inflammatory molecules, cell survival proteins, and drug resistance proteins, CUR has been described as a multi-target drug [20].

Abou-Elkhair, et al. [21], reported that CUR can be used as a feed additive in poultry to improve their growth performance. The free radical scavenging, anti-inflammatory activities, and immune response boosting are just a few of the therapeutic and pharmacological effects of dietary CUR [22–24]. According to the above-mentioned biological characteristics, dietary CUR has been identified as a possible feed additive to lessen the harmful effects of chronic heat stress in poultry [25]. Various experimental and clinical research data have reported that CUR is pharmacologically considered to be a harmless substance that possesses antioxidant, anti-inflammatory, and antimicrobial consequences [15,26,27].

Neonicotinoids are a group of globally used insecticides with systemic properties that were increasingly utilized from early 2000 onwards and are approved in 120 countries [28]. Besides, imidacloprid (IMI) has been established as a novel insecticide due to its molecular properties and distinct effect on pests [29]. Undesirable impacts on non-target species resulted from a wide spectrum of neonicotinoids [30]. Additionally, exposure to neonicotinoids has been linked to sub-lethal effects in birds, including neurobehavioral alterations, immunotoxicity, poor growth and development, and decreased reproductive efficiency [31,32]. Cestonaro, et al. [33], reported that the immune system could be challenged by neonicotinoids. Due to the association with decreased fitness and survival probability in birds, immunotoxicity is one of their notable sub-lethal impacts [34]. Neonicotinoids pesticides target nicotinic-acetylcholine receptors, which are found in several immune system components [35,36]. This may contribute to the immune suppression seen in bees, rodents, and birds [37–39].

Birds appear to be particularly susceptible to adverse impacts from neonicotinoids, together with IMI being the most utilized pesticide worldwide [40] and the most toxic insecticide to avian varieties [32,41]. Exposure to IMI through water or food occurs frequently as broiler chickens are the most common source of animal protein and are frequently raised using traditional farming practices, particularly in developing nations [42]. IMI is regularly found in food samples and drinking water samples at levels as high as 4.49 ng/g and 8.622 ng/L, respectively; this is due to its high water solubility and extended persistence [43,44]. IMI is applied to control insects that attack poultry farms and damage crops [45]. To combat the intense presence of insects, IMI spray is applied for utensil cleaning and wall painting [46]. Although IMI appears to be safe for birds to consume and selectively kills insects, it can still be harmful to birds because the safe dosage levels are unknown, and the chance of its ingesting through feed and water are high [47,48]. The breakdown products of IMI can also potentially cause immunosuppression directly or indirectly through triggering stress responses and the neuroendocrine system [49].

Dietary supplements containing natural products with antioxidant activities offer excellent possibilities for mitigating neonicotinoid toxicity since mitochondrial oxidative stress (OS) is a significant factor in neonicotinoid-induced toxicity [50]. Free radicals implicated in lipid peroxidation and OS are produced in large quantities as a result of IMI toxicity [51]. Osman et al. [52], found that birds exposed to IMI regularly exhibited disturbance of their antioxidative status, inflammation, and immunosuppression. Moreover, levels of liver-related indices (alkaline phosphate and transaminase), lipids (cholesterol and triglycerides), and hematological indices were altered in these birds [53]. Previous studies stated that feed supplements with vitamin E, selenium, and silymarin were found to reduce the harmful effects of IMI exposure in Japanese quails and chickens [46,54,55]. In layers, the hepatic tissue levels of GSH were dropped while TBARS were increased following exposure to IMI [56]. In addition to teratogenic concerns in white leghorn chicken [57], IMI exposure has an impact on embryonic development and chicks' survivability in bobwhite quails [58]. Following IMI exposure, OS and lipid peroxidation were prompted in the RBCs, liver, kidney, and testes of white leghorn cockerels [59]. Therefore, it is advised to use natural antioxidants to restore the antioxidative ability, lessen lipid peroxidation, and control the physiological and metabolic processes inside the birds' body [51,53]. In light of the aforementioned problems, the goal of the current study was to assess the effectiveness of pro and/or concurrent dietary additions of CUR to the diets of Ross 308 broiler chickens that had been exposed to IMI by evaluating the chickens' growth performance, hematological indices, phagocytosis, immune and oxidative status, and mRNA expression profiling of immune-related genes.

2. Materials and Methods

2.1. Test Compounds and Chemical Reagents

Imidacloprid (IMI) (CAS No. 138261-41-3), analytical standard, purity grade (100%) PESTANAL®, Curcumin (CUR) (CAS: 458-37-7) with purity determined by HPLC to be more than 98% were obtained from Sigma-Aldrich Laborchemikalien GmbH; Germany. The total *RNA* extraction reagent was Trizol™ (Invitrogen; Thermo Fisher Scientific, Inc., Waltham, MA, USA), and the HiSenScript™ RH (-) cDNA Synthesis Kit was also used (iNtRON Biotechnology Co., Seongnam, Kyonggi-do, Republic of Korea).

2.2. Experimental Birds, Design, and Diet Preparation

The protocol of the study complied with the principles and regulations approved by Zagazig University's Faculty of Veterinary Medicine's Institutional Animal Care and Use Committee (IACUC) (ZU-IACUC/2/f/75/2022).

One hundred and fifty chicks (one-day-old) of a meat type (Ross 308) with an average body weight of 45 ± 5 g and provided by a commercial chicks' producer (Dakahlia Poultry, Mansoura, Egypt) were used for the current study. On arrival, they were weighed then equally divided randomly into five experimental groups. Each group contained 30 chicks (three replicates/treatment, and 10 birds/replicate). Study groups included the first control group (C), fed a normal control diet; the second group (CUR), the curcumin group, fed a supplemented diet with 450 mg/kg of CUR, according to Cheng et al. [60]; the third imidacloprid group (IMI), fed on control diet for 14 days then fed on a supplemented diet with a dose of IMI 50 mg/kg diet following Ravikanth et al. [61]; the fourth group, CUR+IMI co-treated, fed the control diet for 14 days then fed a supplemented diet with CUR+IMI until the end of the experiment; the fifth group, CUR+IMI pro/co-treated, curcumin + imidacloprid protected/co-treated group fed a supplemented diet with CUR for 14 days then fed a supplemented diet with CUR+IMI until end of the experiment (4 weeks). Experimental groups and the treatment design are shown in Figure 1. Birds were raised in an open home with natural ventilation in the Faculty of Veterinary Medicine at Zagazig University's animal research unit. Birds were reared in batteries with an automatic water system, ban feed in front of birds, and at a density of 10 birds/m^2. Lighting regime was 24 h from days 1 to 3 and then 23 h lighting was applied up to the end of the experiment. The starting temperature was adjusted to 33 ± 1 °C for the first 3 days and then decreased by 3 °C each week until it reached 24 °C at the end of the experimental period according to the Aviagen guidelines [62]. Humidity was maintained at around 60% throughout the whole experiment.

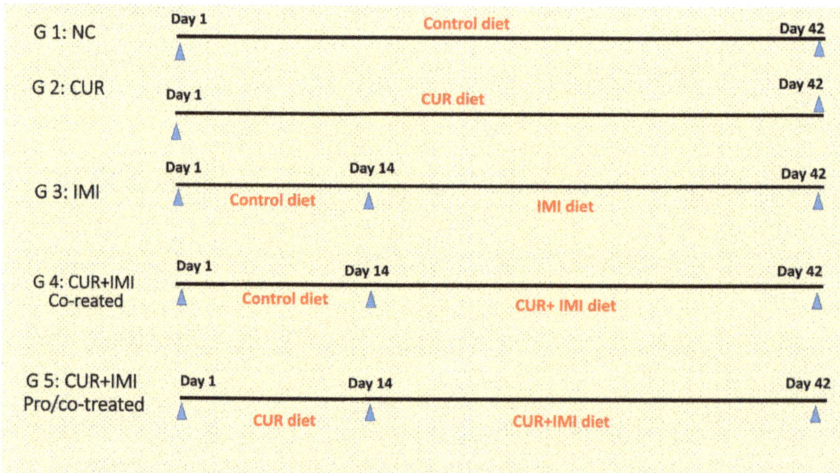

Figure 1. Experimental groups, doses, durations, and treatments: CUR (450 mg/kg diet) and IMI (50 mg/kg diet) in Ross 308 broilers.

The basal isocaloric and isonitrogenous diets were formulated following Ross Broiler-Pocket Guide specifications from Aviagen [63]. The chemical composition and nutrient concentrations of the basal diets are listed in Table 1. The experiment lasted for seven weeks. Diets for the starter stage (1–10 days), grower stage (11–20 days), and finisher stage (21–42 days) were available throughout the experiment. The utilized feedstuffs and the experimental diets' proximate chemical analyses (for moisture, crude protein, and ether extracts) were conducted following AOAC [64] and are shown in Table 2. Birds received vaccinations against Newcastle disease at 7 and 14 days of age and against Gumboro disease at 11 and 22 days of age, according to Giambrone et al. [65]. Birds of all groups were monitored for any disease challenge or mortalities over the experimental period.

Table 1. The ingredients and nutrient contents of basal diet.

Ingredient, %	Starter (1–10 Days)	Grower (11–20 Days)	Finisher (21–35 Days)
Yellow corn	57.8	61	65.2
Soybean meal, 48%	34.8	30.3	25.6
	1.2	1.2	1.2
Soybean oil	0	0	0
Calcium carbonate	1.8	3.2	3.7
Calcium diphasic phosphate	1.2	1.2	1.2
Common salt	1.2	1.2	1.2
Premix [1]	0.3	0.3	0.3
L-Lysine HCL, 78%	0.8	0.8	0.8
DL-Methionine, 99%	0.35	0.3	0.3
Choline chloride	0.20	0.20	0.20
Anti-mycotoxin	0.10	0.10	0.10
Calculated composition			
Metabolizable energy (Kcal/Kg)	3013	3130	3200
Crude protein, %	23.02	21.00	19.22
Ether extract, %	4.31	5.76	6.35
Crude fiber, %	2.64	2.54	2.47
Calcium, %	1.09	1.08	1.07
Available phosphorous, %	0.47	0.44	0.48
Lysine, %	1.45	1.29	1.17
Methionine, %	0.60	0.53	0.51

[1] Vitamin premix supplied per kilogram of diet: tocopheryl acetate, 80 mg; cholecalciferol, 5000 IU; retinol, 20.000 IU; menadione, 2.9 mg; thiamine, 4.5 mg; riboflavin, 5.5 mg; pantothenate, 10 mg; niacin, 450 mg; folate, 2.5 mg; pyridoxine, 8 mg; biotin, 250 µg; Fe (sulphate), 40 mg; cyanocobalamine, 17 µg; Se (selenate), 0.3 mg; I (iodide), 1.50 mg; Cu (sulphate), 8 mg; Zn (sulphate and oxide), 120 mg; Mn (sulphate and oxide), 120 mg.

Table 2. Chemical composition (%) of feedstuffs used in formulation of the experimental diets (air dry basis).

Ingredient	Nutrient (%)								
	Moisture	CP	EE	* CF	* Calcium	* AP [1]	* Lysine	* Methionine	* ME [2]
yellow corn	8	8.9	3.7	2.3	0.05	0.08	0.26	0.18	3350
Soybean meal, 48%	10.6	47.8	1.1	3.7	0.25	0.27	2.92	0.67	2440
Corn gluten, 60%	11	59.4	2.4	1.8	0.07	0.14	1.03	1.78	3720
Soybean oil	-	-	98	-	-	-	-	-	8800
Calcium carbonate	-	-	-	-	38	-	-	-	-
Calcium dibasic phosphate	-	-	-	-	26	18	-	-	-
premix	-	-	-	-	26	-	-	-	-
Lysine, HcL, 78%	-	118	-	-	-	-	78	-	4600
DL-Methionine, 98%	-	58	-	-	-	-	-	98	3600

[1] Available phosphorus; [2] Metabolizable energy Kcal/kg; * Calculated according to Council [66]. Moisture, CP (crude protein), EE (ether extract), CF (crude fiber) were chemically analyzed according to procedures of AOAC [67].

2.3. Total Growth Performance Related Indices

To obtain the average initial body weight (IBW), each bird was weighed separately on the first day of life. The body weight was then calculated each week by dividing the total bird weights by the number of birds in each group. According to procedures outlined by Kishawy, et al. [68] and Ibrahim, et al. [69], the total body weight gain (TBWG), total feed intake (TFI), total feed conversion ratio (TFCR), and final body weight (FBW) per each replicate for the entire experimental period were estimated.

2.4. Collection of Samples

Six birds per group were randomly chosen at the end of the 42-days feeding study, fasted overnight, and weighed. At the end of the experimental period, blood from each group was aseptically collected from the wing vein and separated as follows: one part was collected into clean and dry 15 mL falcon tubes without the use of an anticoagulant, allowed to clot at room temperature, and then centrifuged for five minutes at 3000 rpm for serum separation and kept at −20 °C until biochemically analyzed for protein and lipid profiles, liver functions, and immunological markers. Another part of blood was collected in sterile tubes containing dipotassium Ethylene di amine tetra acetic acid salt (EDTA) for hematological examination. The third part of blood was collected in heparinized tubes for phagocytosis assay.

Splenic tissues (1 g) were collected, cleaned with an ice-cold 0.85% NaCl solution, and homogenized in 9 mL of ice-cold phosphate buffer saline (PBS, pH 7.5). For the purpose of estimating oxidative stress-related indices, the homogenate was spun in a cooled centrifuge for 15 min at 3000 rpm. The supernatant was then collected into Eppendorf tubes and maintained at −80 °C.

Small parts of splenic tissues were dissected for molecular analysis immediately after scarification and maintained in TRIzol reagent at −80 °C until further examination by the RT-qPCR assay of immune-related genes including Toll-Like Receptor 4 (*TLR-4*), Interleukin 1 Beta (*IL-1β*), and Interleukin 10 (*IL-10*). Other splenic tissues were stored for histopathological and immunohistochemical analysis in neutral buffered formalin (10%) at room temperature.

2.5. Hematological Analysis and Phagocytosis Assay

Haematological parameters were measured using Hemascreen 18 Automatic Cell Counter (Hospitex Diagnostics, Sesto Fiorentino, Italy), on the basis of Harrison and Harrison [70], including red blood cells (RBCs), hemoglobin (Hb), hematocrit value (Hct), total leukocyte counts (WBCs), and differential leukocyte counts were determined as described by Nengsih and Mustika [71].

The phagocytic assay was carried out as described by Bos and de Souza [72], with some adjustments. Blood was collected quickly followed by the extraction of a peripheral blood mononuclear cell layer, washing, re-suspension in Roswell Park Memorial Institute (RPMI-164) medium, and the addition of 15% fetal calf serum (FCS). Then, 5×10^6 mononuclear cells were seeded in a 1 mL volume for culture in chambers with coverslips; these were stained and incubated for 1 h at 37 °C with 5% CO_2 and 99% humidity to create a monolayer of macrophages. After washing three times to eliminate non-adherent cells, adherent macrophages were treated for 24 h with 1 mL of *Candida albicans* (10^7/mL of RPMI with 15% FCS) before being washed three times, fixed, and stained. In order to calculate the percentage of phagocytic macrophages (number of phagocytic macrophages/total number of macrophages), 100 macrophages were counted.

2.6. Biochemical Measurements of the Serum and Splenic Tissue

The serum lysozyme activities of broilers were determined according to Ellis [73]. Serum IgG levels were determined with chicken immunoglobulin (IgG) *ELISA* kits obtained from MyBioSource with Catalog number: MBS260043.

Colorimetric diagnostic kits from Sigma Aldrich were used for estimation of serum total cholesterol (TC), triglycerides (TG), high-density lipoprotein-cholesterol (HDL-C), low-density lipoprotein-cholesterol (LDL-C), and very low-density lipoprotein (VLDL) levels, with product number MAK043 for TC, TR0100 for TGs, and MAK045 for HDL and LDL/VLDL assay Kits, following the manufacturer's instructions. The serum levels of albumin and total protein (TP) were determined by ready-made diagnostic kits provided by Agappe diagnostics kits, Code No: 51001002. The serum globulin (Gl.) levels were calculated mathematically by subtracting albumin values from total proteins as described by Doumas, et al. [74]. Serum levels of aspartate aminotransferase (AST) and alanine aminotransferase (ALT) were determined by ready-made diagnostic kits provided by Agappe diagnostics kits, Product. NO.: 51408002 and 51409002, respectively.

Splenic levels of total antioxidant capacity (TAC), catalase (CAT) activity, Superoxide dismutase (SOD) activity, and Glutathione peroxidase (GPx) was determined by colorimetric determination method by ready-made diagnostic kits provided by Bio-diagnostic, Egypt CAT. NO. TA 25 13, CA 25 17, SD 25 21, GP 2524, respectively. Malondialdehyde (MDA) levels were determined by enzymatic colorimetric method by using ready diagnostic kits provided by Bio-diagnostic, Egypt, CAT. No. MD 25 29.

2.7. Transcriptional Analysis of Immune-Related Genes IL-1β, TLR-4, and IL-10 in Spleen Tissue Using Quantitative Real-Time PCR

Splenic tissue samples were used for detecting the mRNA expression levels of immune-related genes. Extraction of total RNA was completed via the QIAamp RNeasy Mini kit (Cat. No. 51304; Qiagen, Hilden, Germany) following the instructions of the manufacturer. The extracted RNA concentration was detected at 260 nm and the clarity of RNA was detected by Spectrostar NanoDrop TM 2000 spectrophotometer (Cat. No. ND-2000; Thermo Fisher, Santa Clara, CA, USA). The Stratagene MX3005P real-time PCR machine (Cat. No. PF1457N; Thermo Fisher, Santa Clara, CA, USA) was utilized for one-step RT-qPCR amplification, in triplicate, via a Quanti Tect SYBR Green RT-PCR Kit (Cat. No. 204243; Qiagen, Hilden, Germany) according to the protocol of the manufacturer. All PCR amplifications were verified via melting curve analysis. The housekeeping gene, namely *β-actin*, was used as an endogenous control to normalize the transcripts' expression levels. The sequences of the primers utilized in RT-qPCR assays are presented in Table 3. The $2^{-\Delta\Delta CT}$ method was used to assess the relative mRNA expression outcomes of the examined genes [75].

Table 3. Primer Oligonucleotide Sequences for target gene RT-PCR analysis.

Gene	Forward Primer (5′–3′)	Reverse Primer (5′–3′)	Gene Bank Accession No.	Product Size
TLR-4	GTTCTTCTGTGACCCGTGAGA	GTGAGGAGCGTTGCGCTTT	FJ915520.1	129
IL-1β	TGCCTGCAGAAGAAGCCTCG	CTCAGGTCGCTGTCAGCAAAG	NM_204524.2	173
IL-10	TTGGGGTGGCATTTCTCCTTG	GTTAGACTGCCTCAAACAGCG	EU999771.1	89
actin-b	GTGGATCAGCAAGCAGGAGT	ATCCTGAGTCAAGCGCCAAA	NM_205518.2	182

TLR-4: Toll-Like Receptor 4, *IL-1β*: Interleukin 1 Beta, *IL-10*: Interleukin 10.

2.8. Histopathological and Immunohistochemical Investigations

At the end of the experimental period, ten birds per group were randomly selected, euthanized by cervical dislocation, and necropsied. Representative tissue samples from the brains and spleens of all birds were harvested, fixed in 10% neutral buffered formalin for 24 h, processed for paraffin technique, sectioned at 5-μm thickness and stained with hematoxylin and eosin [76], and examined microscopically to evaluate any histological alterations. Next, quantitative lesion scoring was carried out in ten randomly selected splenic (10×) microscopic fields per bird. The investigated cerebral lesions were included (neuronal pyknosis, and necrosis, perineuronal vacuolations, gliosis, neuropil vacuolations, vascular congestions, thrombosis, hemorrhages, and leukocytic infiltrations) while the investigated splenic lesions were included, lymphoid depletion, and necrosis, vascular congestions, endothelial hypertrophy, and thrombosis. Finally, the results were expressed as percentages (means ± SEM) using the formula—Lesion FQ (%) = N lesion/N total × 100, where (N lesion) is the number of images exhibited a lesion and (N total) is the total number of images per group.

Successive formalin-fixed, paraffin-embedded, 5 μm thick splenic tissue sections were prepared and immunohistochemically stained following the protocol developed by Hsu, et al. [77]. The splenic tissue sections were stained for (1) TNF-α using the rabbit monoclonal anti-TNF-α primary antibody [TNF/1500R] (ab270264) (abcam, INC, London, UK) at 8 μg/mL dilution with the goat anti-rabbit IgG H&L (HRP) secondary antibody (ab205718) (abcam, INC) at 1/20,000 dilution, and (2) TLR4 using the mouse monoclonal anti-TLR4 primary antibody [76B357.1] (ab22048) (abcam, INC) at (1/100) dilution with the goat anti-mouse IgG H&L (HRP) secondary antibody (ab205719) (abcam, INC) at (1/10,000) dilution. The immune reactions were visualized using 3,3′-Diaminobenzidine (DAB) chromogen and the nuclei were counterstained with Harris hematoxylin. The degree of immunoexpression of the splenic TNF-α and TLR4 were quantified by calculating the percentages of the area fractions of the positively stained brown color concerning the total areas of the images using the image analyzing software, Image J version 1.33, in ten randomly selected (40×) microscopic fields for each marker; the results were expressed as percentages (means ± SEM).

2.9. Statistical Analysis of Data

Statistical tests were performed using a one-way analysis of variance (ANOVA) in SPSS version 21 for Windows (SPSS, Inc., Chicago, IL, USA). The regularly distributed nature of the data was established, followed by post hoc Tukey HSD multiple comparisons to determine the statistically significant variations among the various parameters in all experimental replicates. A *p*-value of <0.05 was considered statistically significant. Data were shown as means ± standard error mean (SEM). All graphs were generated using GraphPad Prism 8. Version 8.0.2 (263) (GraphPad Software Inc., San Diego, CA, USA).

3. Results

3.1. Effect of Dietary Supplementation of CUR, IMI, and Their Combinations on Overall Performance-Related Indices of Ross 308 Broiler Chickens

The results regarding the modulating effects of dietary supplementation of CUR, IMI, and their combinations on the growth performance-related indices (TFI, TBWG, TFCR, and FBW) of Ross 308 broiler chickens are shown in Table 4. The obtained data showed that there were no significant differences ($p < 0.05$) in IBW among all experimental groups. CUR dietary exposure significantly ($p < 0.05$) decreased TFI and TFCR in birds fed CUR by 3.14% and 6.56%, respectively, compared to birds of the C group, but significantly ($p < 0.05$) increased TBWG and FBW by 3.15% and 3.09%, respectively, in birds fed CUR compared to birds of the C group. IMI dietary exposure induced a non-significant ($p < 0.05$) decrease in TFI (0.77% decrease) and a significant increase in TFCR (17.49% increase) in birds fed an IMI-supplemented diet compared to birds of the C group. Additionally, IMI significantly ($p < 0.05$) decreased TBWG and FBW by 15.45% and 15.08%, respectively, in birds fed an IMI-supplemented diet compared to birds of the C group. Supplementation of CUR significantly ($p < 0.05$) decreased TFI by 5.95% and 4.17% in the (CUR+IMI co-treated) and (CUR+IMI pro/co-treated) groups, respectively, and decreased TFCR by 0% and 1.09% in the (CUR+IMI co-treated) and (CUR+IMI pro/co-treated) groups, respectively, compared to birds of the IMI-exposed group.

Table 4. Effect of dietary supplementation of imidacloprid (IMI), curcumin (CUR), and their combinations on overall performance of Ross 308 broiler chickens.

Parameter / Group	IBW (g)	TFI (g)	TBWG (g)	TFCR	FBW (g)
1st group C	45.20 ± 0.80	4300 ± 8.097 ^{a}	2349 ± 8.84 ^{b}	1.83 ± 0.01 ^{b}	2394 ± 8.79 ^{b}
2nd group CUR	46.00 ± 0.84	4133 ± 18.25 ^{b}	2423 ± 9.67 ^{a}	1.71 ± 0.01 ^{c}	2468 ± 9.50 ^{a}
3rd group IMI-treated	44.00 ± 1.30	4267 ± 11.40 ^{a}	1986 ± 36.46 ^{d}	2.15 ± 0.04 ^{a}	2033 ± 36.17 ^{e}
4th group CUR+IMI Co-treated	44.20 ± 0.86	4013 ± 23.74 ^{c}	2196 ± 2.88 ^{c}	1.83 ± 0.01 ^{b}	2242 ± 2.59 ^{d}
5th group CUR+IMI pro/co-treated	45.40 ± 0.51	4089 ± 12.20 ^{b}	2259 ± 5.51 ^{c}	1.81 ± 0.01 ^{b}	2303 ± 5.24 ^{c}

Total feed intake (TFI), Total body weight gain (TBWG), Total feed conversion ratio (TFCR), and Final body weight (FBW). Values are mean ± SEM of six birds per experimental group. Means within the same column carrying different superscripts were significantly different at ($p < 0.05$).

3.2. Effect of Dietary Supplementation of CUR, IMI, and Their Combinations on Blood Hematological-Related Indices of Ross 308 Broiler Chickens

The results regarding the modulating effects of dietary supplementation of CUR, IMI, and their combinations on the blood hematological indices (R.B.Cs, Hb, hematocrit, W.B.Cs, heterophils, and lymphocytes) of Ross 308 broiler chickens are shown in Table 5. The obtained data showed that CUR dietary supplementation induced a significant ($p < 0.05$) decrease in total R.B.C count, Hb content, and Hct value by 11.11, 11.25, and 12.35%, respectively, compared to birds of the C group. IMI dietary exposure induced a significant ($p < 0.05$) decrease in total R.B.Cs count, Hb content, and Hct values by 21.94, 21.22, and 22.58%, respectively, in birds fed IMI when compared to birds of the C group. Supplementation of CUR restored the decrease in total R.B.Cs count, Hb content, and Hct value to decrease of 15.67, 16.78, and 17.74%, respectively, in the (CUR+IMI co-treated) group and to a decrease of 21.37, 19.05, and 21.52%, respectively, in the (CUR+IMI pro/co-treated) group ($p < 0.05$) when compared to birds of the IMI-exposed group.

Table 5. Effect of dietary supplementation of imidacloprid (IMI), curcumin (CUR), and their combinations on blood hematological-related indices of Ross 308 broiler chickens.

Group / Parameters	RBCs ($\times 10^6$ mL^3)	Hb (g/dL)	Hct (%)	TLC ($\times 10^9$/L)	Heterophils %	Lymphocytes %
1st group C	3.51 ± 0.13 ^{a}	10.13 ± 0.34 ^{a}	31.00 ± 0.73 ^{a}	10.20 ± 1.62 ^{abc}	31.83 ± 1.14 ^{ab}	68.17 ± 1.14 ^{a}
2nd group CUR	3.12 ± 0.02 ^{b}	8.99 ± 0.04 ^{b}	27.17 ± 0.11 ^{b}	12.80 ± 0.42 ^{a}	32.00 ± 0.58 ^{a}	68.00 ± 0.58 ^{a}
3rd group IMI-treated	2.74 ± 0.14 ^{d}	7.98 ± 0.29 ^{b}	24.00 ± 0.84 ^{c}	5.96 ± 0.63 ^{d}	37.66 ± 1.02 ^{c}	62.33 ± 1.02 ^{b}
4th group CUR+IMI Co-treated	2.96 ± 0.02 ^{bc}	8.43 ± 0.05 ^{b}	25.50 ± 0.18 ^{ab}	8.50 ± 0.55 ^{bcd}	35.00 ± 0.68 ^{bc}	65.00 ± 0.68 ^{ab}
5th group CUR+IMI Pro/co-treated	2.76 ± 0.10 ^{bc}	8.20 ± 0.12 ^{b}	24.33 ± 0.59 ^{c}	9.50 ± 0.37 ^{bc}	33.83 ± 1.11 ^{b}	66.17 ± 1.11 ^{a}

Red blood cells (R.B.Cs.); hemoglobin (Hb), hematocrit value (Hct), total leukocytic count (TLC). Values are mean ± SEM of six birds per experimental group. Means within the same column carrying different superscripts were significantly different at ($p < 0.05$).

Dietary supplementation of CUR induced a non-significant ($p < 0.05$) increase of W.B.Cs counts and heterophils % by (25.49 and 0.53% increase, respectively) in birds fed diet supplemented with CUR when compared to birds of the C group. IMI dietary exposure induced a significant ($p < 0.05$) decrease in W.B.Cs counts and lymphocytes % (decrease by 41.57 and 8.57%, respectively) but significantly increased heterophils % (increased by 18.32%) in birds fed IMI-supplemented diet when compared to birds fed control diet. Supplementation of CUR non-significantly ($p > 0.05$) restored the decreased W.B.Cs counts and lymphocytes % (decreased by 16.67 and 4.65%) and restored the heterophils % (increased by 9.96%) in the (CUR+IMI co-treated) birds unlike birds exposed to IMI-and non-treated. Moreover, CUR in the (CUR+IMI pro/co-treated) group, significantly ($p < 0.05$) restored the decreased W.B.Cs count and lymphocytes % to (6.68 and 2.93% decrease) and restored the heterophils % (increased by 6.82%) in comparison with birds exposed to IMI-and non-treated.

3.3. Effect of Dietary Supplementation of CUR, IMI, and Their Combinations on Phagocytosis %, Phagocytic Index, Intracellular Killing Capacity, Lysozyme Activity, and IgG of Ross 308 Broiler Chickens

The results regarding the modulating effects of dietary supplementation of CUR, IMI, and their combinations on phagocytosis, phagocytic index, intracellular killing capacity, lysozyme activity, and IgG of Ross 308 broiler chickens are shown in Figure 2. The obtained data showed that CUR dietary supplementation induced a significant ($p < 0.05$) increase in phagocytic % by 17.18% and a non-significant increase in PhI and IKC by 7.62 and 12.67%, respectively, in birds fed a diet supplemented with CUR when compared to birds of the C group. IMI dietary exposure induced a significant ($p < 0.05$) decrease in phagocytic %, PhI, and IKC by 66.67, 49.33, and 56.36% decrease, respectively, in birds fed a diet supplemented with IMI when compared to birds of the C group. Supplementation of CUR significantly ($p < 0.05$) restored the decreased phagocytic %, PhI, and IKC to a decrease of 34.33, 37.22

and 36.63%, respectively, in the (CUR+IMI co-treated) group and to a decrease of 12.12, 13.45, and 21.12%, respectively, in the (CUR+IMI pro/co-treated) group when compared to birds of the IMI-exposed group.

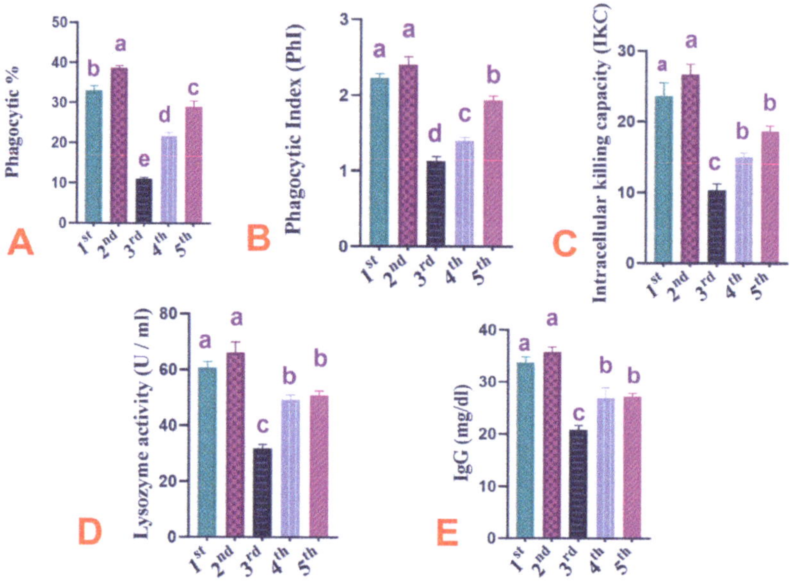

Figure 2. Effect of dietary supplementation of CUR, IMI, and their combinations on Phagocytosis, lysozyme activity, and IgG of Ross 308 broiler chickens. 1st group C, 2nd group CUR, 3rd group IMI-treated, 4th group CUR+IMI Co-treated, 5th group CUR+IMI Pro/co-treated. (**A**): Phagocytosis % (Ph %). (**B**): Phagocytic index (PhI). (**C**): Intracellular killing capacity (ICK). (**D**): Lysozyme activity (LYZ). (**E**): Immunoglobulin G (IgG). Values are shown as mean ± SEM of (6) birds per experimental group. Means bearing different superscripts are significantly different at $p < 0.05$.

The obtained data showed that dietary supplementation of CUR induced a non-significant ($p > 0.05$) increase of LYZ and IgG serum levels % (increased by 9.07 and 6.05% respectively) in birds fed diet supplemented with CUR if compared to birds of the C group. IMI dietary exposure induced a significant ($p < 0.05$) reduction of LYZ and IgG serum levels (decreased by 47.39 and 38.33% respectively) in birds fed diet supplemented with IMI if compared with birds of the C group. Supplementation of CUR significantly ($p < 0.05$) restored the decreased LYZ and IgG levels to (decreased by 18.86 and 20.25%, respectively) in the CUR+IMI co-treated group and to 16.22 and 19.27% decrease, respectively, in the CUR+IMI pro/co-treated group when compared to birds of the IMI-exposed group.

3.4. *Effect of Dietary Supplementation of CUR, IMI, and Their Combinations on Serum Biochemical Measurements of Ross 308 Broiler Chickens*

The modulatory impact of dietary supplementation of CUR, IMI, and their combinations on blood protein profile and liver function indices (ALT, AST, TP, Album, Gl., and A/G ratio) of Ross 308 broiler chickens is shown in Table 6. The obtained data showed that CUR dietary supplementation induced a significant ($p < 0.05$) decrease in ALT serum levels by 13.74%, but the decrease was non-significant for AST levels (decreased by 19.19%). Also, CUR non-significantly increased TP, albumin, globulin, and A/G ratio by 4.66, 7.79, 0.8 and 9.76%, respectively, in birds fed diet supplemented with CUR when compared to birds of the C group. IMI dietary exposure induced a significant ($p < 0.05$) increase in ALT and AST serum levels (increased by 24.14% and 1-fold, respectively), but significantly decreased TP, albumin, and globulin by 37.28, 39.61, and 34.4%, respectively, in birds fed IMI when compared with birds of C group. Supplementation of CUR significantly reduced the increased AST serum levels by 6.50% and non-significantly ($p > 0.05$) reduced the increased ALT, TP, albumin, globulin, and A/G ratio to 12.05, 27.24, 24.03, 31.20 and 8.13%, respectively, in the (CUR+IMI co-treated) group when compared to birds of the IMI-exposed group. Also, CUR supplementation in the (CUR+IMI pro/co-treated) group significantly ($p < 0.05$) restored the increased ALT and AST levels to 1.59 and 32.66%, respectively, and non-significantly reduced the increased TP, albumin, globulin, and A/G ratio to (decreased to 25.09, 21.43, 29.6 and 15.45%, respectively) unlike birds in the IMI-exposed group.

Table 6. Effect of dietary supplementation of imidacloprid (IMI), curcumin (CUR), and their combinations on serum biochemical measurements (liver function, protein profile, and lipid profile) of Ross 308 broiler chickens.

Group \ Parameter	ALT (U/L)	AST (U/L)	TP (g/dL)	Albumin (g/dL)	Globulin (g/dL)	A/G Ratio	TG (mg/dL)	TC (mg/dL)	HDL (mg/dL)	LDL (mg/dL)	VLDL (mg/dL)
1st group C	20.67 $\pm 0.92^{b}$	215.33 $\pm 24.58^{b}$	2.79 $\pm 0.16^{ab}$	1.54 $\pm 0.09^{a}$	1.25 $\pm 0.07^{a}$	1.23 ±0.01	43.00 $\pm 1.32^{b}$	115.33 $\pm 3.75^{c}$	78.33 $\pm 1.12^{ab}$	34.60 $\pm 1.27^{c}$	10.07± 0.22^{b}
2nd group CUR	17.83 $\pm 0.60^{c}$	174.00 $\pm 20.10^{b}$	2.92 $\pm 0.17^{a}$	1.66 $\pm 0.07^{a}$	1.26 $\pm 0.11^{a}$	1.35 ±0.10	24.00 $\pm 0.73^{c}$	101.33 $\pm 2.74^{d}$	82.67 $\pm 1.65^{a}$	11.07 $\pm 1.00^{d}$	7.60± 0.48^{b}
3rd group IMI-treated	25.66 $\pm 0.56^{a}$	438.33 $\pm 55.56^{a}$	1.75 $\pm 0.09^{b}$	0.93 $\pm 0.04^{d}$	0.82 $\pm 0.05^{b}$	1.16 ±0.05	77.04 $\pm 2.01^{a}$	147.00 $\pm 4.21^{a}$	55.00 $\pm 2.39^{c}$	76.57 $\pm 1.44^{a}$	15.43± 0.39^{a}
4th group CUR+IMI Co-treated	23.16 $\pm 0.70^{ab}$	229.33 $\pm 8.83^{b}$	2.03 $\pm 0.11^{b}$	1.17 $\pm 0.08^{cd}$	0.86 $\pm 0.05^{b}$	1.33 ±0.08	49.50 $\pm 1.78^{b}$	128.33 $\pm 2.79^{b}$	71.67 $\pm 4.59^{b}$	46.00 $\pm 4.05^{b}$	10.67± 0.22^{b}
5th group CUR+IMI Pro/co-treated	21.00 $\pm 0.73^{b}$	285.67 $\pm 16.61^{b}$	2.09 $\pm 0.16^{bc}$	1.21 $\pm 0.09^{bcd}$	0.88 $\pm 0.08^{b}$	1.42 ±0.11	44.33 $\pm 2.76^{b}$	121.00 $\pm 1.32^{bc}$	76.00 $\pm 2.03^{ab}$	34.67 $\pm 3.17^{c}$	10.33± 0.28^{b}

Alanine aminotransferase (ALT), Aspartate aminotransferase (AST), Total protein (TP), Albumin (Album), Globulin (Gl.), Albumin/Globulin ratio (A/G ratio), Triglycerides (TGs), Total Cholesterol (TC), High-density lipoprotein (HDL), Low density lipoprotein (LDL), and Very low-density lipoprotein (VLDL). Values are mean ± SEM of six birds per experimental group. Means within the same column carrying different superscripts were significantly different at ($p < 0.05$).

The modulatory influence of dietary supplementation of CUR, IMI, or their combinations on blood lipid profile (TGs, TC, HDL, LDL, and VLDL) of Ross 308 broiler chickens is shown in Table 6. The obtained data showed that CUR dietary supplementation induced a significant ($p < 0.05$) decrease of TG, TC, LDL, and VLDL serum levels by 44.19, 12.14, 68.01, and 24.53%, respectively, but non-significantly increased HDL serum levels (increased by 5.54%) when compared to the C group. IMI dietary exposure induced a significant ($p < 0.05$) increase of TG, TC, LDL, and VLDL serum levels by 79.17%, 27.46%, 1 fold, and 53.23%, respectively, but significantly decreased HDL serum levels by 29.78% in birds fed IMI when compared with birds of the C group. Supplementation of CUR significantly reduced the increased TG, TC, LDL, and VLDL serum levels to 15.12, 11.27, 32.95, and 5.95%, respectively, and significantly ($p < 0.05$) restored the decreased HDL to 8.50% in the CUR+IMI co-treated group, unlike IMI-exposed group. Also, CUR supplementation in the CUR+IMI pro/co-treated group significantly ($p < 0.05$) reduced the increased TG, TC, LDL, and VLDL serum levels to 3.09, 5.20, 0.20, and 2.58%, respectively and significantly ($p < 0.05$) restored the decreased HDL levels to 2.97% in comparison with birds exposed to IMI.

3.5. Effect of Dietary Supplementation of CUR, IMI, and Their Combinations on Oxidative Stress-Related Indices in Spleen of Ross 308 Broiler Chickens

The impact of dietary supplementation of CUR, IMI, or their combinations on serum antioxidant-related parameters (TAC, SOD, CAT, GPx, and MDA) in the spleen of Ross 308 broiler chickens is shown in Figure 3. The obtained data showed that CUR dietary supplementation induced a non-significant ($p > 0.05$) increase of TAC, SOD, CAT, and GPx levels in the spleen by 11.32, 0.59, 7.32, and 18.64%, respectively, and non-significantly decreased MDA levels in the spleen by 9.29% when compared to the C group. IMI dietary exposure induced a significant ($p < 0.05$) decrease of TAC, SOD, CAT, and GPx spleen levels by 54.72, 15.78, 65.06, and 49.73%, respectively, and significantly increased MDA spleen levels by 78.89% in birds fed IMI when compared with birds of the C group. Supplementation of CUR non-significantly elevated the decreased TAC spleen levels by 47.17%. CUR significantly elevated the decreased SOD, CAT, and GPx spleen levels (10.07, 30.12, and 27.12% decrease, respectively) and significantly ($p < 0.05$) reduced the increased MDA levels by 24.89% in the CUR+IMI co-treated group when compared to the IMI-exposed group. Also, CUR supplementation in the CUR+IMI pro/co-treated group significantly ($p < 0.05$) elevated the decreased TAC, SOD, CAT, and GPx spleen levels to 28.30, 5.56, 16.81, and 25.42%, respectively, and significantly ($p < 0.05$) reduced the increased MDA levels to 19.82% when compared to the IMI-exposed group.

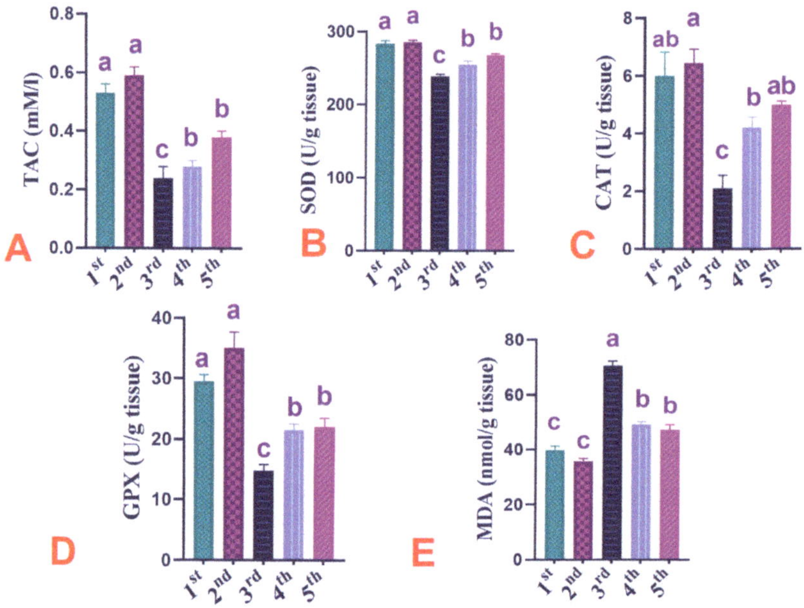

Figure 3. Effect of dietary supplementation of CUR, IMI, and their combinations on Phagocytosis, lysozyme activity, and IgG of Ross 308 broiler chickens. 1st group C, 2nd group CUR, 3rd group IMI-treated, 4th group CUR+IMI Co-treated, 5th group CUR+IMI Pro/co-treated. (**A**): Total antioxidant capacity (TAC). (**B**): Superoxide dismutase (SOD). (**C**): Catalase (CAT). (**D**): Glutathione peroxidase (GPx). (**E**): Malondialdehyde (MDA). Values are shown as mean ± SEM of (6) birds per experimental group. Means bearing different superscripts are significantly different at $p < 0.05$.

3.6. Effect of Dietary Supplementation of CUR, IMI, and Their Combinations on mRNA Expression of IL-1β, TLR-4, and IL-10 Genes in Spleen of Ross 308 Broiler Chickens

The effects of dietary supplementation of CUR, IMI, or their combinations on mRNA expression of *IL-1β*, *TLR-4*, and *IL-10* genes in splenic tissues of Ross 308 broiler chickens are shown in Figure 4. The obtained data showed that CUR dietary exposure non-significantly ($p > 0.05$) modulated the *IL-1β* and *TLR-4* mRNA expression by 11 and 6%, respectively, but significantly increased spleen *IL-10* mRNA expression by 17% in the birds fed CUR-supplemented diet compared to the birds of the C group. IMI dietary exposure significantly ($p < 0.05$) up-regulated *IL-1β* and *TLR-4* mRNA expression levels (increased by 1-fold and 1 fold %, respectively), but significantly down-regulated *IL-10* mRNA expression levels (decreased by 74%) in splenic tissues of birds fed diet supplemented with IMI if compared with birds of the C group. Supplementation of CUR significantly ($p < 0.05$) restored the up-regulated *IL-1β* mRNA expression levels to 61%, and non-significantly ($p > 0.05$) restored the up-regulated *TLR-4* mRNA expression levels (increased by 78%). CUR non-significantly restored the down-regulated *IL-10* mRNA expression levels to 61% in splenic tissues in the CUR co-treated group when compared with birds of the IMI-exposed group. Supplementation of CUR significantly ($p < 0.05$) restored the up-regulated *IL-1β* and *TLR-4* mRNA expression levels to 32 and 33%, respectively, and significantly restored the down-regulated *IL-10* mRNA expression levels by 23% in the CUR pro/co-treated group when compared with birds of the IMI-exposed group.

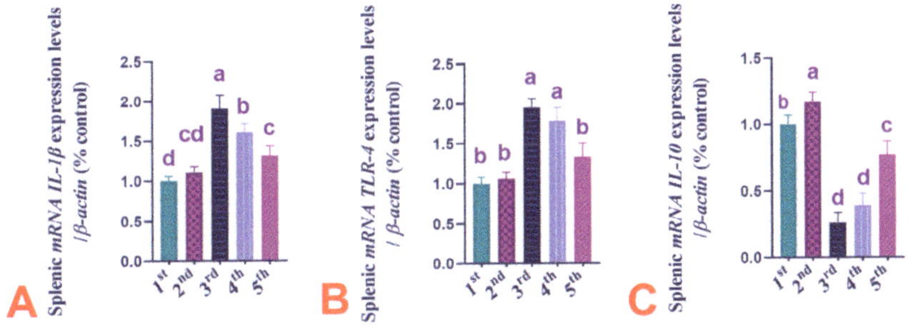

Figure 4. Effect of dietary supplementation of CUR, IMI, and their combinations on *mRNA* expression of *IL-1β*, *TLR-4*, and *IL-10* genes in spleen of Ross 308 broiler chickens. 1st group C, 2nd group CUR, 3rd group IMI-treated, 4th group CUR+IMI Co-treated, 5th group CUR+IMI Pro/co-treated. (**A**): Interleukin 1 Beta (*IL-1β*). (**B**): Toll-Like Receptor 4 (*TLR-4*). (**C**): Interleukin 10 (*IL-10*). Values are shown as mean ± SEM of three birds per experimental group. Means bearing different superscripts are significantly different at $p < 0.05$.

3.7. Histopathological and Immunohistochemical Findings

The investigated splenic lesions included lymphoid depletion and necrosis, vascular congestion, endothelial hypertrophy, and thrombosis. The results were expressed as percentages (means ± SEM) and are shown in Table 7. The negative control and CUR-treated groups showed normal histology in Figure 5A, B, whereas the IMI-exposed group manifested some structural alterations such as lymphoid depletion, vascular congestion, and thrombosis (Figure 5C). The response of the splenic tissue to the CUR supplementation in the birds exposed to IMI was reduced in the extent and frequencies of the IMI-induced splenic lesions that were noticed in all CUR-supplemented groups (co-treated or pro/co-treated). The most encountered lesions in these groups were expressed by vascular congestion and lymphoid depletion (Figure 5D, E). The quantitative lesion scoring in the splenic tissue sections of all groups is shown in Table 7.

Table 7. Effect of dietary supplementation of IMI, CUR, and their combinations on the splenic histology, and the immuno-expression of the splenic TNF-α and TLR-4 of Ross 308 broiler chickens.

Parameters / Groups	1st Group C	2nd Group CUR	3th Group IMI-treated	4th Group CUR+IMI Co-Treated	5th Group IMI+CUR Pro/Co-Treated
Lymphoid depletion	0.00 ± 0.00 ^{c}	0.00 ± 0.00 ^{c}	32.00 ± 2.91 ^{a}	8.00 ± 2.00 ^{b}	9.00 ± 1.79 ^{b}
Lymphoid necrosis	0.00 ± 0.00 ^{b}	0.00 ± 0.00 ^{b}	6.00 ± 1.63 ^{a}	2.00 ± 1.33 ^{ab}	4.00 ± 1.63 ^{ab}
Vascular congestion	0.00 ± 0.00 ^{c}	0.00 ± 0.00 ^{c}	16.00 ± 1.63 ^{a}	5.00 ± 1.66 ^{bc}	7.00 ± 1.52 ^{b}
Vascular thrombosis	0.00 ± 0.00 ^{a}	0.00 ± 0.00 ^{a}	2.00 ± 1.33 ^{a}	0.00 ± 0.00 ^{a}	1.00 ± 0.10 ^{a}
Endothelial hypertrophy	0.00 ± 0.00 ^{a}	0.00 ± 0.00 ^{a}	5.00 ± 1.66 ^{a}	2.00 ± 1.33 ^{a}	3.00 ± 2.13 ^{a}
TNF-α Immuno-positive area fraction	0.48 ± 0.06 ^{c}	0.47 ± 0.04 ^{c}	7.49 ± 0.43 ^{a}	3.63 ± 0.13 ^{b}	4.38 ± 0.22 ^{b}
TLR4 immuno-positive area fraction	0.43 ± 0.07 ^{d}	0.46 ± 0.08 ^{d}	8.18 ± 0.44 ^{a}	4.01 ± 0.11 ^{bc}	4.62 ± 0.14 ^{b}

Values are mean ± SEM of 10 birds per experimental group. Means within the same row carrying different superscripts were significantly different at ($p < 0.05$). TNF-α and TLR-4 splenic immuno-reactivity.

The data analysis obtained from Image J software (version. 1.32j, http://rsb.info.nih.gov/ij, accessed on 20 November 2023) declared that exposure to IMI significantly upregulated the immunoexpression of the TNF-α and TLR4 in the splenic tissues of the IMID-treated group compared to the control and CUR groups. CUR supplementation either in the CUR co-treated group or CUR pro/co-treated significantly down-regulated the immunoexpression of both the TNF-α and TLR4 in the splenic tissue. The levels of immunoreactivity of the splenic TNF-α and TLR4 among all groups are shown in Figures 6 and 7, respectively, and statistically summarized in Table 7.

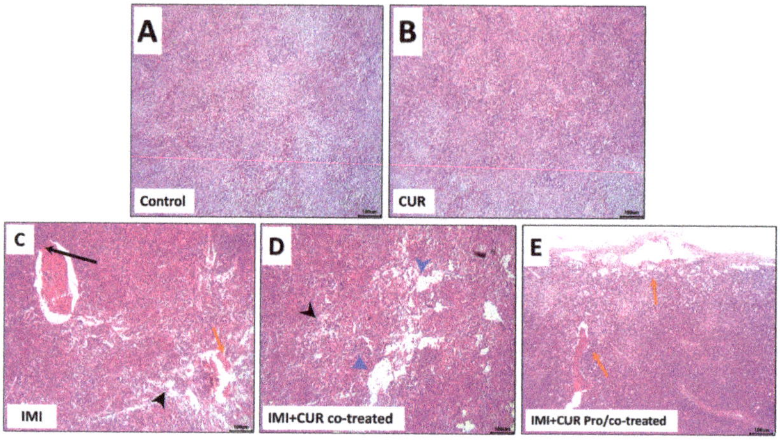

Figure 5. Representative photomicrographs of H&E-stained splenic tissue sections for the effect of dietary supplementation of CUR, IMI, and their combinations splenic tissue structure showing normal histology in the control (**A**) and the CUR (**B**) groups. Histopathological alterations in the IMI-treated group (**C**), with reduction of these splenopathic alterations in the CUR co-treated group or CUR pro/co-treated group. (**D**,**E**). The symbols in the images denote black arrowhead; lymphoid depletion, blue arrowhead; lymphoid necrosis, black arrow; thrombus, red arrow; vascular congestion. (Scale bar is 100 μm).

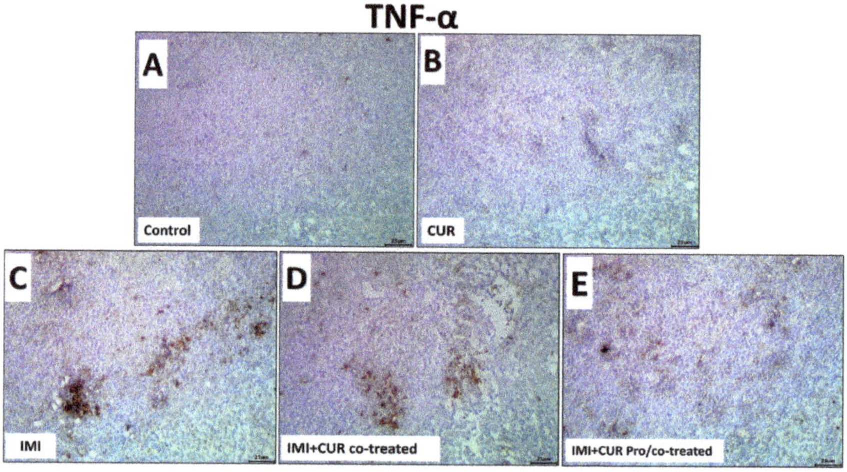

Figure 6. Representative photomicrographs of the TNF-α immuno-stained splenic tissue sections for the effect of dietary supplementation of CUR, IMI, and their combinations in spleen of Ross 308 broiler chickens. (**A**,**B**): control and CUR groups for TNF-α showing weak expression in splenic tissue. (**C**): showing up-regulation of the TNF-α expression in the IMI-treated group in splenic tissue. (**D**,**E**): CUR-supplemented groups, showed down-regulation of TNF-α expression in the CUR co-treated group or CUR pro/and co-treated groups. (Scale bar is 25 μm).

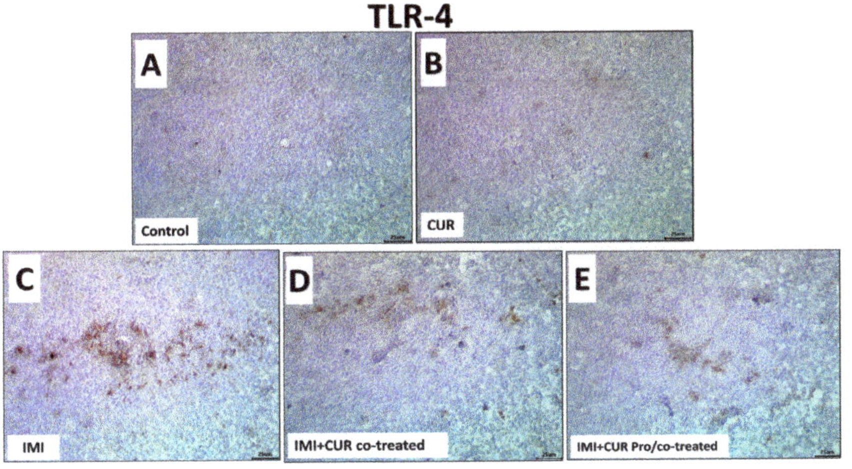

Figure 7. Representative photomicrographs of the TLR-4 immuno-stained splenic tissue sections for the effect of dietary supplementation of CUR, IMI, and their combinations in spleen of Ross 308 broiler chickens. (**A**,**B**): control and CUR groups for TLR-4 showing weak expression in splenic tissue. (**C**): showing up-regulation of the TLR-4 expression in the IMI-treated group in splenic tissue. (**D**,**E**): CUR- supplemented groups, showed down-regulation of TLR-4 expression in the CUR-treated group or CUR pro/and co-treated groups. (Scale bar is 25 μm).

4. Discussion

Optimizing the farming practices of chickens is essential for preserving their productivity and assuring the production of high-quality food for human consumption because chickens are a valued source of protein [78,79]. Considering the indiscriminate use of insecticides, birds are frequently exposed to IMI through different sources, and there is a need to search for herbal growth promoters and antioxidative medication to be used in the poultry industry. The purpose of the current study was to assess the impact of dietary supplementation of CUR in ameliorating IMI-induced effects on immune-related indices of Ross 308 broiler chickens.

Regarding the growth performance-related indices, the obtained data revealed that IMI induced a significant increase in TFCR, and significantly decreased TFI, TBWG, and FBW in birds fed the IMI-supplemented diets compared to the C group and the CUR-supplemented group. The obtained outcomes are consistent with those reported by Osman, Shaaban and Ahmed [52], Adegoke et al. [80], and Abotaleb, et al. [81]. In the IMI-fed groups, there was a correlation between the observed lower TFI and lower TBWG and FBW. IMI's hazardous potential could be the reason for the broilers' lower feed intake because the pesticides have detrimental toxic effects on the broilers' gross performance measures, which causes appetite loss and decreased body weight [82]. Additionally, FCR was significantly elevated owing to the reduced weight gain in IMI-exposed birds. Additionally, IMI's detrimental effects on health status can be related to its effects on the digestion and absorption of feed in the birds' stomachs, which resulted in poor growth performances [48]. Moreover, IMI exposure resulted in a weakened state of health due to abnormal metabolic and physiological reactions resulting from OS [50,83]. Furthermore, IMI exposure has been linked to a drop in cumulative body gain in birds, as reported by Gibbon et al. [31] and Lopez-Antia et al. [84].

In contrast, birds fed the CUR-supplemented diets in the CUR+IMI co-treated and CUR+IMI pro/co-treated groups showed a significantly decreased TFI and TFCR with an increased TBWG and FBW compared to birds of the C group or the IMI-exposed group. These results were consistent with those reported by Hafez et al. [85], Khodadadi et al. [86], Rajput et al. [87], and Yadav et al. [88]. Hafez et al. [85] reported that CUR dietary supplementation (200 mg or 100 mg) for 42 days significantly enhanced BW and FCR of Cobb 500 chicks during the finisher phase. This may be linked to CUR's ability to boost bile production, intestinal villi length, cecal width, and gastric digestion fluid, which contributed to better fat digestion. In addition, these advantages were attributed to feeding CUR for a longer period, which improved nutrient absorption during the mature stage [23].

Additionally, CUR boosted intestinal sucrose and maltase activity [89]; up-regulated pancreatic lipase; increased trypsin, amylase, and chymotrypsin; and up-regulated trypsin, amylase, and chymotrypsin. These effects lead to an improved FCR in CUR-supplemented birds. Moreover, the carcass quality was significantly enhanced after adding turmeric powder to the diet of broiler chickens at levels of 500 and 750 mg/kg. In addition, a significant effect of dietary turmeric on BW was discovered at week 3 and later ages concerning desirable biological activities according to Khodadadi et al. [86].

Concerning hematological indices, the obtained results of the current study showed that birds exposed to IMI- had decreased values of RBCs, Hb, Hct, and TLC. These birds showed reduced lymphocytes and increased heterophils. The obtained results are consistent with those of Ravikanth et al. [55], Eid, et al. [90], Sankhala, et al. [91]. Gul et al. [54] reported that birds exposed to IMI showed decreased values of RBCs, Hb, Hct, and WBCs. Oxidative stress, weakened immunity, and metabolic failure in birds exposed to IMI could be responsible for these effects [50,83]. Stressed birds that have been physiologically exposed to insecticides showed disruption in feed digestion and metabolism, which resulted in abnormal values of hematological indices [92]. Additionally, the decline in the mean values of RBC count, Hb, and Hct values may be caused by the direct toxic effects of IMI on the bone marrow, liver, and kidneys, which may have a crucial effect on the production of hemopoiesis and erythropoietin in these organs [55]. The considerable decrease in total leukocytic count observed in the present study was consistent with the results reported by Babu et al. [56] regarding laying birds. The pathological lesions found in the splenic tissues of birds exposed to IMI supported the hypothesis that the lymphocytic depletion seen in the current investigation was caused by splenic hemorrhages.

Regarding the mitigating impact of CUR dietary supplementation, the obtained results showed that birds fed CUR-supplemented diets in the CUR+IMI co-treated or CUR+IMI pro/co-treated groups significantly improved all hematological indices unlike IMI-exposed birds, which are in agreement with those of Adegoke et al. [80], Hafez et al. [85], and Abd El-Samie et al. [93]. This beneficial effect may be linked to CUR's anti-inflammatory and antioxidant properties, which boosted the metabolism and, in turn, improved iron absorption and utilization, and subsequently RBC formation and Hb concentration. Dietary CUR at the levels of 200 mg or 100 mg for 42 days in Cobb 500 chicks enhanced all hematological indices, along with an improvement in the antioxidant defense system of broiler raised at high stocking density [89]. On the other hand, when broiler birds were supplemented with turmeric powder, Kafi, et al. [94] and Shohe, et al. [95] observed that there were no significant variations in the Hb and PCV levels. Furthermore, broilers fed a basal diet containing 400 g/100 kg CUR exhibited no appreciable changes in PCV, RBCs, or Hb with the exception of WBCs [80]. Ali, et al. [96], demonstrated that a variety of factors, including age, country, temperature, environment, production level, and maintenance system, might affect the variations of erythrocyte count. One type of white blood cell, lymphocytes, can strengthen the immune system and attack pathogens that enter the body [97]. Chickens exposed to excessive stress resulted in higher cortisol hormone production, which in turn resulted in suppression of the immune system, causing lymphoid organs to contract and reduced lymphocyte numbers. In the same line, higher blood levels of cortisol hormone account for the prevention of lymphocyte formation [98,99]. Moreover, Puvadolpirod and Thaxton [99] explained that heat or environmental stress can have an impact on the number of lymphocytes because it reduces the weight of the thymus and bursa Fabricius, two lymphoid organs, which in turn affects the lymphocytes number [100]. In contrast, turmeric extract can serve as an immunomodulator via stimulating lymphocyte formation causing more lymphocyte production [101]. Therefore, in the current investigation, the broilers' immune system appeared to be strengthened by the increased proportion of lymphocytes, suggesting that dietary CUR can activate T and B lymphocyte cells [102].

Concerning phagocytosis-related indices, the obtained results of the present experiment revealed that birds fed the IMI-supplemented diets had significantly declined Ph % and PhI and IKC values. In contrast, birds fed the diets supplemented with CUR in either the CUR+IMI co-treated group or the CUR+IMI pro/co-treated group showed improved phagocytosis-related indices when compared to IMI-exposed birds. The first immune system activity, known as phagocytic activity, is responsible for engulfing and destroying foreign pathogens before presenting them to the remainder of the immune system for pathogen neutralization [103]. In the present study, IMI dietary exposure markedly decreased Ph % and PhI, indicating IMI-mediated nonspecific adverse effects on cellular immunity. Our outcomes are consistent with those reported by [Abou-Zeid, et al. [104], Mohany, et al. [105], Walderdorff, et al. [106]]. The decrease in phagocytic activity could be brought on by several factors, including the impact of the pesticide used on hematopoietic organs, the uptake prevention of macrophage-arming factor, and an increase in migration inhibitory factor (MIF) brought on by IMI, which inhibits the mobility of neutrophils and macrophages and impairs their capacity to reach inflammatory sites [105]. Additionally, OS may alter receptor-mediated phagocytosis and membrane fluidity; these are essential for innate and adaptive immune responses [107]. Similar results have been reported in domestic chickens exposed to thiamethoxam, a different neonicotinoid, at sub-lethal dosages, which resulted in impaired humoral and cellular immunity [108]. Similar results of decreased phagocytic activity of leukocytes have also has been reported by Mohany et al. [105] and Gawade et al. [109]. In a previous study, old domestic chickens (1–4 weeks old) exposed to IMI at the level of 0.05 mg/kg/d for 37 days experienced a reduction in humoral and cellular immune responses and histopathological changes in the spleen and bursa of Fabricius [39]. Moreover, the results are in agreement with Franzen-Klein, et al. [48]. Neonicotinoid-related immunotoxicity in birds [39,84,110] and the decreased percentages of killed *E. coli* and *C. albicans* after oral exposure may be a sign of immune suppression induced by IMI [48]. Similarly, Khayal, et al. [111] mentioned that IMI decreased phagocytic activity, PhI, and LYZ activity in rats. The observed CUR immune-enhancing effect is consistent with the results described by Farag et al. [112], which may be alluded to the activation of neutrophils and macrophages to produce ROS [113]. Dietary CUR elevated WBCs and phagocytic activity and resulted in greater expression of immune-related cytokines [114].

Humoral and cell-mediated immunity are the two main components of the immune system. According to the current study, there was a significant drop in blood IgG levels of broilers, which may indicate immunosuppression after IMI exposure. Similarly, chickens given IMI showed a marked reduction in serum levels of total immunoglobulin and circulating immune complexes on day 45 [39]. Additionally, the decrease in LYZ activity following IMI exposure is consistent with [Attia, et al. [115], Rahman, et al. [116]]. According to Hafez et al. [85], CUR prevents the decline of Ig synthesis induced by the high stocking density (HSD). Likewise, Isroli, et al. [117] revealed that turmeric could elevate the globulin concentration in broilers. Current outcomes are parallel to the results of Shawky, et al. [118], who stated that turmeric powder (5 g/kg diet) enhanced levels of IgM and IgG in broilers. Similar findings were described by Arshami, et al. [119], who mentioned that the IgM and IgG titers were elevated by various concentrations of CUR powder (0.25 to 0.75%).

Regarding serum biochemical parameters, the obtained results of the present study showed that IMI dietary exposure considerably elevated serum AST and ALT levels. The obtained results are in agreement with those reported by Abu Zeid et al. [41], Eid et al. [90], Mia, et al. [83], Sankhala et al. [91], and Xu et al. [50]. This demonstrates the pathological abnormalities induced by IMI in various essential organs, including the liver and kidneys. Interestingly, Akter, et al. [120] reported that the hepatic serum enzymes AST and ALT were noticeably elevated in rabbits exposed to IMI, which indicated liver injury. Our findings are in the same line with the results reported by Emam et al. [46], who discovered that birds exposed to IMI had higher ALT and AST levels. Lipid peroxidation may be the cause of the unregulated release of ALT and AST after IMI exposure. The overproduction of ROS implicated in OS caused by pesticide exposure leads to increased MDA levels [52]. When MDA levels are higher than the capacity of the body's defenses against oxidation, ROS severely damage cellular DNA [121]. Therefore, increased MDA levels may be responsible for the change in the metabolism, physiological responses, immunological responses, and growth rate of birds exposed to IMI poisoning. The outcomes of this study revealed that birds exposed to IMI had elevated MDA levels. Indeed, IMI-induced ROS overproduction leads to high LPO and inflammatory responses [122]. CUR supplementation in the diet reduced ALT and AST activities in birds, demonstrating CUR's capacity to scavenge and neutralize free radicals to protect liver cells from attack by free radicals [85,123]. The observed decline in liver enzymes' activities in the present experiment confirmed the improved liver functions and showed the antioxidant-modulating effect of CUR supplementation and its role in preventing liver cell damage induced by free radicals.

The drop in albumin, globulin, and total protein levels found in broilers' blood after IMI exposure was parallel to results reported by Abu Zeid et al. [41]. This might be caused by competitive inhibition of phenylalanine-t-RNA synthesis, which prevents amino-acylation and peptide elongation and inhibits hepatic protein synthesis at the post-transcriptional stage [124]. Reducing the downstream absorption of digested amino acids from birds' guts to the blood is considered one of the IMI-induced impacts on blood protein reductions [47,48]. Additionally, Nebbia [125] reported that the liver tissue predominantly detoxifies and eliminates xenobiotics that are harmful to birds.

The observed effect of IMI in increasing TC in our investigation is consistent with findings showed that stressors elevate blood cholesterol concentrations in broiler chickens. In comparison to birds fed a control diet, we noticed that adding CUR to broiler chickens' diets reduced TG, TC, LDL-C, and VLDL-C levels, while increasing HDL levels. Hafez et al. [85] discovered that feeding broilers CUR lowered their blood's TC compared to those fed a control diet. Furthermore, it has been reported the impact of dietary CUR supplementation on TC and LDL in rats [126].

Notably, IMI induced a decrease in SOD, CAT, GPx, and TAC levels; this is consistent with Zhang, et al. [127], who found that the concentrations of T-AOC, SOD, GSH, and GSH-Px were reduced, but the levels of MDA were elevated in renal tissue of mice given (10 mg/L,) IMI for 30 days in drinking water when compared with the control mice. This is supported by the fact that CUR therapy reversed the elevated MDA levels and decreased T-AOC, SOD, GSH, and GSH-Px concentrations in the current study in contrast, exposure to IMI reduced the antioxidants levels, resulting in an accumulation of lipid peroxide, which led to inflammatory reactions.

According to Kammon et al. [39], exposure of birds to IMI had negative effects on biochemical and immune system indices and induced OS-related biomarkers. The hepatic tissue of laying birds fed IMI showed a considerable decline in GSH levels and raised levels of thiobarbituric acid reactive compounds (TBARS) [56]. In RBCs, liver, kidney, and testes of cockerels, IMI induced oxidative stress, reduced CAT, and increased lipid peroxidation [59]. In agreement with Ravikanth et al. [61] and Subha [128], IMI-exposed birds had significantly lower levels of antioxidant-related biomarkers and higher lipid peroxidation levels in the splenic tissue.

Similar to our findings, Salah et al. [89] reported that dietary supplementation of CUR in chickens reduced the TBA (thiobarbituric acid) and enhanced the activities of antioxidant enzymes. CUR prevents OS by increasing the antioxidant enzyme activity including SOD, CAT, and GPx enzymes. On the other hand, CUR could antagonize OS induced by IMI in broilers' spleen, which is consistent with the findings of Cheng, et al. [60]. Similarly, Li, et al. [129], reported that CUR mitigated the AFB1-induced changes in GSH, SOD, CAT, and MDA levels. This might be a result of CUR's capacity to neutralize free radicals by boosting the activities of antioxidant enzymes and decreasing OS [130]. Additionally, earlier studies reported by [Nayak and Sashidhar [131], Zhang, et al. [132]] have shown that CUR has antioxidant properties against hepatic damage induced by AFB1in rats and chicks.

In the current investigation, IMI-exposed broilers showed up-regulated expression levels of *IL1β* and *TLR-4* in splenic tissues and, in contrast, down-regulated *IL-10* mRNA expression levels. The spleen is a peripheral lymphoid organ that plays a crucial role in the body's innate and adaptive immune responses against systemically acquired antigens [133, 134].To the best of our knowledge, this is the first study that reported that IMI-induced up-regulated the expression level of the *TLR-4* gene in the spleen of IMI-exposed broilers. Similar findings were obtained by Farag, et al. [135], who found that the Toll-like receptor 2 (*TLR2*) gene was up-regulated in the brains of rats after IMI exposure, while *TLR2* had a strong immunopositive response in the brains of IMI-treated rats. Toll-like receptor is activated by molecules generated from pathogens, which causes the production of inflammatory mediators including TNF-α [136]. Lipopolysaccharide (LPS), a crucial part of Gram-negative bacteria's cell walls, ligates *TLR4* to start an inflammatory response in organs [137]. There is evidence that IL-1β, TNFα, and interferon (INFγ) expression levels are increased in the blood and brain after sub-lethal exposure to insecticides such as acephate [138]. The identification of endogenous damage-associated molecular patterns (DAMPs) and exogenous pathogen-associated molecular patterns (PAMPs) is a critical function of *TLRs* [139]. Stimulation of *TLRs* by PAMPs or DAMPs results in the release of chemokines and cytokines, which intensifies inflammatory responses [140]. Inflammation and OS have complicated interactions. Cell injury as a result of redox stress brought on by ROS can activate *TLR2/4* and the downstream gene *NF-B*, producing inflammation and organ damage [141]. Our obtained outcomes are in disagreement with those of Pandit et al. [142], who reported that there was a non-significant fold increase in the expression of *TLR-4* and *TNFα* mRNA following the oral administration of IMI.

Similarly, Farag, et al. [143] observed that oxidative damage was significantly enhanced by thiacloprid, including elevated protein carbonyl, MDA content, and DNA damage in the brain of exposed chicken embryos. Additionally, proinflammatory cytokine induction is a primary indicator of the inflammatory process [143]. High levels of nitric oxide (NO) can trigger pro-inflammatory cytokine (*IFN-γ*, *TNF-α*, and *IL-1β*) overexpression. According to the current research, IMI exposure caused splenic tissues to become oxidatively damaged, which, in turn, induced or encouraged subsequent inflammatory responses that were probably mediated by the NF-κB signaling system. Herein, the observed up-regulation of *IL-1β* mRNA expression served as evidence for this hypothesis.

Curcumin supplementation markedly decreased the mRNA expression patterns of *IL-1β*, mucin 2, *COX-2*, and *p38 MAPK* in the ileal mucosa [144] and serum *TNF-α* concentration [145]. CUR predominantly alters the *p38-MAPK* pathway and thus suppresses the downstream activation of *IL-1β*, *IL-6*, and *TNF-α* genes.

The histopathological alterations observed in the current study were consistent with those of Gupta and Deepika [146], who reported that 14 day old broiler chicks exposed to IMI showed congestion in the spleen. Additionally, splenic tissues of rats treated with IMI displayed low numbers of lymphocytes, and thymus tissues showed lymphocytic depletion with pyknotic nuclei [105,147]. The intense immunopositive reactivity of TLR2 and TNFα in the liver found in this study could be explained by the up-regulation of TLR4 and TNFα in the spleen in this study. The obtained results are in agreement with those of Alhusaini, et al. [148], who reported that acetamiprid-treated rats showed detectable TLR4 protein expression in the glomeruli that were mainly localized to podocytes, moderately expressed along the proximal tubule and strongly expressed along the distal tubule

5. Conclusions

Herein, the current study provided potent evidence that the consumption of CUR improved the broiler chicken's immune system. Curcumin counteracts IMI-induced detrimental effects on growth performance, hematological associated indices, oxidative status, and mRNA expression of immune-related genes (*IL-1β*, *TLR-4*, and *IL-10*) in 308 Ross broiler chickens. Thus, CUR has the potential for utilization as a remedy in biomedical and pharmaceutical products, especially as antioxidant supplements constructing a precise antidote owing to its unique properties for numerous biomedical applications. Finally, our results provide new insight into IMI-induced immuno-toxicity in broiler chickens, moreover, for the first time, CUR preserves an in vivo protective effect against IMI principally in the pro/concurrent-supplementation compared with the con-current supplementation only.

Author Contributions: Conceptualization, E.H.A. and N.Z.E.; methodology, N.Z.E. and E.H.A.; software, D.I. and A.A.E.-S.; validation, E.H.A., A.A.E.-S., E.M.Y. and D.I.; formal analysis, E.H.A.; investigation, D.I.; resources, A.A.E.-S. and A.A.A.; data curation, E.H.A. and S.J.D.; writing—original draft preparation, E.H.A. and D.I.; writing—review and editing, A.A.E.-S.; visualization, M.M.M.M.; supervision, E.H.A., N.Z.E. and D.I.; funding acquisition, A.A.E.-S. All authors have read and agreed to the published version of the manuscript.

Funding: This work was funded by the researchers supporting project number (RSPD2023R700), King Saud University, Riyadh, Saudi Arabia.

Institutional Review Board Statement: The birds growing practices and samples collection techniques were performed according to the guidelines and rules of the Institutional Animal Care and Use Committee of the Faculty of Veterinary Medicine at Zagazig University (ZU-IACUC/2/F/75/2022). Date: 7 June 2022–7 June 2025.

Informed Consent Statement: Not applicable.

Data Availability Statement: The data depicted in this work are available upon asking from the corresponding author.

Acknowledgments: This work was supported by the researches supporting project number (RSPD2023R700), King Saud University, Riyadh, Saudi Arabia.

Conflicts of Interest: The authors declare no conflict of interest.

References

1. Nabi, F.; Arain, M.A.; Rajput, N.; Alagawany, M.; Soomro, J.; Umer, M.; Soomro, F.; Wang, Z.; Ye, R.; Liu, J. Health benefits of carotenoids and potential application in poultry industry: A review. *J. Anim. Physiol. Anim. Nutr.* **2020**, *104*, 1809–1818. [CrossRef] [PubMed]
2. Abd El-Hack, M.E.; El-Saadony, M.T.; Salem, H.M.; El-Tahan, A.M.; Soliman, M.M.; Youssef, G.B.; Taha, A.E.; Soliman, S.M.; Ahmed, A.E.; El-Kott, A.F. Alternatives to antibiotics for organic poultry production: Types, modes of action and impacts on bird's health and production. *Poult. Sci.* **2022**, *101*, 101696. [CrossRef] [PubMed]
3. Abou-Kassem, D.E.; El-Abasy, M.M.; Al-Harbi, M.S.; Abol-Ela, S.; Salem, H.M.; El-Tahan, A.M.; El-Saadony, M.T.; Abd El-Hack, M.E.; Ashour, E.A. Influences of total sulfur amino acids and photoperiod on growth, carcass traits, blood parameters, meat quality and cecal microbial load of broilers. *Saudi J. Biol. Sci.* **2022**, *29*, 1683–1693. [CrossRef] [PubMed]
4. Alagawany, M.; Elnesr, S.S.; Farag, M.R.; El-Naggar, K.; Taha, A.E.; Khafaga, A.F.; Madkour, M.; Salem, H.M.; El-Tahan, A.M.; El-Saadony, M.T. Betaine and related compounds: Chemistry, metabolism and role in mitigating heat stress in poultry. *J. Therm. Biol.* **2022**, *104*, 103168. [CrossRef] [PubMed]
5. Righi, F.; Pitino, R.; Manuelian, C.L.; Simoni, M.; Quarantelli, A.; De Marchi, M.; Tsiplakou, E. Plant feed additives as natural alternatives to the use of synthetic antioxidant vitamins on poultry performances, health, and oxidative status: A review of the literature in the last 20 years. *Antioxidants* **2021**, *10*, 659. [CrossRef] [PubMed]
6. Ibrahim, D.; Ismail, T.A.; Khalifa, E.; El-Kader, A.; Shaimaa, A.; Mohamed, D.I.; Mohamed, D.T.; Shahin, S.E.; El-Hamid, A.; Marwa, I. Supplementing Garlic Nanohydrogel Optimized Growth, Gastrointestinal Integrity and Economics and Ameliorated Necrotic Enteritis in Broiler Chickens Using a Clostridium perfringens Challenge Model. *Animals* **2021**, *11*, 2027. [CrossRef] [PubMed]
7. Ibrahim, D.; Eldemery, F.; Metwally, A.S.; Abd-Allah, E.M.; Mohamed, D.T.; Ismail, T.A.; Hamed, T.A.; Al Sadik, G.M.; Neamat-Allah, A.N.; El-Hamid, A. Dietary Eugenol Nanoemulsion Potentiated Performance of Broiler Chickens: Orchestration of Digestive Enzymes, Intestinal Barrier Functions and Cytokines Related Gene Expression with a Consequence of Attenuating the Severity of *E. coli* O78 Infection. *Front. Vet. Sci.* **2022**, *9*, 847580. [CrossRef] [PubMed]
8. Ibrahim, D.; Shahin, S.; Alqahtani, L.; Hassan, Z.; Althobaiti, F.; Albogami, S.; Soliman, M.; El-Malt, R.; Al-Harthi, H.; Alqadri, N. Exploring the Interactive Effects of Thymol and Thymoquinone: Moving towards an Enhanced Performance, Gross Margin, Immunity and Aeromonas sobria Resistance of Nile Tilapia (*Oreochromis niloticus*). *Animals* **2022**, *12*, 3034. [CrossRef] [PubMed]

9. Ibrahim, D.; Khater, S.I.; Abdelfattah-Hassan, A.; Alqahtani, L.S.; Metwally, A.S.M.; Bazeed, S.M.; Elgamal, A.; Sheraiba, N.I.; Hussein, E.M.; Alasmary, F.A. Prospects of new targeted nanotherapy combining liponiosomes with berberine to combat colorectal cancer development: An in vivo experimental model. *Int. J. Pharm.* **2023**, *647*, 123511. [CrossRef] [PubMed]
10. El-Ghareeb, W.R.; Kishawy, A.T.; Anter, R.G.; Aboelabbas Gouda, A.; Abdelaziz, W.S.; Alhawas, B.; Meligy, A.M.; Abdel-Raheem, S.M.; Ismail, H.; Ibrahim, D. Novel Antioxidant Insights of Myricetin on the Performance of Broiler Chickens and Alleviating Experimental Infection with Eimeria spp.: Crosstalk between Oxidative Stress and Inflammation. *Antioxidants* **2023**, *12*, 1026. [CrossRef]
11. Ibrahim, D.; Arisha, A.H.; Khater, S.I.; Gad, W.M.; Hassan, Z.; Abou-Khadra, S.H.; Mohamed, D.I.; Ahmed Ismail, T.; Gad, S.A.; Eid, S.A. Impact of Omega-3 Fatty Acids Nano-Formulation on Growth, Antioxidant Potential, Fillet Quality, Immunity, Autophagy-Related Genes and Aeromonas hydrophila Resistance in Nile Tilapia (*Oreochromis niloticus*). *Antioxidants* **2022**, *11*, 1523. [CrossRef]
12. Ibrahim, D.; Moustafa, A.; Metwally, A.S.; Nassan, M.A.; Abdallah, K.; Eldemery, F.; Tufarelli, V.; Laudadio, V.; Kishawy, A.T. Potential Application of Cornelian Cherry Extract on Broiler Chickens: Growth, Expression of Antioxidant Biomarker and Glucose Transport Genes, and Oxidative Stability of Frozen Meat. *Animals* **2021**, *11*, 1038. [CrossRef] [PubMed]
13. Cheng, Y.; Du, M.; Xu, Q.; Chen, Y.; Wen, C.; Zhou, Y. Dietary mannan oligosaccharide improves growth performance, muscle oxidative status, and meat quality in broilers under cyclic heat stress. *J. Therm. Biol.* **2018**, *75*, 106–111. [CrossRef] [PubMed]
14. Andrew, R.; Izzo, A.A. Principles of pharmacological research of nutraceuticals. *Br. J. Pharmacol.* **2017**, *174*, 1177. [CrossRef] [PubMed]
15. Alhawas, B.; Abd El-Hamid, M.I.; Hassan, Z.; Ibrahim, G.A.; Neamat-Allah, A.N.; El-Ghareeb, W.R.; Alahmad, B.A.-H.Y.; Meligy, A.M.; Abdel-Raheem, S.M.; Ismail, H.A.-M.A. Curcumin loaded liposome formulation: Enhanced efficacy on performance, flesh quality, immune response with defense against Streptococcus agalactiae in Nile tilapia (*Orechromis niloticus*). *Fish Shellfish Immunol.* **2023**, *138*, 108776. [CrossRef] [PubMed]
16. Dono, N.D. Turmeric (*Curcuma longa* Linn.) supplementation as an alternative to antibiotics in poultry diets. *WARTAZOA. Indones. Bull. Anim. Vet. Sci.* **2014**, *23*, 41–49. [CrossRef]
17. Ashraf, K. A comprehensive review on *Curcuma longa* Linn.: Phytochemical, pharmacological, and molecular study. *Int. J. Green Pharm.* **2017**, *11*, S671–S685. [CrossRef]
18. Choudhury, D. Study on the nutrient composition of local variety of turmeric (*Curcuma longa*). *J. Pharm. Innov.* **2019**, *8*, 205–207.
19. Attia, Y.A.; Al-Harthi, M.A.; Hassan, S.S. Turmeric (*Curcuma longa* Linn.) as a phytogenic growth promoter alternative for antibiotic and comparable to mannan oligosaccharides for broiler chicks. *Rev. Mex. Cienc. Pecu.* **2017**, *8*, 11–21. [CrossRef]
20. Zhong, W.; Qian, K.; Xiong, J.; Ma, K.; Wang, A.; Zou, Y. Curcumin alleviates lipopolysaccharide induced sepsis and liver failure by suppression of oxidative stress-related inflammation via PI3K/AKT and NF-κB related signaling. *Biomed. Pharmacother.* **2016**, *83*, 302–313. [CrossRef]
21. Abou-Elkhair, R.; Ahmed, H.; Selim, S. Effects of black pepper (*Piper nigrum*), turmeric powder (*Curcuma longa*) and coriander seeds (Coriandrum sativum) and their combinations as feed additives on growth performance, carcass traits, some blood parameters and humoral immune response of broiler chickens. *Asian-Australas. J. Anim. Sci.* **2014**, *27*, 847. [PubMed]
22. Amalraj, A.; Pius, A.; Gopi, S.; Gopi, S. Biological activities of curcuminoids, other biomolecules from turmeric and their derivatives–A review. *J. Tradit. Complement. Med.* **2017**, *7*, 205–233. [CrossRef] [PubMed]
23. Nawab, A.; Li, G.; Liu, W.; Lan, R.; Wu, J.; Zhao, Y.; Kang, K.; Kieser, B.; Sun, C.; Tang, S. Effect of dietary curcumin on the antioxidant status of laying hens under high-temperature condition. *J. Therm. Biol.* **2019**, *86*, 102449. [CrossRef] [PubMed]
24. Pulido-Moran, M.; Moreno-Fernandez, J.; Ramirez-Tortosa, C.; Ramirez-Tortosa, M. Curcumin and health. *Molecules* **2016**, *21*, 264. [CrossRef] [PubMed]
25. Liu, W.; Yuan, Y.; Sun, C.; Balasubramanian, B.; Zhao, Z.; An, L. Effects of dietary betaine on growth performance, digestive function, carcass traits, and meat quality in indigenous yellow-feathered broilers under long-term heat stress. *Animals* **2019**, *9*, 506. [CrossRef] [PubMed]
26. Moniruzzaman, M.; Min, T. Curcumin, curcumin nanoparticles and curcumin nanospheres: A review on their pharmacodynamics based on monogastric farm animal, poultry and fish nutrition. *Pharmaceutics* **2020**, *12*, 447. [CrossRef] [PubMed]
27. Paw, M.; Gogoi, R.; Sarma, N.; Pandey, S.K.; Borah, A.; Begum, T.; Lal, M. Study of anti-oxidant, anti-inflammatory, genotoxicity, and antimicrobial activities and analysis of different constituents found in rhizome essential oil of Curcuma caesia Roxb., collected from north east India. *Curr. Pharm. Biotechnol.* **2020**, *21*, 403–413. [CrossRef] [PubMed]
28. Wood, T.J.; Goulson, D. The environmental risks of neonicotinoid pesticides: A review of the evidence post 2013. *Environ. Sci. Pollut. Res.* **2017**, *24*, 17285–17325. [CrossRef]
29. Lu, C.; Lu, Z.; Lin, S.; Dai, W.; Zhang, Q. Neonicotinoid insecticides in the drinking water system–Fate, transportation, and their contributions to the overall dietary risks. *Environ. Pollut.* **2020**, *258*, 113722. [CrossRef]
30. Anadón, A.; Ares, I.; Martínez, M.; Martínez-Larrañaga, M.-R.; Martínez, M.-A. Neurotoxicity of neonicotinoids. *Adv. Neurotoxicology* **2020**, *4*, 167–207.
31. Gibbons, D.; Morrissey, C.; Mineau, P. A review of the direct and indirect effects of neonicotinoids and fipronil on vertebrate wildlife. *Environ. Sci. Pollut. Res.* **2015**, *22*, 103–118. [CrossRef] [PubMed]

32. Mineau, P.; Palmer, C. The Impact of the Nation's Most Widely Used Insecticides on Birds. Neonicotinoid Insecticides and Birds. Report by *American Bird Conservancy*. 2013. Available online: www.abcbirds.org/abcprograms/policy/toxins/Neonic_FINAL.pdf (accessed on 23 November 2023).
33. Cestonaro, L.V.; Macedo, S.M.D.; Piton, Y.V.; Garcia, S.C.; Arbo, M.D. Toxic effects of pesticides on cellular and humoral immunity: An overview. *Immunopharmacol. Immunotoxicol.* **2022**, *44*, 816–831. [CrossRef] [PubMed]
34. Fairbrother, A.; Smits, J.; Grasman, K.A. Avian immunotoxicology. *J. Toxicol. Environ. Health Part B* **2004**, *7*, 105–137. [CrossRef] [PubMed]
35. Jeschke, P.; Nauen, R.; Schindler, M.; Elbert, A. Overview of the status and global strategy for neonicotinoids. *J. Agric. Food Chem.* **2011**, *59*, 2897–2908. [CrossRef]
36. Kawashima, K.; Fujii, T. Extraneuronal cholinergic system in lymphocytes. *Pharmacol. Ther.* **2000**, *86*, 29–48. [CrossRef] [PubMed]
37. Badgujar, P.C.; Jain, S.; Singh, A.; Punia, J.; Gupta, R.; Chandratre, G.A. Immunotoxic effects of imidacloprid following 28 days of oral exposure in BALB/c mice. *Environ. Toxicol. Pharmacol.* **2013**, *35*, 408–418. [CrossRef] [PubMed]
38. Brandt, A.; Gorenflo, A.; Siede, R.; Meixner, M.; Büchler, R. The neonicotinoids thiacloprid, imidacloprid, and clothianidin affect the immunocompetence of honey bees (*Apis mellifera* L.). *J. Insect Physiol.* **2016**, *86*, 40–47. [CrossRef]
39. Kammon, A.; Brar, R.; Banga, H.; Sodhi, S. Ameliorating effects of vitamin E and selenium on immunological alterations induced by imidacloprid chronic toxicity in chickens. *J. Environ. Anal. Toxicol. S* **2012**, *4*. [CrossRef]
40. Macaulay, S.J.; Hageman, K.J.; Piggott, J.J.; Matthaei, C.D. Time-cumulative effects of neonicotinoid exposure, heat waves and food limitation on stream mayfly nymphs: A multiple-stressor experiment. *Sci. Total Environ.* **2021**, *754*, 141941. [CrossRef]
41. Abu Zeid, E.H.; Alam, R.T.; Ali, S.A.; Hendawi, M.Y. Dose-related impacts of imidacloprid oral intoxication on brain and liver of rock pigeon (*Columba livia domestica*), residues analysis in different organs. *Ecotoxicol. Environ. Saf.* **2019**, *167*, 60–68. [CrossRef]
42. Mo, Q.; Kulyar, M.F.-e.-A.; Ding, Y.; Zhang, Y.; Pan, H.; Li, J. Thiram induces myocardial oxidative damage and apoptosis in broilers via interfering their cardiac metabolism. *Ecotoxicol. Environ. Saf.* **2022**, *247*, 114225. [CrossRef] [PubMed]
43. Chen, Q.; Zhang, Y.; Su, G. Comparative study of neonicotinoid insecticides (NNIs) and NNI-Related substances (r-NNIs) in foodstuffs and indoor dust. *Environ. Int.* **2022**, *166*, 107368. [CrossRef] [PubMed]
44. Mahai, G.; Wan, Y.; Xia, W.; Wang, A.; Shi, L.; Qian, X.; He, Z.; Xu, S. A nationwide study of occurrence and exposure assessment of neonicotinoid insecticides and their metabolites in drinking water of China. *Water Res.* **2021**, *189*, 116630. [CrossRef] [PubMed]
45. Simon-Delso, N.; Amaral-Rogers, V.; Belzunces, L.P.; Bonmatin, J.-M.; Chagnon, M.; Downs, C.; Furlan, L.; Gibbons, D.W.; Giorio, C.; Girolami, V. Systemic insecticides (neonicotinoids and fipronil): Trends, uses, mode of action and metabolites. *Environ. Sci. Pollut. Res.* **2015**, *22*, 5–34. [CrossRef] [PubMed]
46. Emam, H.; Ahmed, E.; Abdel-Daim, M. Antioxidant capacity of omega-3-fatty acids and vitamin E against imidacloprid-induced hepatotoxicity in Japanese quails. *Environ. Sci. Pollut. Res.* **2018**, *25*, 11694–11702. [CrossRef] [PubMed]
47. Conte, F.M.; Cestonaro, L.V.; Piton, Y.V.; Guimarães, N.; Garcia, S.C.; da Silva, D.D.; Arbo, M.D. Toxicity of pesticides widely applied on soybean cultivation: Synergistic effects of fipronil, glyphosate and imidacloprid in HepG2 cells. *Toxicol. In Vitro* **2022**, *84*, 105446. [CrossRef] [PubMed]
48. Franzen-Klein, D.; Jankowski, M.; Roy, C.L.; Nguyen-Phuc, H.; Chen, D.; Neuman-Lee, L.; Redig, P.; Ponder, J. Evaluation of neurobehavioral abnormalities and immunotoxicity in response to oral imidacloprid exposure in domestic chickens (*Gallus gallus domesticus*). *J. Toxicol. Environ. Health Part A.* **2020**, *83*, 45–65. [CrossRef]
49. Rios, F.M.; Wilcoxen, T.E.; Zimmerman, L.M. Effects of imidacloprid on Rana catesbeiana immune and nervous system. *Chemosphere* **2017**, *188*, 465–469. [CrossRef]
50. Xu, X.; Wang, X.; Yang, Y.; Ares, I.; Martínez, M.; Lopez-Torres, B.; Martinez-Larranaga, M.-R.; Wang, X.; Anadón, A.; Martinez, M.-A. Neonicotinoids: Mechanisms of systemic toxicity based on oxidative stress-mitochondrial damage. *Arch. Toxicol.* **2022**, *96*, 1493–1520. [CrossRef]
51. Naiel, M.A.; Shehata, A.M.; Negm, S.S.; Abd El-Hack, M.E.; Amer, M.S.; Khafaga, A.F.; Bin-Jumah, M.; Allam, A.A. The new aspects of using some safe feed additives on alleviated imidacloprid toxicity in farmed fish: A review. *Rev. Aquac.* **2020**, *12*, 2250–2267. [CrossRef]
52. Osman, K.A.; Shaaban, M.M.; Ahmed, N.S. Biomarkers of imidacloprid toxicity in Japanese quail, Coturnix coturnix japonica. *Environ. Sci. Pollut. Res.* **2023**, *30*, 5662–5676. [CrossRef] [PubMed]
53. Khandia, R.; Pathe, C.S.; Vishwakarma, P.; Dhama, K.; Munjal, A. Evaluation of the ameliorative effects of Phyllanthus niruri on the deleterious insecticide imidacloprid in the vital organs of chicken embryos. *J. Ayurveda Integr. Med.* **2020**, *11*, 495–501. [CrossRef] [PubMed]
54. Gul, S.T.; Khan, R.L.; Saleemi, M.K.; Ahmad, M.; Hussain, R.; Khan, A. Amelioration of toxicopathological effects of thiamethoxam in broiler birds with vitamin E and selenium. *Toxin Rev.* **2022**, *41*, 218–228. [CrossRef]
55. Ravikanth, V.; Lakshman, M.; Madhuri, D.; Kalakumar, B. Haematological alterations in broilers administered with imidacloprid and spinosad and its amelioration with Vitamin E and Silymarin. *Int. J. Curr. Microbiol. App. Sci* **2017**, *6*, 496–500.
56. Sasidhar Babu, N.; Kumar, A.; Reddy, A.; Amaravathi, P.; Hemanth, I. Chronic experimental feeding of imidacloprid induced oxidative stress and amelioration with vitamin C and Withania somnifera in layer birds. *Int. J. Sci. Environ. ISSN Technol.* **2014**, *3*, 1679–1684.
57. Hussein, M.; Singh, V. Effect on chick embryos development after exposure to neonicotinoid insecticide imidacloprid. *J. Anat. Soc. India* **2016**, *65*, 83–89. [CrossRef]

58. Gobeli, A.; Crossley II, D.; Johnson, J.; Reyna, K. The effects of neonicotinoid exposure on embryonic development and organ mass in northern bobwhite quail (*Colinus virginianus*). *Comp. Biochem. Physiol. Part C Toxicol. Pharmacol.* **2017**, *195*, 9–15. [CrossRef]
59. Gupta, M.; Singh, S.P.; Pankaj, N.K. Ameliorative effect of Spirulina platensis and Erythrina variegata on oxidative stress in imidacloprid intoxicated white leghorn cockerels. *Toxicol. Int* **2017**, *24*, 171–177. [CrossRef]
60. Cheng, P.; Ishfaq, M.; Yu, H.; Yang, Y.; Li, S.; Li, X.; Fazlani, S.A.; Guo, W.; Zhang, X. Curcumin ameliorates duodenal toxicity of AFB1 in chicken through inducing P-glycoprotein and downregulating cytochrome P450 enzymes. *Poult. Sci.* **2020**, *99*, 7035–7045. [CrossRef]
61. Ravikanth, V.; Lakshman, M.; Madhuri, D.; Kalakumar, B. Effect of spinosad and imidacloprid on Serum Biochemical alterations in male broilers and Its Amelioration with vitamin E and Silymarin. *Int. J. Curr. Microbiol. App. Sci.* **2018**, *7*, 2186–2192. [CrossRef]
62. Aviagen, W.R. *308: Broiler's Management and Nutrition Specification*; AOAC International Aviagen Inc.: Huntsville, AL, USA, 2018; Available online: http://en.aviagen.com/assets/Tech_Center/Ross_Broiler/Ross-BroilerHandbook2018-EN.pdf (accessed on 1 January 2018).
63. Aviagen, W.R. *308: Broiler's Management and Nutrition Specification*; 308 Broiler Nutrition Specifications; Aviagen, W.R., Ed.; Aviagen: Huntsville, AL, USA, 2014.
64. Horwitz, W.; Latimer, G. *AOAC Official Methods of Analysis of AOAC International. AOAC Official Methods of Analysis of AOAC International*; AOAC International: Gaithersburg, MD, USA, 2005.
65. Giambrone, J.; Clay, R.P. Vaccination of day-old broiler chicks against Newcastle disease and infectious bursal disease using commercial live and/or inactivated vaccines. *Avian Dis.* **1986**, *30*, 557–561. [CrossRef]
66. Council, N.R. *Nutrient Requirements of Poultry: 1994*; National Academies Press: Cambridge, MA, USA, 1994.
67. AOAC. *Official Method of Analysis: Association of Analytical Chemists*, 19th ed.; AOAC: Washington, DC, USA, 2012; pp. 121–130.
68. Kishawy, A.T.; Al-Khalaifah, H.S.; Nada, H.S.; Roushdy, E.M.; Zaglool, A.W.; Ahmed Ismail, T.; Ibrahim, S.M.; Ibrahim, D. Black pepper or radish seed oils in a new combination of essential oils modulated broiler chickens' performance and expression of digestive enzymes, lipogenesis, immunity, and autophagy-related genes. *Vet. Sci.* **2022**, *9*, 43. [CrossRef] [PubMed]
69. Ibrahim, D.; El-Sayed, H.I.; Mahmoud, E.R.; El-Rahman, G.I.A.; Bazeed, S.M.; Abdelwarith, A.A.; Elgamal, A.; Khalil, S.S.; Younis, E.M.; Kishawy, A.T. Impacts of Solid-State Fermented Barley with Fibrolytic Exogenous Enzymes on Feed Utilization, and Antioxidant Status of Broiler Chickens. *Vet. Sci.* **2023**, *10*, 594. [CrossRef] [PubMed]
70. Harrison, G.J.; Harrison, L.R. *Clinical Avian Medicine and Surgery, Including Aviculture*; W. B. Saunders co.: Philadelphia, WB, USA, 1986.
71. Nengsih, R.F.; Mustika, A. Evaluasi Gambaran Darah dan Marker Stres (Rasio H/L) Ayam Pedaging yang Diberi Daun Bangun-Bangun selama 28 Hari. *Acta Vet. Indones.* **2020**, *8*, 9–15. [CrossRef]
72. Bos, H.; de Souza, W. Phagocytosis of yeast: A method for concurrent quantification of binding and internalization using differential interference contrast microscopy. *J. Immunol. Methods* **2000**, *238*, 29–43. [CrossRef] [PubMed]
73. Ellis, A.E. Lysozyme assays. *Tech. Fish Immunol.* **1990**, *1*, 101–103.
74. Doumas, B.T.; Biggs, H.G.; Arends, R.L.; Pinto, P.V. Determination of serum albumin. In *Standard Methods of Clinical Chemistry*; Elsevier: Amsterdam, The Netherlands, 1972; Volume 7, pp. 175–188.
75. Livak, K.J.; Schmittgen, T.D. Analysis of relative gene expression data using real-time quantitative PCR and the $2^{-\Delta\Delta CT}$ method. *Methods* **2001**, *25*, 402–408. [CrossRef] [PubMed]
76. Suvarna, K.S.; Layton, C.; Bancroft, J.D. *Bancroft's Theory and Practice of Histological Techniques E-Book*; Elsevier Health Sciences: Amsterdam, The Netherlands, 2018; ISBN 0702068861.
77. Hsu, S.-M.; Cossman, J.; Jaffe, E.S. A comparison of ABC, unlabeled antibody and conjugated immunohistochemical methods with monoclonal and polyclonal antibodies—An examination of germinal center of tonsils. *Am. J. Clin. Pathol.* **1983**, *80*, 429–435. [CrossRef]
78. Romero-Garay, M.G.; Montalvo-González, E.; Hernández-González, C.; Soto-Domínguez, A.; Becerra-Verdín, E.M.; García-Magaña, M.D.L. Bioactivity of peptides obtained from poultry by-products: A review. *Food Chem. X* **2022**, *13*, 100181. [CrossRef]
79. Alandiyjany, M.N.; Kishawy, A.T.; Abdelfattah-Hassan, A.; Eldoumani, H.; Elazab, S.T.; El-Mandrawy, S.A.; Saleh, A.A.; ElSawy, N.A.; Attia, Y.A.; Arisha, A.H. Nano-silica and magnetized-silica mitigated lead toxicity: Their efficacy on bioaccumulation risk, performance, and apoptotic targeted genes in Nile tilapia (*Oreochromis niloticus*). *Aquat. Toxicol.* **2022**, *242*, 106054. [CrossRef]
80. Adegoke, A.; Abimbola, M.; Sanwo, K.; Egbeyale, L.; Abiona, J.; Oso, A.; Iposu, S. Performance and blood biochemistry profile of broiler chickens fed dietary turmeric (*Curcuma longa*) powder and cayenne pepper (*Capsicum frutescens*) powders as antioxidants. *Vet. Anim. Sci.* **2018**, *6*, 95–102. [CrossRef] [PubMed]
81. Abotaleb, A.; AboSalem, M.; Elshewy, E.A.; Abdeen, A. Alleviation of imidacloprid-induced oxidative stress and immune damage by Spirulina platensis in broiler chickens. *Benha Vet. Med. J.* **2021**, *40*, 144–148. [CrossRef]
82. Li, J.; Bi, D.; Pan, S.; Zhang, Y. Effect of diet with thiram on liver antioxidant capacity and tibial dyschondroplasia in broilers. *Br. Poult. Sci.* **2007**, *48*, 724–728. [CrossRef]
83. Miao, Z.; Miao, Z.; Wang, S.; Wu, H.; Xu, S. Exposure to imidacloprid induce oxidative stress, mitochondrial dysfunction, inflammation, apoptosis and mitophagy via NF-kappaB/JNK pathway in grass carp hepatocytes. *Fish Shellfish Immunol.* **2022**, *120*, 674–685. [CrossRef]
84. Lopez-Antia, A.; Ortiz-Santaliestra, M.E.; Mougeot, F.; Mateo, R. Imidacloprid-treated seed ingestion has lethal effect on adult partridges and reduces both breeding investment and offspring immunity. *Environ. Res.* **2015**, *136*, 97–107. [CrossRef] [PubMed]

85. Hafez, M.H.; El-Kazaz, S.E.; Alharthi, B.; Ghamry, H.I.; Alshehri, M.A.; Sayed, S.; Shukry, M.; El-Sayed, Y.S. The impact of curcumin on growth performance, growth-related gene expression, oxidative stress, and immunological biomarkers in broiler chickens at different stocking densities. *Animals* **2022**, *12*, 958. [CrossRef] [PubMed]
86. Khodadadi, M.; Sheikhi, N.; Nazarpak, H.H.; Brujeni, G.N. Effects of dietary turmeric (*Curcuma longa*) on innate and acquired immune responses in broiler chicken. *Vet. Anim. Sci.* **2021**, *14*, 100213. [CrossRef] [PubMed]
87. Rajput, N.; Muhammad, N.; Yan, R.; Zhong, X.; Wang, T. Effect of dietary supplementation of curcumin on growth performance, intestinal morphology and nutrients utilization of broiler chicks. *J. Poult. Sci.* **2013**, *50*, 44–52. [CrossRef]
88. Yadav, S.; Teng, P.-Y.; Dos Santos, T.S.; Gould, R.L.; Craig, S.W.; Fuller, A.L.; Pazdro, R.; Kim, W.K. The effects of different doses of curcumin compound on growth performance, antioxidant status, and gut health of broiler chickens challenged with Eimeria species. *Poult. Sci.* **2020**, *99*, 5936–5945. [CrossRef] [PubMed]
89. Salah, A.S.; Mahmoud, M.A.; Ahmed-Farid, O.A.; El-Tarabany, M.S. Effects of dietary curcumin and acetylsalicylic acid supplements on performance, muscle amino acid and fatty acid profiles, antioxidant biomarkers and blood chemistry of heat-stressed broiler chickens. *J. Therm. Biol.* **2019**, *84*, 259–265. [CrossRef]
90. Eid, Y.Z.; Omara, Y.; Ragab, A.; Ismail, A.; Zommara, M.; Dawood, M.A. Mitigation of Imidacloprid Toxicity in Poultry Chicken by Selenium Nanoparticles: Growth Performance, Lipid Peroxidation, and Blood Traits. *Biol. Trace Elem. Res.* **2023**, *201*, 5379–5388. [CrossRef] [PubMed]
91. Sankhala, L.; Ranjan, A.; Suvidhi, L.K.; Tripathi, S. Evaluation of ameliorative effect of cow urine distillate on serum biochemical parameters in imidacloprid intoxicated white leghorn broilers. *J. Pharm. Innov.* **2022**, *11*, 263–266.
92. Pang, S.; Lin, Z.; Zhang, Y.; Zhang, W.; Alansary, N.; Mishra, S.; Bhatt, P.; Chen, S. Insights into the toxicity and degradation mechanisms of imidacloprid via physicochemical and microbial approaches. *Toxics* **2020**, *8*, 65. [CrossRef] [PubMed]
93. Abd EL-Samie, L. Comparative study on effect of turmeric powder, probiotic and prebiotic supplementation on broiler performance and immunity. *Assiut Vet. Med. J.* **2019**, *65*, 143–151.
94. Kafi, A.; Uddin, M.N.; Uddin, M.J.; Khan, M.M.H.; Haque, M.E. Effect of Dietary Supplementation of Turmeric *(Curcuma longa)*, Ginger *(Zingiber officinale)* and Their Combination as Feed Additives on Feed Intake, Growth Performance and Economics of Broiler. *Int. J. Poult. Sci.* **2017**, *16*, 257–265. [CrossRef]
95. Shohe, A.; Vidyarthi, V.; Zuyie, R. Performance of broiler chicken on diet supplemented with Turmeric powder (*Curcuma longa*). *Livest. Res. Int.* **2019**, *7*, 77–82.
96. Ali, A.; Ismoyowati, I.; Indrasanti, D. Jumlah eritrosit, kadar hemoglobin dan hematokrit pada berbagai jenis itik lokal terhadap penambahan probiotik dalam ransum. *J. Ilm. Peternak.* **2013**, *1*, 1001–1013.
97. Yosi, F.; Sandi, S. Meat quality, blood profile, and fecal ammonia concentration of broiler supplemented with liquid smoke. *Media Peternak.* **2014**, *37*, 169–174. [CrossRef]
98. Davis, A.; Maney, D.; Maerz, J. The use of leukocyte profiles to measure stress in vertebrates: A review for ecologists. *Funct. Ecol.* **2008**, *22*, 760–772. [CrossRef]
99. Puvadolpirod, S.; Thaxton, J. Model of physiological stress in chickens 1. Response parameters. *Poult. Sci.* **2000**, *79*, 363–369. [CrossRef]
100. Pimson, C.; Bakban, P.; Suwanrat, S.; Chanutsa, N. The effect of curcumin on growth performance, blood biochemistry and antioxidant activities in boiler chickens. *Vet. Integr. Sci.* **2018**, *16*, 95–107.
101. Ma'rifah, B.; Isroli, I.; Sartono, T.A. Pengaruh air rebusan kunyit (*Curcuma domestica*) dalam air minum terhadap daya tahan dan perfromans karkas ayam broiler. *J. Ris. Agribisnis Dan Peternak.* **2020**, *5*, 7–12. [CrossRef]
102. Agustanti, L. *Gambaran sel Darah Putih dan Indeks Stres Ayam Broiler Yang Diberi Jamu Bagas Waras (jahe, kunyit, dan kencur) Melalui Air Minum*. Skripsi. Institut Pertanian Bogor. Bogor. 2014. Available online: https://repository.ipb.ac.id/handle/123456789/72263 (accessed on 23 November 2023).
103. Ramadan, A.; Mansour, U. Cytotoxic Effect of Some Commercial Neonicotinoids on Sheep Phagocytic Cells Activity In vitro. *Res. Rev. J. Vet. Sci.* **2018**, *4*, 2.
104. Abou-Zeid, S.M.; Aljuaydi, S.H.; AbuBakr, H.O.; Tahoun, E.A.; Di Cerbo, A.; Alagawany, M.; Khalil, S.R.; Farag, M.R. Astaxanthin mitigates thiacloprid-induced liver injury and immunotoxicity in male rats. *Mar. Drugs* **2021**, *19*, 525. [CrossRef]
105. Mohany, M.; Badr, G.; Refaat, I.; El-Feki, M. Immunological and histological effects of exposure to imidacloprid insecticide in male albino rats. *Afr. J. Pharm. Pharmacol.* **2011**, *5*, 2106–2114. [CrossRef]
106. Walderdorff, L.; Laval-Gilly, P.; Wechtler, L.; Bonnefoy, A.; Falla-Angel, J. Phagocytic activity of human macrophages and Drosophila hemocytes after exposure to the neonicotinoid imidacloprid. *Pestic. Biochem. Physiol.* **2019**, *160*, 95–101. [CrossRef]
107. Julius, A.; Abernathy, L.; Yung, R. Defective Dendritic Cell Phagocytic Function in Aging (134.36). *J. Immunol.* **2009**, *182*, 134–136. [CrossRef]
108. Gul, S.T.; Khan, A.; Ahmad, M.; Ahmad, H.; Saleemi, M.K.; Naseem, M.N.; Bilal, M. Immuno-toxicological effects of different sub-lethal doses of thiamethoxam (TMX) in broiler birds. *Toxin Rev.* **2018**, *38*, 200–205. [CrossRef]
109. Gawade, L.; Dadarkar, S.S.; Husain, R.; Gatne, M. A detailed study of developmental immunotoxicity of imidacloprid in Wistar rats. *Food Chem. Toxicol.* **2013**, *51*, 61–70. [CrossRef]
110. Lopez-Antia, A.; Ortiz-Santaliestra, M.E.; Mougeot, F.; Mateo, R. Experimental exposure of red-legged partridges (Alectoris rufa) to seeds coated with imidacloprid, thiram and difenoconazole. *Ecotoxicology* **2013**, *22*, 125–138. [CrossRef] [PubMed]

111. Khayal, E.E.-S.; Alabiad, M.A.; Elkholy, M.R.; Shalaby, A.M.; Nosery, Y.; El-Sheikh, A.A. The immune modulatory role of marjoram extract on imidacloprid induced toxic effects in thymus and spleen of adult rats. *Toxicology* **2022**, *471*, 153174. [CrossRef] [PubMed]
112. Farag, M.R.; Alagawany, M.M.; Dhama, K. Antidotal effect of turmeric (*Curcuma longa*) against endosulfan-induced cytogenotoxicity and immunotoxicity in broiler chicks. *Int. J. Pharmacol.* **2014**, *10*, 429–439. [CrossRef]
113. Jagetia, G.C.; Aggarwal, B.B. "Spicing up" of the immune system by curcumin. *J. Clin. Immunol.* **2007**, *27*, 19–35. [CrossRef] [PubMed]
114. Gao, X.; Kuo, J.; Jiang, H.; Deeb, D.; Liu, Y.; Divine, G.; Chapman, R.A.; Dulchavsky, S.A.; Gautam, S.C. Immunomodulatory activity of curcumin: Suppression of lymphocyte proliferation, development of cell-mediated cytotoxicity, and cytokine production in vitro. *Biochem. Pharmacol.* **2004**, *68*, 51–61. [CrossRef]
115. Attia, A.; El-Saadawy, H.; El-Belbasi, H.; Abd El-Hameed, S. Ameliorative effect of azolla pinnata on imidacloprid induced hepatorenal toxicity, oxidative stress and immunosuppression in nile tilapia. *J. Anim. Health Prod.* **2021**, *9*, 1–6. [CrossRef]
116. Rahman, A.N.A.; Mohamed, A.A.-R.; Mohammed, H.H.; Elseddawy, N.M.; Salem, G.A.; El-Ghareeb, W.R. The ameliorative role of geranium (*Pelargonium graveolens*) essential oil against hepato-renal toxicity, immunosuppression, and oxidative stress of profenofos in common carp, *Cyprinus carpio* (L.). *Aquaculture* **2020**, *517*, 734777. [CrossRef]
117. Isroli, I.; Yudiarti, T.; Widiastuti, E.; Sugiharto, S. Effect of decocted turmeric on performance, hematological parameters and carcass traits of broiler chickens. *J. Indones. Trop. Anim. Agric.* **2017**, *42*, 263–269. [CrossRef]
118. Shawky, S.; Fathalla, S.; Orabi, S.; El-Mosalhi, H.; Abu-Alya, I. Turmeric Powder Supplementation in Broiler Diet Improves Growth Performance and Immunity via Increasing mRNA Expression of Growth Hormone, Insulin Like Growth Factor-1, Interferon Gamma and Interleukin12. *Res. Sq.* **2022**, 1–13. [CrossRef]
119. Arshami, J.; Pilevar, M.; Azghadi, M.A.; Raji, A.R. Hypolipidemic and antioxidative effects of curcumin on blood parameters, humoral immunity, and jejunum histology in Hy-line hens. *Avicenna J. Phytomed.* **2013**, *3*, 178.
120. Akter, L.; Kobir, M.A.; Nasrin, M.; Siddiqi, M.N.H.; Pervin, M.; Karim, M.R. Effects of exposure to imidacloprid contaminated feed on the visceral organs of adult male rabbits (*Oryctolagus cuniculus*). *Saudi J. Biol. Sci.* **2023**, *30*, 103684. [CrossRef] [PubMed]
121. Lei, Y.; Zhang, W.; Gao, M.; Lin, H. Mechanism of evodiamine blocking Nrf2/MAPK pathway to inhibit apoptosis of grass carp hepatocytes induced by DEHP. *Comp. Biochem. Physiol. Part C Toxicol. Pharmacol.* **2023**, *263*, 109506. [CrossRef] [PubMed]
122. Guimarães, A.R.d.J.S.; Bizerra, P.F.V.; Miranda, C.A.; Mingatto, F.E. Effects of imidacloprid on viability and increase of reactive oxygen and nitrogen species in HepG2 cell line. *Toxicol. Mech. Methods* **2022**, *32*, 204–212. [CrossRef] [PubMed]
123. Laganá, C.; Saldanha, E.S.B.; Sartori, J.R.; Turco, P.H.N.; Gonzales, E.; Luciano, R.L.; Zanatta, G.; Fascina, V.B. Turmeric on poultry production: A Review. *Agric. Sci.* **2019**, *10*, 1592. [CrossRef]
124. Vettorazzi, A.; van Delft, J.; de Cerain, A.L. A review on ochratoxin A transcriptomic studies. *Food Chem. Toxicol.* **2013**, *59*, 766–783. [CrossRef] [PubMed]
125. Nebbia, C. Biotransformation enzymes as determinants of xenobiotic toxicity in domestic animals. *Vet. J.* **2001**, *161*, 238–252. [CrossRef]
126. Kim, M.; Kim, Y. Hypocholesterolemic effects of curcumin via up-regulation of cholesterol 7a-hydroxylase in rats fed a high fat diet. *Nutr. Res. Pract.* **2010**, *4*, 191–195. [CrossRef]
127. Zhang, D.; Wu, C.; Ba, D.; Wang, N.; Wang, Y.; Li, X.; Li, Q.; Zhao, G. Ferroptosis contribute to neonicotinoid imidacloprid-evoked pyroptosis by activating the HMGB1-RAGE/TLR4-NF-κB signaling pathway. *Ecotoxicol. Environ. Saf.* **2023**, *253*, 114655. [CrossRef]
128. Subha, G. Long term exposure to chemicals, insecticides and heavy metals causing toxicity: A review. *Int. J. Pharm. Res. Bio-Sci.* **2013**, *2*, 333–342.
129. Li, S.; Muhammad, I.; Yu, H.; Sun, X.; Zhang, X. Detection of Aflatoxin adducts as potential markers and the role of curcumin in alleviating AFB1-induced liver damage in chickens. *Ecotoxicol. Environ. Saf.* **2019**, *176*, 137–145. [CrossRef]
130. El-Bahr, S. Effect of curcumin on hepatic antioxidant enzymes activities and gene expressions in rats intoxicated with aflatoxin B1. *Phytother. Res.* **2015**, *29*, 134–140. [CrossRef] [PubMed]
131. Nayak, S.; Sashidhar, R. Metabolic intervention of aflatoxin B1 toxicity by curcumin. *J. Ethnopharmacol.* **2010**, *127*, 641–644. [CrossRef] [PubMed]
132. Zhang, N.-Y.; Qi, M.; Zhao, L.; Zhu, M.-K.; Guo, J.; Liu, J.; Gu, C.-Q.; Rajput, S.A.; Krumm, C.S.; Qi, D.-S. Curcumin prevents aflatoxin B1 hepatoxicity by inhibition of cytochrome P450 isozymes in chick liver. *Toxins* **2016**, *8*, 327. [CrossRef] [PubMed]
133. Abdul-Careem, M.; Hunter, D.; Lambourne, M.; Barta, J.; Sharif, S. Ontogeny of cytokine gene expression in the chicken spleen. *Poult. Sci.* **2007**, *86*, 1351–1355. [CrossRef] [PubMed]
134. Mebius, R.E.; Kraal, G. Structure and function of the spleen. *Nat. Rev. Immunol.* **2005**, *5*, 606–616. [CrossRef]
135. Farag, M.R.; Abou-EL Fotoh, M.F.; EL-Sayed, G.G.; EL-Sayed, E.W. Modulatory effect of ginger aqueous extract against imidacloprid-induced neurotoxicity in rats. *Zagazig Vet. J.* **2019**, *47*, 432–446. [CrossRef]
136. Alves-Filho, J.C.; Freitas, A.; Souto, F.O.; Spiller, F.; Paula-Neto, H.; Silva, J.S.; Gazzinelli, R.T.; Teixeira, M.M.; Ferreira, S.H.; Cunha, F.Q. Regulation of chemokine receptor by Toll-like receptor 2 is critical to neutrophil migration and resistance to polymicrobial sepsis. *Proc. Natl. Acad. Sci. USA* **2009**, *106*, 4018–4023. [CrossRef]
137. Sugiyama, K.-I.; Muroi, M.; Tanamoto, K.-I. A novel TLR4-binding peptide that inhibits LPS-induced activation of NF-κB and in vivo toxicity. *Eur. J. Pharmacol.* **2008**, *594*, 152–156. [CrossRef]

138. Singh, A.; Jiang, Y. Lipopolysaccharide (LPS) induced activation of the immune system in control rats and rats chronically exposed to a low level of the organothiophosphate insecticide, acephate. *Toxicol. Ind. Health* **2003**, *19*, 93–108. [CrossRef]
139. Nemati, M.; Larussa, T.; Khorramdelazad, H.; Mahmoodi, M.; Jafarzadeh, A. Toll-like receptor 2: An important immunomodulatory molecule during Helicobacter pylori infection. *Life Sci.* **2017**, *178*, 17–29. [CrossRef]
140. Cui, J.; Chen, Y.; Wang, H.Y.; Wang, R.-F. Mechanisms and pathways of innate immune activation and regulation in health and cancer. *Hum. Vaccines Immunother.* **2014**, *10*, 3270–3285. [CrossRef] [PubMed]
141. Gill, R.; Tsung, A.; Billiar, T. Linking oxidative stress to inflammation: Toll-like receptors. *Free Radic. Biol. Med.* **2010**, *48*, 1121–1132. [CrossRef] [PubMed]
142. Pandit, A.A.; Choudhary, S.; Singh, B.; Sethi, R. Imidacloprid induced histomorphological changes and expression of TLR-4 and TNFα in lung. *Pestic. Biochem. Physiol.* **2016**, *131*, 9–17. [CrossRef] [PubMed]
143. Farag, M.R.; Khalil, S.R.; Zaglool, A.W.; Hendam, B.M.; Moustafa, A.A.; Cocco, R.; Di Cerbo, A.; Alagawany, M. Thiacloprid induced developmental neurotoxicity via ROS-oxidative injury and inflammation in chicken embryo: The possible attenuating role of chicoric and rosmarinic acids. *Biology* **2021**, *10*, 1100. [CrossRef] [PubMed]
144. Liu, Y.; Song, M.; Che, T.; Lee, J.; Bravo, D.; Maddox, C.; Pettigrew, J. Dietary plant extracts modulate gene expression profiles in ileal mucosa of weaned pigs after an Escherichia coli infection. *J. Anim. Sci.* **2014**, *92*, 2050–2062. [CrossRef] [PubMed]
145. Liu, Y.; Che, T.; Song, M.; Lee, J.; Almeida, J.; Bravo, D.; Van Alstine, W.; Pettigrew, J. Dietary plant extracts improve immune responses and growth efficiency of pigs experimentally infected with porcine reproductive and respiratory syndrome virus. *J. Anim. Sci.* **2013**, *91*, 5668–5679. [CrossRef] [PubMed]
146. Gupta, R.; Deepika, L. Clinico-pathological studies of imidacloprid toxicity in broiler chickens. *Haryana Vet.* **2016**, *55*, 163–165.
147. Kammon, A.M.; Brar, R.S.; Banga, H.S.; Sodhi, S. Patho-biochemical studies on hepatotoxicity and nephrotoxicity on exposure to chlorpyrifos and imidacloprid in layer chickens. *Vet. Arh.* **2010**, *80*, 663–672.
148. Alhusaini, A.; Fadda, L.M.; Ali, H.M.; Hasan, I.H.; Ali, R.A.; Zakaria, E.A. Mitigation of acetamiprid—Induced renotoxicity by natural antioxidants via the regulation of ICAM, NF-kB and TLR 4 pathways. *Pharmacol. Rep.* **2019**, *71*, 1088–1094. [CrossRef]

animals

MDPI

Article

Protective Role of Bergamot Polyphenolic Fraction (BPF) against Deltamethrin Toxicity in Honeybees (*Apis mellifera*)

Roberto Bava [1], Fabio Castagna [1,2], Stefano Ruga [1], Rosamaria Caminiti [1], Saverio Nucera [1], Rosa Maria Bulotta [1], Clara Naccari [1], Domenico Britti [1], Vincenzo Mollace [1,3,4] and Ernesto Palma [1,3,4,*]

1 Department of Health Sciences, University of Catanzaro Magna Graecia, 88100 Catanzaro, Italy; roberto.bava@unicz.it (R.B.); fabiocastagna@unicz.it (F.C.); rugast1@gmail.com (S.R.); rosamariacaminiti4@gmail.com (R.C.); saverio.nucera@hotmail.it (S.N.); rosamaria.bulotta@gmail.com (R.M.B.); c.naccari@unicz.it (C.N.); britti@unicz.it (D.B.); mollace@unicz.it (V.M.)
2 Mediterranean Ethnobotanical Conservatory, Sersale (CZ), 88054 Catanzaro, Italy
3 Department of Health Sciences, Institute of Research for Food Safety & Health (IRC-FSH), University of Catanzaro Magna Graecia, 88100 Catanzaro, Italy
4 Nutramed S.c.a.r.l., Complesso Ninì Barbieri, Roccelletta di Borgia, 88021 Catanzaro, Italy
* Correspondence: palma@unicz.it

Simple Summary: The inappropriate use of pesticides is one of the underlying causes of the extensive honeybee die-off that is taking place worldwide. Pesticides can cause acute, sub-acute, and chronic toxicity, in the latter case leading to physiological and behavioral changes in honeybees. Acute pesticide toxicity is exacerbated by nutritional deficiencies and poor immune system fitness. Studies have shown that polyphenols extracted from many botanical species have been shown to possess protective properties against acute and chronic pesticide intoxication. In this study, we wanted to test the protective role of the bergamot polyphenolic fraction (BPF) against deltamethrin intoxication in honeybees. The semi-filed toxicity tests showed that, when administered in combination with deltamethrin, BPF was able to protect against pesticide toxicity. In particular, survival indices were improved, and the honeybees showed a reduction in abnormal behavior compared to the positive control group treated with deltamethrin alone.

Abstract: Pesticide-induced poisoning phenomena are a serious problem for beekeeping and can cause large losses of honeybee populations due to acute and sub-acute poisoning. The reduced responsiveness of honeybees to the damage caused by pesticides used in agriculture can be traced back to a general qualitative and quantitative impoverishment of the nectar resources of terrestrial ecosystems. Malnutrition is associated with a decline in the functionality of the immune system and the systems that are delegated to the detoxification of the organism. This research aimed to verify whether bergamot polyphenolic extract (BPF) could have protective effects against poisoning by the pyrethroid pesticide deltamethrin. The studies were conducted with caged honeybees under controlled conditions. Sub-lethal doses of pesticides and related treatments for BPF were administered. At a dose of 21.6 mg/L, deltamethrin caused mortality in all treated subjects (20 caged honeybees) after one day of administration. The groups where BPF (1 mg/kg) was added to the toxic solution recorded the survival of honeybees by up to three days. Comparing the honeybees of the groups in which the BPF-deltamethrin association was added to the normal diet (sugar solution) with those in which deltamethrin alone was added to the normal diet, the BPF group had a statistically significant reduction in the honeybee mortality rate ($p \leq 0.05$) and a greater consumption of food. Therefore, it can be argued that the inclusion of BPF and its constituent antioxidants in the honeybee diet reduces toxicity and oxidative stress caused by oral intake of deltamethrin. Furthermore, it can be argued that BPF administration could compensate for metabolic energy deficits often induced by the effects of malnutrition caused by environmental degradation and standard beekeeping practices.

Keywords: honeybee (*Apis mellifera*); natural products (NPs); bergamot polyphenolic fraction (BPF); deltamethrin; pyrethroid

1. Introduction

The honeybee die-off that has occurred in recent years is due to numerous factors [1,2]. Among these, pesticide poisoning is particularly important [3,4]. The term pesticides is generally used to indicate all products that are employed to combat harmful organisms, especially in agriculture [5]. Unfortunately, it is not only the organisms targeted by pesticide treatments that suffer but very often also the useful ones [6,7]. Honeybees can be exposed to pesticides through a variety of routes, with contact or ingestion being the main two [8]. In addition to the usual way, contact between honeybees and pesticides can also occur in ways that are not easily predictable. For example, the treatment of the seeds of various crops with some insecticides, in particular neonicotinoids, can pose a danger to honeybees comparable to that of spray formulations [9]. During sowing, the abrasion of the film covering the seed in the hopper of the seeder produces dust that is dispersed in the surrounding environment, which can form a deadly cloud for the bees in flight that cross it or cause, after being deposited, intoxications at a later time [9,10]. Contamination can also occur at a considerable distance from the treated field due to the drift effect caused by the wind or through indirect contamination [11,12]. According to Krupke et al. (2012) [13], the main sources of hive contamination for adults and larvae are nectar, recently stored pollen, and bee bread [13]. When forager honeybees collect contaminated pollen, nectar, honeydew, or water, they may die immediately, or if the dosages are not fatal, the contaminants may be carried into the hive. During the most crucial times, when honeybees need to utilize their food reserves, they are likely to consume these contaminants [13]. Therefore, moderate levels of pesticides can still pose a serious threat to the honeybee colony, leading to a gradual decline in the population. Paradoxically, direct treatments of honeybees with very toxic substances can have less impact, as by killing or preventing the foragers from returning to the hive, they do not act on the brood and the queen's fecundity. In these cases, families can recover quickly by replacing the foragers, even if there is an irreversible loss of harvest. Most pesticides have different levels of toxicity based on a variety of variables, such as the exposure method, the age of the honeybees, the fitness of the colonies or honeybee subspecies, and the nutritional requirement [8,14,15]. The research studies revealed significant levels of pesticide toxicity and the related detrimental consequences for honeybees [16–18]. For example, research attention has been focused on neonicotinoid pesticides [19–21], and nowadays their use has been limited due to their negative effects on honeybees and growing resistance to them in treated pest populations [22].

Today, pesticides commonly used in agriculture belong to the class of pyrethroids [23,24]. Their insecticidal activity is due to the lipophilic keto-alcoholic esters of chrysanthemum and pyrethroic acid [25]. First- and second-generation pyrethroids are distinguished. Compared to second-generation (Type II) pyrethroids, first-generation (Type I) pyrethroids are less dangerous to mammals [26]. The voltage-dependent sodium channels are the major target of pyrethroid pesticides. Because of their low environmental persistence and toxicity, the pyrethroid family of insecticides is employed as alternatives to organochlorines, organophosphates, and neonicotinoids in pest-control programs [27,28]. Deltamethrin is a Type II pyrethroid characterized by a broad spectrum of activity that is widely used in professional agriculture, forestry, and hobby farming [29]. Its use is not free from the dangers of pollinating insects. Deltamethrin disrupts physiology in honeybees by causing memory disturbances, hypofertility, hypothermia, alterations in body and intestinal development, and altering normal dances and foraging activity [30–33]. It is also important to emphasize that pesticides exacerbate their effects when the body's defenses are poor.

In the last few years, the modification of the landscape caused by human activity has led to a decrease in the quality of bee food [34]. As agriculture becomes more intensive, the landscape changes and the availability of bee food supplies progressively decreases, which reduces environmental sustainability. Consequently, the variety of flowering plants has decreased [35]. Low species diversity of flowering plants results in a reduction in the variety and availability of macro- and micro-elements in bee nutrition, which ultimately has a detrimental impact on honeybee populations [18]. Ineffective beekeeping techniques also contribute to nutritional deficiency; when winter supplies need to be replenished, bees are sometimes given little more than a solution of sugar and synthetic pollen replacements. The majority of the time, these food supplements are deficient in nutrients that are present in honeybees' normal diets [36,37]. The number of honeybee colonies may be declining as a direct consequence of poor nutrition, which may also increase susceptibility to diseases and pesticides [38]. Many studies have demonstrated that the dietary consumption of phenolic compounds and flavonoids can increase the body's ability to respond to pesticide injuries and pathogens [18,39]. Depending on food sources, the quantity and intake of phenolic compounds and flavonoids could change considerably [40]. The phenolic acids, flavonoids, and their derivatives are often abundant and diverse in honeybees' natural diets [41], and it is these varying concentrations and ratios that affect the detoxifying effects [42]. Natural products (NPs) have been shown to have several properties [43–47]. Supplementing the diet with NPs and/or their compounds, such as polyphenols, could help honeybees respond better to the injuries that pesticides pose to their normal physiology. *Citrus Bergamia* Risso and Poiteau, commonly known as bergamot, is a shrub native to the Calabrian area of Southern Italy [48]. Its juice and albedo both exhibit a distinctive flavonoid and flavonoid glycoside profile. The composition and especially the high flavonoid concentration of bergamot set it apart from other citrus fruits [48]. Researchers have found that BPF, a polyphenol-rich fraction produced from bergamot juice and albedo, possesses antioxidant, anti-inflammatory, lipid-lowering, and hypoglycemic properties [49–55]. Bergamot requires particular cultivation conditions, such as alluvial, clayey, and calcareous soils. Calabria is the world's largest producer. Over 90% of the world's bergamot production comes from this region [56]. Among the flavonoids and flavonoid glycosides present in bergamot, there are neoerocitrin, neoesperidin, naringin, rutin, neodesmin, roifolin, and poncirin [53]. A total of 95% of flavonoids are represented by flavanones. It also features carbohydrates, pectins, and other compounds [53]. Our research aims to shed more light on the intricate and subtle impacts that pesticides could have on honeybee behavior and health. This study's primary objective was to ascertain the impact of polyphenols on the mortality of honeybees poisoned by deltamethrin, one of the most popular pyrethroids. The polyphenol fraction of bergamot, also known as BPF, was chosen for the food supplementation. To assess the positive effect of polyphenol intake, the mortality rate of the honeybees fed BPF-deltamethrin in sugar solution was monitored over time and compared with that of honeybees taking only the pesticide in sugar solution. Furthermore, the abnormal honeybee behavior of the experimental groups as well as food consumption were assessed.

2. Materials and Methods

This investigation was carried out in the summer of 2023 at the Interregional Research Center for Food Safety and Health (IRC-FSH), Department of Health Science, University "Magna Graecia" of Catanzaro (Italy). The experimental honeybees came from one healthy honeybee colony. The honeybees used for the experiment belonged to the subspecies *A. mellifera ligustica*. The colony was conducted using conventional beekeeping methods. To ensure that the colony was healthy and free from parasitic or infectious infestations, established inspection procedures were used. As established by the standard methods for toxicological research, to obtain individuals of the same age, honeycombs of brood with hatching honeybees were placed in an incubator (35 °C and 65–80% relative humidity), and emerging honeybees were collected after 12 h [15].

After brushing the frames, all the honeybees were mixed and split into the experimental groups. Disposable cages have been used for toxicological studies because it is difficult to remove chemical residues [15]. Only one feeder (a plastic syringe with the tip cut off to enable solution flow) was given to each test cage [57].

Therefore, the young honeybees were moved into cages (20 per cage). To introduce the honeybees into the cages and administer the treatments, routine procedures without anesthesia were used [15,58]. After honeybees were introduced, cages were kept at 33 ± 2 °C and 50–70% RH in a dark chamber. Before the trial started on Day 0, the 1 day old emerged honeybees were kept in cages for one day (from Day −1 to Day 0) and fed with a sucrose solution (50% (*w*/*v*)) to give them time to become accustomed to the test conditions.

Subsequently, they were fed with the treatment solutions. Five experimental replicates were performed for each treatment under study.

Tests were conducted on the individual effects of deltamethrin (Sigma Aldrich—Schnelldorf, BO, Germany) and BPF, as well as the protective impact of BPF when administered in association with deltamethrin. Two doses of deltamethrin and one of BPF were chosen for administration. The doses were chosen for preliminary studies. Specifically, deltamethrin dosages were combined with the sucrose solution at two distinct concentrations: 2.16 mg/L and 21.6 mg/L; five control groups (dose of 0 mg/mL honeybee) were also devised. BPF dosage (1 mg/kg) was evaluated in conjunction with each sublethal dose of deltamethrin in the combined deltamethrin and BPF therapy. The effects of the treatments on honeybee survival (1–72 h) and the frequency of aberrant behavior in honeybees (1–4, 24, 48, and 72 h after treatment) were recorded.

The organization of the experimental groups is summarized below:

1. Deltamethrin treatment 1 (DTM 1): a low concentration of deltamethrin (2.16 mg/L) in a 50% *w*/*v* sugar solution;
2. Deltamethrin treatment 2 (DTM 2): deltamethrin at a high dose (21.6 mg/L) in a 50% *w*/*v* sugar solution;
3. Bergamot polyphenolic fraction treatment 1 (BPF-1): a BPF (1 mg/kg) combination in a 50% *w*/*v* sugar solution with the lower dose of deltamethrin (2.16 mg/L);
4. Bergamot polyphenolic fraction treatment 2 (BPF-2): a combination of BPF (1 mg/kg) in a 50% *w*/*v* sugar solution with a higher concentration of deltamethrin (21.6 mg/L);
5. Bergamot polyphenolic fraction (BPF): BPF (1 mg/kg) dose in a 50% *w*/*v* sugar solution;
6. Control treatment: sucrose solution (50% *w*/*v*).

2.1. BPF Preparation

For the study, fruits of the *Citrus bergamia* Risso and Poiteau varieties were collected in the area between Bianco and Reggio Calabria (Calabria Region, Italy). Subsequently, squeezing was carried out to extract the juice from the peeled citrus fruits.

The juice underwent oil fraction depletion by stripping, clarification by ultra-filtration, and loading onto an appropriate polystyrene resin column capable of absorbing polyphenol chemicals with molecular weights between 300 and 600 Da (Mitsubishi).

A solution of 1 mM KOH was used to elute the polyphenol fractions. To lower the amount of furocoumarin, the basic eluate was incubated on a rocking platform. According to the quantity of furocoumarin impurities, the shaking duration was modified. The phytocomplex left over from the procedure used to extract furocoumarins was then neutralized by filtering cationic resin at an acidic pH. To obtain BPF powder, it was vacuum dried and then chopped to the appropriate particle size [48]. The BPF was subjected to physical, microbiological, and compositional analyses. In particular, the power was analyzed in search of flavonoids, furocoumarin, and other polyphenols. The amount of polyphenols in BPF powder was analyzed using HPLC.

2.2. Feeding Solutions

Deltamethrin and BPF stock solutions were created using deionized water and kept at a temperature of 4 °C. By combining the stock solutions of deltamethrin and BPF with 50% (*w*/*v*) water sugar solutions, the final treatment solutions were created.

The BPF treatment had concentrations of 1 mg/kg. Deltamethrin treatments were prepared at concentrations of 2.16 mg/L and 21.6 mg/L. The above detailed deltamethrin concentrations were mixed with BPF concentrations to verify the protective effect of the polyphenolic extract. The honeybees received feeding solutions ad libitum from the beginning of the experiment and were supplied with new ones every 24 h. At least once every three days, the feeding dilutions were made, carefully wrapped in aluminum foil to shield them from light deterioration, and kept at a temperature of 6 to 2 °C. No precipitation was ever seen in feeding solutions.

2.3. Behavior

The OECD's established guidelines were used to categorize and quantify behavioral disorders [58]. Depending on the pesticide dosage, the percentage of honeybees displaying aberrant behaviors across time (1, 2, 4, 24, 48, and 72 h after treatment) and the number of improperly behaving honeybees per cage were evaluated. The following behaviors were taken into account: a curved-down abdomen, hyperactivity, apathy, motion coordination impairments, and moribundness [17]. These types of anomalous behaviors are based on ecotoxicological recommendations. We monitored each honeybee for 6 s (up to 120 s for a cage with 20 honeybees), with the cage serving as the unit of replication.

2.4. Food Composition

The cages were equipped with feeders. The feeders were inserted horizontally into the bottom of the cage. The feeders were sterile 2.5 mL disposable syringes with capped ends. A notch was made at the top of the syringe, near the capped end, creating a slit through which the bees fed. Food consumption was recorded daily.

2.5. Data Analysis

The statistical analysis was conducted using GraphPad PRISM software (version 9.0, GraphPad Software Inc., La Jolla, CA, USA). To estimate the survival function from the data obtained, the Kaplan–Meier estimator was employed. Once the analysis was obtained, the Longrank test was performed to compare the survival of the different treated groups. The difference between the experimental groups was considered significant for p-values of $\leq$0.05.

3. Results

3.1. Bergamot Polyphenolic Fraction (BPF) Analysis

The results of the analysis, including the chemical characteristics, active ingredients, heavy metals, and microbiological evaluation, are shown in Table 1 [59,60].

Toxicological tests ruled out the existence of any harmful substances. Microbiological standard testing found no bacteria or mycotoxin. Neoeriocitrin (370 ppm), naringin (520 ppm), and neohesperidin (310 ppm) were the primary flavonoids found in BPF.

3.2. Honeybee Survival and Mortality

Results for honeybee survival are depicted in Figure 1.

In the control groups, survival remained essentially unchanged over the three days of the trial, suffering a slight deflection on the third day. The same trend was found for the groups treated with BPF, deltamethrin 2.16 mg/L, and deltamethrin 2.16 in association with BPF. The deaths that occurred in the above mentioned groups can be associated with a physiological death that was not statistically significant when compared to the control group. Since deltamethrin 2.16 mg/mL and BPF1 were found to be non-toxic, the combination was also found to be non-toxic and safe.

Honeybees treated with deltamethrin (21.6 mg/L) had a survival probability of 38% compared to the control (sugar syrup) at 1 day of treatment. There was therefore a reduced survival, which was statistically significant ($p \leq 0.001$) compared to the control group, already from day one of treatment. Even at day two, the difference between the two groups was statistically significant ($p \leq 0.001$); on day three, in the deltamethrin-treated group, all subjects had died. The groups fed BPF plus deltamethrin (21.6 mg/mL) after one day of treatment had a survival probability of 86%. At two days post-treatment, the survival probability was 72%, and at three days, it stood at 46%. Therefore, the combination with BPF statistically increased the survival of honeybees compared to those in the group fed deltamethrin at 21.6 mg/mL ($p \leq 0.001$).

Table 1. Results of the bergamot polyphenolic fraction (BPF) analysis.

Description	Specifications	Methods
Chemical Characteristics		
pH	3.0–4.0	
Average Mesh Size	Pass 70 mesh	IM (0.5% in water) at 25 °C
Mass Density	30–70 g/100 mL	Sieve: (CQ-MO-023)
Water Content	<10.0%	PT CHIM 65 rev 0 2011
Organic Solvent Residue	None	ISTISAN 96/34
Soluble in 40 °C H_2O	Good	GC: (CQ-MO-168)
Soluble in 50% H_2O + EtOH	Good	visual: (CQ-MO-148)
Active Ingredient Strength	HPLC	visual: (CQ-MO-148)
Pesticides Residue	Negative	PT CHIM 69rev 02 011
Active Ingredients	Unit	Range
Polyphenols (neoeriocitrin, naringin, neohesperidin, melitidin, bruteridin, and hesperetin)	%	38%
Heavy Metals		
Arsenic	ppm	<2.0
Lead	ppm	<2.0
Heavy Metal Tot. Quantity	ppm	<20.0
Microbiological Evaluation		
Aerobic Plate Count	<1000 CFU/g	ISO 4833-1:2013 [61]
Yeast and Mold Count	<100 CFU/g	ISO 21527-1:2008 [61]
E. coli	Negative	ISO 16694-2:2001 [61]
Coliform	Negative	ISO 4832:2006 [61]
Salmonella	Negative	UNI EN ISO 6579:2000 [61]
Staphilococcus aureus	Negative	UNI EN ISO 6888-2:2004 [61]
Streptococci	Negative	UNI EN ISO 7218:2007—PT BAT26 rev0 02012 [61]
Product Treatment		
Extraction Solvents	Water + KOH	
Drying Method	Spydry	

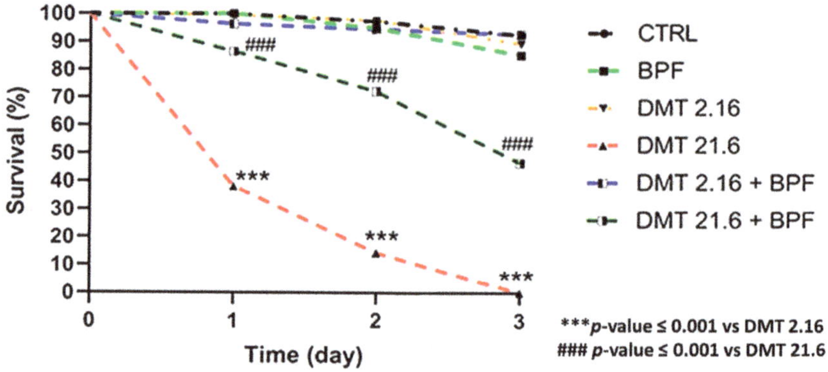

Figure 1. Honeybee survival curve.

3.3. Abnormal Behavior

The overall percentage of abnormal behavior throughout the duration of the experiment was taken as the basis for recording this data. Figure 2 depicts the trend in abnormal behavior for the various experimental groups.

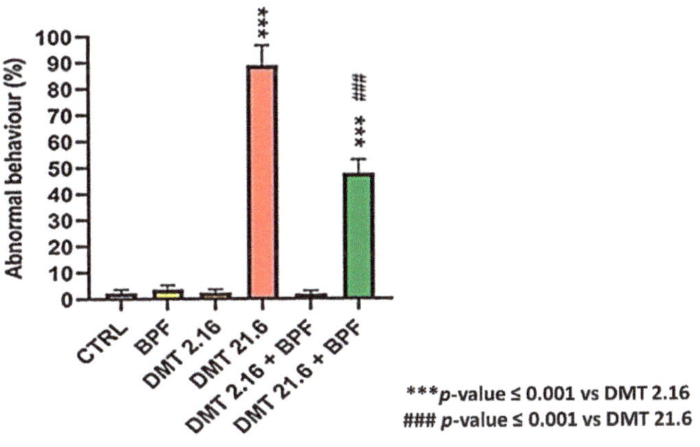

Figure 2. Abnormal behavior.

The BPF, deltamethrin 2.16, and deltamethrin 2.16 in combination with BPF groups did not present significant abnormal behaviors compared to the control group. Subjects in the deltamethrin 21.6 groups exhibited the highest percentage of abnormal behavior, involving precisely 88% of all subjects under treatment. The data was statistically significant compared to the control group ($p \leq 0.001$). BPF not only increased survival but also reduced the percentage of abnormal behaviors exhibited in a statistically significant manner compared to the deltamethrin 21.6 group ($p \leq 0.001$).

3.4. Feeding Solution Consumption

The results relating to the average consumption of the experimental groups recorded in the three days of treatment are depicted in Figure 3.

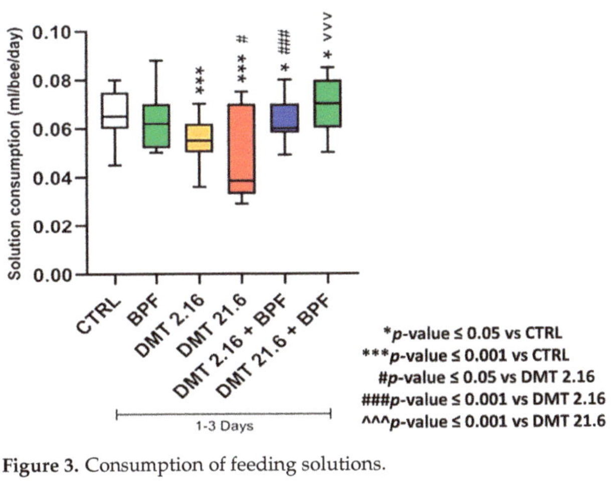

Figure 3. Consumption of feeding solutions.

The consumption was calculated by dividing the quantity of solution consumed by the number of surviving bees. Except for the BPF group, all experimental groups drank less solution than the control. The deltamethrin 21.6 group consumed food solution significantly less ($p \leq 0.05$) compared to deltamethrin 2.16. The deltamethrin 2.16 group, in association with BPF, resulted in significantly higher food consumption than the deltamethrin 2.16 group ($p \leq 0.001$). The groups with deltamethrin 21.6 in combination with BPF consumed more solution than both the control and deltamethrin 21.6 groups, with a statistical significance of less than 0.05 and 0.001, respectively.

4. Discussion

Beekeepers often utilize artificial food in the form of candies or syrup during the winter or to encourage the queen to oviposit. When the addition of food supplements to the normal diet is not dictated by management practices, they are dutifully necessary in ecosystems increasingly modified by man. Overbuilding, intensive agriculture, and increasingly monocultured land reduce the availability of food for honeybees, resulting in a shortage of nectar and pollen. Therefore, nowadays, honeybees' normal diet is often altered. The majority of the time, the food replacements employed lack some essential nutritious elements that make up the normal diet of these pollinating insects. Along with macronutrients (carbohydrates and proteins), honeybees' diets should also include trace elements and other substances, such as phenolic compounds, that have a significant influence on their capacity for detoxification. Phenolic compounds are among the components in honey that contribute most significantly to its antioxidant action [62]. The therapeutic qualities of honey are attributed to the phenolic chemicals found in honey, particularly the flavonoids and phenolic acid, which are important natural antioxidants of medicinal relevance [63]. Previous research has shown a considerable correlation between the antioxidant capabilities of honey derived from different floral sources and their phenolic content [64]. Numerous research investigations have also emphasized the benefits of including compounds with high nutritional value and rich in certain phenolic components. The molecular processes behind pesticide-induced toxicity entail the formation of free radicals, lipid peroxidation induction, and disruption of the body's overall antioxidant capacity [65]. There is a strong correlation between pesticide exposure, elevated reactive oxygen species, and oxidative stress induction. According to Uchendu et al. (2018) [66], deltamethrin and chlorpyrifos (CPF), which are classified as pyrethroid and organophosphate (OP) pesticides, respectively, cause oxidative stress by changing antioxidant defense systems and producing free radicals. The authors used a combination of pyrethroid and OP insecticides, which are often applied by farmers and kept close to cereals in certain nations, such as Nigeria [66]. Rats exposed to CPF and deltamethrin, either alone or in combination, exhibited considerably higher levels of malondialdehyde and significantly lower levels of catalase, superoxide dismutase, and glutathione peroxidase than the control group [66]. Citrus fruits have been widely reported for their strong bioactivities, such as antioxidant, anti-inflammatory, antimicrobial, etc., activities [67–70]. Over 40% of BPF is made up of flavonoids; the remaining 60% is made up of various chemicals, fatty acids, carbohydrates, pectins, and maltodextrins, which are added to facilitate exsiccation [71]. The flavonoids and flavonoid glycosides present in BPF are neoeriocitrin, naringin, neohesperidin, melitidin, bruteridin, and hesperetin. These flavonoids have a wide range of positive effects on animals, including anti-inflammatory, anti-allergic, antibacterial, and anti-apoptotic capabilities. Analyzing how Naringin interacts with pesticides in animal models has drawn more attention recently. Mani et al. (2015) [72] experimented to learn more about the ameliorating benefits of naringin (100 mg/kg BW by gavage, 21 days) against hepato-pathological and hematological impairments (12.8 mg/kg BW by gavage, 21 days) in rats intoxicated by deltamethrin. The researchers discovered that the percentages of neutrophils, eosinophils, monocytes, and white blood cells in the serum, as well as the degree of tissue damage, lipid peroxidation level, lactate dehydrogenase, AST, ALT, and ALP activities in the liver of rats given deltamethrin, were significantly higher than those of the control group. Naringin therapy significantly returned all prior values to normal ranges in deltamethrin-intoxicated rats, indicating that naringin acted as a protective agent against the hematotoxicity and hepatotoxicity associated with deltamethrin exposure. Naringin's efficacy in combating deltamethrin poisoning in rats may be attributed to its capacity to scavenge free radicals, its anti-inflammatory properties, and its immune- and defense-stimulating properties [72]. Positive results were also obtained by Agha et al. (2015) [73], who showed that Hesperidin supplementation before experimental deltamethrin intoxication drastically reduced the frequencies of chromosome aberrations and restored mitotic activity compared to the group treated with deltamethrin alone [73]. A recent study by Hybl et al. (2021) [18] showed that supplementation of phenolic acids and flavonoids to the diet of thiacloprid-intoxicated bees resulted in increased longevity, probably due to the increased detoxification capacity caused by the increased expression level of genes encoding the cytochrome P450 enzyme [18]. The BPF administered in our study could act both by attenuating the consequences of oxidative stress, such as lipid peroxidation, and by increasing the activity of the enzymatic systems deputed to detoxification. The protective results against pesticide intoxication obtained in this study with BPF were achieved in other animal species with other polyphenols of plant origin, such as quercetin, catechin, epicatechin, (−)-epigallocatechin-3-gallate, apigenin, luteolin, and taxifolin. It can be hypothesized that these other plants or their polyphenols may also have a similar protective action [74,75]. Based on the findings of this experimental study, the inclusion of phenolic compounds in the bee diet may, to a certain extent, increase the bees' capacity for detoxification, which is frequently decreased due to malnutrition brought on by environmental degradation and the ensuing loss and contamination of food resources, as well as by factors related to the routine management of beekeeping. The survival data that were recorded in the groups in which deltamethrin was associated with BPF are promising and encourage the integration of polyphenolic substances into the normal diet. In the present study, two doses of deltamethrin were used in connection with preliminary toxicity studies. The dose chosen of 21.6 mg/L was the one that allowed us to cause the death of caged subjects within 48 h, as required by the guidelines for the evaluation of acute toxicity. The lowest dose of 2.16 mg/L was chosen because it was the one that resulted in mild toxic effects, such as behavioral abnormalities. This dose allowed us to appreciate the protective effects of BPF against mild poisoning. The intoxicated subjects with the highest concentration of the pesticide managed to survive one day longer than those who received deltamethrin alone. On the second day, all the honeybees that had been intoxicated with deltamethrin (21.6 mg/mL) had died, while in the intoxicated groups to which BPF had been added, the honeybees remained alive until the third day, with a survival rate of 46%. There was no statistically significant difference regarding survival and mortality data between the control group and the group that had been fed BPF alone. BPF, therefore, proves to be safe. The improvement trend observed with survival is also common with anomalous behaviors. Intoxicated subjects administered BPF show a lower percentage of behavioral anomalies in both groups in which BPF was supplemented at the highest and lowest doses than in the respective groups without BPF supplementation. These described results are preliminary and need to be further developed to give more strength to our evidence; however, it can be asserted that the integration of compounds with high biological value into food substitutes could help honeybees respond better to pesticide-induced stress.

5. Conclusions

The use of pesticides in agriculture is a common practice for the control of insects, pests, and plant pathogens. Often, the compounds used do not have good selectivity for the target but can also harm insects valuable to ecosystems, such as honeybees. In such conditions, the discovery of mixtures and/or compounds that can protect or aid the detoxification of the organism is particularly important. In this study, the BPF was shown to increase the probability of survival of honeybees intoxicated by deltamethrin. BPF may reduce intoxication damage caused by exposure to this pesticide, probably by improving the body's detoxifying abilities. Subsequent studies are needed to better define the mechanisms by which BPF exerts its protective action. However, it can already be said that the addition of BPF as a dietary supplement could be of interest in improving the fitness of hives.

Author Contributions: Conceptualization, R.B. and F.C.; formal analysis, R.B., F.C., S.R., R.C. and S.N.; investigation, R.B., F.C., S.R., R.C. and S.N.; data curation, R.B. and S.R.; writing—original draft preparation, R.B., F.C., S.R., R.C., S.N., R.M.B., C.N., D.B., V.M. and E.P.; writing—review and editing, R.B., F.C., S.R., R.C., S.N., R.M.B., C.N., D.B., V.M. and E.P.; supervision, V.M. and E.P.; project administration, V.M. and E.P. All authors have read and agreed to the published version of the manuscript.

Funding: This research received no external funding.

Institutional Review Board Statement: Not applicable.

Informed Consent Statement: Not applicable.

Data Availability Statement: The data are kept at the University of Magna Græcia of Catanzaro and are available upon request.

Conflicts of Interest: All the authors declare no conflict of interest and that the research was conducted in the absence of any commercial or financial relationships that could be construed as a potential conflict of interest.

References

1. Kaplan, K. Colony collapse disorder a complex buzz. *Am. Bee J.* **2008**, *148*, 8–11.
2. Neumann, P.; Carreck, N.L. Honey bee colony losses. *J. Apic. Res.* **2010**, *49*, 1–6. [CrossRef]
3. Becher, M.A.; Osborne, J.L.; Thorbek, P.; Kennedy, P.J.; Grimm, V. Towards a systems approach for understanding honeybee decline: A stocktaking and synthesis of existing models. *J. Appl. Ecol.* **2013**, *50*, 868–880. [CrossRef] [PubMed]
4. Johnson, R.M.; Ellis, M.D.; Mullin, C.A.; Frazier, M. Pesticides and honey bee toxicity–USA. *Apidologie* **2010**, *41*, 312–331. [CrossRef]
5. Khan, B.A.; Nadeem, M.A.; Nawaz, H.; Amin, M.M.; Abbasi, G.H.; Nadeem, M.; Ali, M.; Ameen, M.; Javaid, M.M.; Maqbool, R. Pesticides: Impacts on agriculture productivity, environment, and management strategies. In *Emerging Contaminants and Plants: Interactions, Adaptations and Remediation Technologies*; Springer: Berlin/Heidelberg, Germany, 2023; pp. 109–134.
6. Kumar, V.; Sharma, N.; Sharma, P.; Pasrija, R.; Kaur, K.; Umesh, M.; Thazeem, B. Toxicity analysis of endocrine disrupting pesticides on non-target organisms: A critical analysis on toxicity mechanisms. *Toxicol. Appl. Pharmacol.* **2023**, *474*, 116623. [CrossRef] [PubMed]
7. Duke, S.O.; Kudsk, P.; Solomon, K.R. *Pesticide Dose: Effects on the Environment and Target and Non-Target Organisms*; American Chemical Society: Washington, DC, USA, 2017; ISBN 0841232113.
8. Rortais, A.; Arnold, G.; Dorne, J.-L.; More, S.J.; Sperandio, G.; Streissl, F.; Szentes, C.; Verdonck, F. Risk assessment of pesticides and other stressors in bees: Principles, data gaps and perspectives from the European Food Safety Authority. *Sci. Total Environ.* **2017**, *587*, 524–537. [CrossRef]
9. Krupke, C.H.; Long, E.Y. Intersections between neonicotinoid seed treatments and honey bees. *Curr. Opin. Insect Sci.* **2015**, *10*, 8–13. [CrossRef]
10. Lundin, O.; Rundlöf, M.; Smith, H.G.; Fries, I.; Bommarco, R. Neonicotinoid insecticides and their impacts on bees: A systematic review of research approaches and identification of knowledge gaps. *PLoS ONE* **2015**, *10*, e0136928. [CrossRef]
11. Davis, B.N.K.; Williams, C.T. Buffer zone widths for honeybees from ground and aerial spraying of insecticides. *Environ. Pollut.* **1990**, *63*, 247–259. [CrossRef]
12. AV, M.; Pandey, R.; Mall, P. Protecting honeybees from pesticides: A call to action. *Biodiversity* **2023**, *24*, 117–123.
13. Krupke, C.H.; Hunt, G.J.; Eitzer, B.D.; Andino, G.; Given, K. Multiple routes of pesticide exposure for honey bees living near agricultural fields. *PLoS ONE* **2012**, *7*, e29268. [CrossRef] [PubMed]
14. Rortais, A.; Arnold, G.; Halm, M.-P.; Touffet-Briens, F. Modes of honeybees exposure to systemic insecticides: Estimated amounts of contaminated pollen and nectar consumed by different categories of bees. *Apidologie* **2005**, *36*, 71–83. [CrossRef]
15. Medrzycki, P.; Giffard, H.; Aupinel, P.; Belzunces, L.P.; Chauzat, M.-P.; Classen, C.; Colin, M.E.; Dupont, T.; Girolami, V.; Johnson, R. Standard methods for toxicology research in *Apis mellifera*. *J. Apic. Res.* **2013**, *52*, 1–60. [CrossRef]
16. Mussen, E.C.; Lopez, J.E.; Peng, C.Y.S. Effects of selected fungicides on growth and development of larval honey bees, *Apis mellifera* L.(Hymenoptera: Apidae). *Environ. Entomol.* **2004**, *33*, 1151–1154. [CrossRef]
17. Tosi, S.; Nieh, J.C. Lethal and sublethal synergistic effects of a new systemic pesticide, flupyradifurone (Sivanto®), on honeybees. *Proc. R. Soc. B* **2019**, *286*, 20190433. [CrossRef]
18. Hýbl, M.; Mráz, P.; Šipoš, J.; Hoštičková, I.; Bohatá, A.; Čurn, V.; Kopec, T. Polyphenols as food supplement improved food consumption and longevity of honey bees (*Apis mellifera*) intoxicated by pesticide thiacloprid. *Insects* **2021**, *12*, 572. [CrossRef]
19. Doublet, V.; Labarussias, M.; de Miranda, J.R.; Moritz, R.F.A.; Paxton, R.J. Bees under stress: Sublethal doses of a neonicotinoid pesticide and pathogens interact to elevate honey bee mortality across the life cycle. *Environ. Microbiol.* **2015**, *17*, 969–983. [CrossRef]
20. Williams, G.R.; Troxler, A.; Retschnig, G.; Roth, K.; Yañez, O.; Shutler, D.; Neumann, P.; Gauthier, L. Neonicotinoid pesticides severely affect honey bee queens. *Sci. Rep.* **2015**, *5*, 14621. [CrossRef]

21. Laurino, D.; Porporato, M.; Patetta, A.; Manino, A. Toxicity of neonicotinoid insecticides to honey bees: Laboratory tests. *Bull. Insectology* **2011**, *64*, 107–113.
22. Gross, M. EU ban puts spotlight on complex effects of neonicotinoids. *Curr. Biol.* **2013**, *23*, R462–R464. [CrossRef]
23. Katsuda, Y. Progress and future of pyrethroids. *Top. Curr. Chem.* **2012**, *314*, 1–30.
24. Tang, W.; Wang, D.I.; Wang, J.; Wu, Z.; Li, L.; Huang, M.; Xu, S.; Yan, D. Pyrethroid pesticide residues in the global environment: An overview. *Chemosphere* **2018**, *191*, 990–1007. [CrossRef]
25. LaForge, F.B.; Gersdorff, W.A.; Green, N.; Schechter, M.S. Allethrin-type esters of cyclopropanecarboxylic acids and their relative toxicities to house flies. *J. Org. Chem.* **1952**, *17*, 381–389. [CrossRef]
26. Rehman, H.; Aziz, A.-T.; Saggu, S.; Abbas, Z.K.; Mohan, A.; Ansari, A.A. Systematic review on pyrethroid toxicity with special reference to deltamethrin. *J. Entomol. Zool. Stud.* **2014**, *2*, 60–70.
27. Palmquist, K.; Salatas, J.; Fairbrother, A. Pyrethroid insecticides: Use, environmental fate, and ecotoxicology. *Insectic. Integr. Pest Manag.* **2012**, 251–278. [CrossRef]
28. Kamrin, M.A. *Pesticide Profiles: Toxicity, Environmental Impact, and Fate*; CRC Press: Boca Raton, FL, USA, 1997; ISBN 1420049224.
29. Abdel-Daim, M.M.; El-Ghoneimy, A. Synergistic protective effects of ceftriaxone and ascorbic acid against subacute deltamethrin-induced nephrotoxicity in rats. *Ren. Fail.* **2015**, *37*, 297–304. [CrossRef] [PubMed]
30. Dai, P.; Wang, Q.; Sun, J.; Liu, F.; Wang, X.; Wu, Y.; Zhou, T. Effects of sublethal concentrations of bifenthrin and deltamethrin on fecundity, growth, and development of the honeybee *Apis mellifera ligustica*. *Environ. Toxicol. Chem. An Int. J.* **2010**, *29*, 644–649. [CrossRef] [PubMed]
31. Decourtye, A.; Devillers, J.; Cluzeau, S.; Charreton, M.; Pham-Delègue, M.-H. Effects of imidacloprid and deltamethrin on associative learning in honeybees under semi-field and laboratory conditions. *Ecotoxicol. Environ. Saf.* **2004**, *57*, 410–419. [CrossRef] [PubMed]
32. Zhang, Z.Y.; Li, Z.; Huang, Q.; Zhang, X.W.; Ke, L.; Yan, W.Y.; Zhang, L.Z.; Zeng, Z.J. Deltamethrin impairs honeybees (*Apis mellifera*) dancing communication. *Arch. Environ. Contam. Toxicol.* **2020**, *78*, 117–123. [CrossRef] [PubMed]
33. Vandame, R.; Belzunces, L.P. Joint actions of deltamethrin and azole fungicides on honey bee thermoregulation. *Neurosci. Lett.* **1998**, *251*, 57–60. [CrossRef]
34. Steffan-Dewenter, I.; Kuhn, A. Honeybee foraging in differentially structured landscapes. *Proc. R. Soc. London. Ser. B Biol. Sci.* **2003**, *270*, 569–575. [CrossRef] [PubMed]
35. Langlois, A.; Jacquemart, A.-L.; Piqueray, J. Contribution of extensive farming practices to the supply of floral resources for pollinators. *Insects* **2020**, *11*, 818. [CrossRef] [PubMed]
36. El Mohandes, S.S.; Nafea, E.A.; Fawzy, A.M. Effect of different feeding diets on the haemolymph of the newly emerged honeybee workers *Apis mellifera* L. *Egypt. Acad. J. Biol. Sci. A, Entomol.* **2010**, *3*, 113–220. [CrossRef]
37. De Jong, D.; da Silva, E.J.; Kevan, P.G.; Atkinson, J.L. Pollen substitutes increase honey bee haemolymph protein levels as much as or more than does pollen. *J. Apic. Res.* **2009**, *48*, 34–37. [CrossRef]
38. Johnson, R.; Resources, Science, and Industry Division. *Recent Honey Bee Colony Declines*; Congressional Research Service; Library of Congress, Congressional Research Service: Washington, DC, USA, 2007.
39. Hybl, M.; Mraz, P.; Sipos, J.; Pridal, A. Effects of phenolic bioactive substances on reducing mortality of bees (*Apis mellifera*) intoxicated by thiacloprid. In Proceedings of the MendelNet Conference, Brno, Czech Republic, 6–7 November 2019; pp. 6–7.
40. Mao, W.; Schuler, M.A.; Berenbaum, M.R. Honey constituents up-regulate detoxification and immunity genes in the western honey bee *Apis mellifera*. *Proc. Natl. Acad. Sci. USA* **2013**, *110*, 8842–8846. [CrossRef] [PubMed]
41. Cianciosi, D.; Forbes-Hernández, T.Y.; Afrin, S.; Gasparrini, M.; Reboredo-Rodriguez, P.; Manna, P.P.; Zhang, J.; Bravo Lamas, L.; Martínez Flórez, S.; Agudo Toyos, P. Phenolic compounds in honey and their associated health benefits: A review. *Molecules* **2018**, *23*, 2322. [CrossRef] [PubMed]
42. Liao, L.-H.; Wu, W.-Y.; Berenbaum, M.R. Impacts of dietary phytochemicals in the presence and absence of pesticides on longevity of honey bees (*Apis mellifera*). *Insects* **2017**, *8*, 22. [CrossRef]
43. Štrbac, F.; Krnjajić, S.; Stojanović, D.; Ratajac, R.; Simin, N.; Orčić, D.; Rinaldi, L.; Ciccone, E.; Maurelli, M.P.; Cringoli, G. *In vitro* and *in vivo* anthelmintic efficacy of peppermint (*Mentha piperita* L.) essential oil against gastrointestinal nematodes of sheep. *Front. Vet. Sci.* **2023**, *10*. [CrossRef]
44. Castagna, F.; Bava, R.; Musolino, V.; Piras, C.; Cardamone, A.; Carresi, C.; Lupia, C.; Bosco, A.; Rinaldi, L.; Cringoli, G. Potential new therapeutic approaches based on *Punica granatum* fruits compared to synthetic anthelmintics for the sustainable control of gastrointestinal nematodes in sheep. *Animals* **2022**, *12*, 2883. [CrossRef] [PubMed]
45. Bava, R.; Castagna, F.; Piras, C.; Palma, E.; Cringoli, G.; Musolino, V.; Lupia, C.; Perri, M.R.; Statti, G.; Britti, D.; et al. *In vitro* evaluation of acute toxicity of five citrus spp. Essential oils towards the parasitic mite *Varroa destructor*. *Pathogens* **2021**, *10*, 1182. [CrossRef]
46. Castagna, F.; Bava, R.; Piras, C.; Carresi, C.; Musolino, V.; Lupia, C.; Marrelli, M.; Conforti, F.; Palma, E.; Britti, D. Green Veterinary Pharmacology for Honey Bee Welfare and Health: *Origanum heracleoticum* L. (Lamiaceae) Essential Oil for the Control of the *Apis mellifera* Varroatosis. *Vet. Sci.* **2022**, *9*, 124. [CrossRef] [PubMed]
47. Bava, R.; Castagna, F.; Palma, E.; Musolino, V.; Carresi, C.; Cardamone, A.; Lupia, C.; Marrelli, M.; Conforti, F.; Roncada, P. Phytochemical Profile of *Foeniculum vulgare* subsp. *piperitum* Essential oils and evaluation of acaricidal efficacy against *Varroa destructor* in *Apis mellifera* by in *vitro* and semi-field fumigation tests. *Vet. Sci.* **2022**, *9*, 684. [CrossRef] [PubMed]

48. Gliozzi, M.; Walker, R.; Muscoli, S.; Vitale, C.; Gratteri, S.; Carresi, C.; Musolino, V.; Russo, V.; Janda, E.; Ragusa, S. Bergamot polyphenolic fraction enhances rosuvastatin-induced effect on LDL-cholesterol, LOX-1 expression and protein kinase B phosphorylation in patients with hyperlipidemia. *Int. J. Cardiol.* **2013**, *170*, 140–145. [CrossRef] [PubMed]
49. Ferro, Y.; Montalcini, T.; Mazza, E.; Foti, D.; Angotti, E.; Gliozzi, M.; Nucera, S.; Paone, S.; Bombardelli, E.; Aversa, I. Randomized clinical trial: Bergamot citrus and wild cardoon reduce liver steatosis and body weight in non-diabetic individuals aged over 50 years. *Front. Endocrinol.* **2020**, *11*, 494. [CrossRef]
50. Musolino, V.; Gliozzi, M.; Carresi, C.; Maiuolo, J.; Mollace, R.; Bosco, F.; Scarano, F.; Scicchitano, M.; Maretta, A.; Palma, E. Lipid-lowering effect of bergamot polyphenolic fraction: Role of pancreatic cholesterol ester hydrolase. *J. Biol. Regul. Homeost. Agents* **2017**, *31*, 1087–1093.
51. Mirarchi, A.; Mare, R.; Musolino, V.; Nucera, S.; Mollace, V.; Pujia, A.; Montalcini, T.; Romeo, S.; Maurotti, S. Bergamot polyphenol extract reduces hepatocyte neutral fat by increasing beta-oxidation. *Nutrients* **2022**, *14*, 3434. [CrossRef]
52. Musolino, V.; Gliozzi, M.; Nucera, S.; Carresi, C.; Maiuolo, J.; Mollace, R.; Paone, S.; Bosco, F.; Scarano, F.; Scicchitano, M.; et al. The effect of bergamot polyphenolic fraction on lipid transfer protein system and vascular oxidative stress in a rat model of hyperlipemia. *Lipids Health Dis.* **2019**, *18*, 115. [CrossRef] [PubMed]
53. Mollace, V.; Sacco, I.; Janda, E.; Malara, C.; Ventrice, D.; Colica, C.; Visalli, V.; Muscoli, S.; Ragusa, S.; Muscoli, C. Hypolipemic and hypoglycaemic activity of bergamot polyphenols: From animal models to human studies. *Fitoterapia* **2011**, *82*, 309–316. [CrossRef]
54. Maiuolo, J.; Mollace, R.; Bosco, F.; Scarano, F.; Oppedisano, F.; Nucera, S.; Ruga, S.; Guarnieri, L.; Macri, R.; Bava, I. The phytochemical synergistic properties of combination of bergamot polyphenolic fraction and *Cynara cardunculus* extract in non-alcoholic fatty liver disease. *Agriculture* **2023**, *13*, 249. [CrossRef]
55. Carresi, C.; Musolino, V.; Gliozzi, M.; Maiuolo, J.; Mollace, R.; Nucera, S.; Maretta, A.; Sergi, D.; Muscoli, S.; Gratteri, S. Anti-oxidant effect of bergamot polyphenolic fraction counteracts doxorubicin-induced cardiomyopathy: Role of autophagy and c-kitposCD45negCD31neg cardiac stem cell activation. *J. Mol. Cell Cardiol.* **2018**, *119*, 10–18. [CrossRef]
56. Ciani, F.; Huggard, J.; Zervas, T. *The Resilience of Bergamot Farmers in the Reggio Calabria Province of Southern Italy*; Dipartimento di Scienze per l'Economia, Universita'degli Studi di Firenze: Firenze, Italy, 2014.
57. Williams, G.R.; Alaux, C.; Costa, C.; Csaki, T.; Doublet, V.; Eisenhardt, D.; Fries, I.; Kuhn, R.; McMahon, D.P.; Medrzycki, P. Standard methods for maintaining adult *Apis mellifera* in cages under *in vitro* laboratory conditions. *J. Apic. Res.* **2013**, *52*, 1–36. [CrossRef]
58. OECD/OCDE OECD Guideline 245 for the Testing of Chemicals. Honey Bee (*Apis mellifera* L.), Chronic Oral Toxicity Test (10-Day Feeding). 2017. Available online: https://www.oecd-ilibrary.org/environment/test-no-245-honey-bee-apis-mellifera-l-chronic-oral-toxicity-test-10-day-feeding_9789264284081-en (accessed on 5 October 2023). [CrossRef]
59. Musolino, V.; Gliozzi, M.; Bombardelli, E.; Nucera, S.; Carresi, C.; Maiuolo, J.; Mollace, R.; Paone, S.; Bosco, F.; Scarano, F. The synergistic effect of *Citrus bergamia* and *Cynara cardunculus* extracts on vascular inflammation and oxidative stress in non-alcoholic fatty liver disease. *J. Tradit. Complement. Med.* **2020**, *10*, 268–274. [CrossRef] [PubMed]
60. Ilari, S.; Lauro, F.; Giancotti, L.A.; Malafoglia, V.; Dagostino, C.; Gliozzi, M.; Condemi, A.; Maiuolo, J.; Oppedisano, F.; Palma, E. The Protective Effect of Bergamot Polyphenolic Fraction (BPF) on Chemotherapy-Induced Neuropathic Pain. *Pharmaceuticals* **2021**, *14*, 975. [CrossRef] [PubMed]
61. Available online: https://www.iso.org/home.html (accessed on 12 October 2023).
62. Yao, L.; Jiang, Y.; D'Arcy, B.; Singanusong, R.; Datta, N.; Caffin, N.; Raymont, K. Quantitative high-performance liquid chromatography analyses of flavonoids in Australian Eucalyptus honeys. *J. Agric. Food Chem.* **2004**, *52*, 210–214. [CrossRef] [PubMed]
63. Gheldof, N.; Wang, X.-H.; Engeseth, N.J. Identification and quantification of antioxidant components of honeys from various floral sources. *J. Agric. Food Chem.* **2002**, *50*, 5870–5877. [CrossRef] [PubMed]
64. Dong, R.; Zheng, Y.; Xu, B. Phenolic profiles and antioxidant capacities of Chinese unifloral honeys from different botanical and geographical sources. *Food bioprocess Technol.* **2013**, *6*, 762–770. [CrossRef]
65. Abdollahi, M.; Ranjbar, A.; Shadnia, S.; Nikfar, S.; Rezaie, A. Pesticides and oxidative stress: A review. *Med. Sci. Monit.* **2004**, *10*, 141–147.
66. Uchendu, C.; Ambali, S.F.; Ayo, J.O.; Esievo, K.A.N. Chronic co-exposure to chlorpyrifos and deltamethrin pesticides induces alterations in serum lipids and oxidative stress in Wistar rats: Mitigating role of alpha-lipoic acid. *Environ. Sci. Pollut. Res.* **2018**, *25*, 19605–19611. [CrossRef]
67. İnan, Ö.; Özcan, M.M.; Aljuhaimi, F. Effect of location and *Citrus* species on total phenolic, antioxidant, and radical scavenging activities of some *Citrus* seed and oils. *J. Food Process. Preserv.* **2018**, *42*, e13555. [CrossRef]
68. Sicari, V.; Pellicanò, T.M.; Giuffrè, A.M.; Zappia, C.; Capocasale, M. Bioactive compounds and antioxidant activity of citrus juices produced from varieties cultivated in Calabria. *J. Food Meas. Charact.* **2016**, *10*, 773–780. [CrossRef]
69. Xi, W.; Zhang, Y.; Sun, Y.; Shen, Y.; Ye, X.; Zhou, Z. Phenolic composition of Chinese wild mandarin (*Citrus reticulata balnco.*) pulps and their antioxidant properties. *Ind. Crops Prod.* **2014**, *52*, 466–474. [CrossRef]
70. Al-Jabri, N.N.; Hossain, M.A. Chemical composition and antimicrobial potency of locally grown lemon essential oil against selected bacterial strains. *J. King Saud Univ.* **2018**, *30*, 14–20. [CrossRef]
71. Salerno, R.; Casale, F.; Calandruccio, C.; Procopio, A. Characterization of flavonoids in *Citrus bergamia* (Bergamot) polyphenolic fraction by liquid chromatography–high resolution mass spectrometry (LC/HRMS). *PharmaNutrition* **2016**, *4*, S1–S7. [CrossRef]

72. Mani, V.M.; Ali, A.L.; Gokulakrishnan, A.; Sadiq, A.M. Pyrethroid deltamethrin induced haematological and hepato-pathological impairment in male Wistar rats and potential attenuation by flavonoid naringin. *Sci. Humanit.* **2015**, *1*, 623–640.
73. Agha, F.E.; Raouf, A.A.; Ahmed, A.A.M. Vitamin C and hesperidin attenuate deltamethrin–induced genotoxicity, sperm abnormalities and biochemical alterations in rats. *World J. Pharm. Res.* **2015**, *4*, 111–135.
74. Hussein, S.A.; El Senosi, Y.A.; Mansour, M.K.; Hassan, M.F. Potential protective effects of Quercetin on metalaxyl-induced oxidative stress, impaired liver functions and hepatotoxicity in rat. *Benha Vet. Med. J.* **2017**, *33*, 517–532. [CrossRef]
75. Afolabi, O.K.; Aderibigbe, F.A.; Folarin, D.T.; Arinola, A.; Wusu, A.D. Oxidative stress and inflammation following sub-lethal oral exposure of cypermethrin in rats: Mitigating potential of epicatechin. *Heliyon* **2019**, *5*, e02274. [CrossRef]

animals

MDPI

Article

Vitamin B_{12} Ameliorates Pesticide-Induced Sociability Impairment in Zebrafish (*Danio rerio*): A Prospective Controlled Intervention Study

Madalina Andreea Robea [1], Ovidiu Dumitru Ilie [2], Mircea Nicusor Nicoara [3,4,*], Gheorghe Solcan [5], Laura Ecaterina Romila [6], Dorel Ureche [7,*] and Alin Ciobica [3,8,9]

1 Doctoral School of Biology, Faculty of Biology, "Alexandru Ioan Cuza" University of Iasi, Bd. Carol I, 20A, 700505 Iasi, Romania; madalina.robea11@gmail.com
2 Department of Mother and Child, Faculty of Medicine, University of Medicine and Pharmacy "Grigore T. Popa", University Street No. 16, 700115 Iasi, Romania; ovidiuilie90@yahoo.com
3 Department of Biology, Faculty of Biology, "Alexandru Ioan Cuza" University of Iasi, Bd. Carol I, 20A, 700505 Iasi, Romania; alin.ciobica@uaic.ro
4 Doctoral School of Geosciences, Faculty of Geography and Geology, "Alexandru Ioan Cuza" University of Iasi, 700505 Iasi, Romania
5 Internal Medicine Clinic, Faculty of Veterinary Medicine, Ion Ionescu de la Brad Iasi University of Life Sciences, 700489 Iasi, Romania; gsolcan@yahoo.com
6 Preclinical Department, Apollonia University, Pacurari Street 11, 700511 Iasi, Romania; laura_ekaa@yahoo.com
7 Department of Biology, Ecology and Environmental Protection, Faculty of Sciences, University "Vasile Alecsandri" of Bacau, Calea Marasesti Street, No. 157, 600115 Bacau, Romania
8 Academy of Romanian Scientists, 54, Independence Street, Sector 5, 050094 Bucharest, Romania
9 Center of Biomedical Research, Romanian Academy, Iasi Branch, Teodor Codrescu 2, 700481 Iasi, Romania
* Correspondence: mirmag@uaic.ro (M.N.N.); dureche@ub.ro (D.U.)

Simple Summary: Dietary vitamin supplementation is frequently mentioned as an alternative therapy for people with autism but is still controversial due to a lack of studies. The current study described a hypothetical real-life situation and evaluated the effect of vitamin B_{12} on the behavior of zebrafish. Vitamin-treated fish showed behavioral improvements after 14 days of daily exposure. In addition, the presence of the vitamin improved the redox state, leading to increased activity of antioxidant enzymes.

Abstract: Constant exposure to a variety of environmental factors has become increasingly problematic. A variety of illnesses are initiated or aided by the presence of certain perturbing factors. In the case of autism spectrum disorder, the environmental component plays an important part in determining the overall picture. Moreover, the lack of therapies to relieve existing symptoms complicates the fight against this condition. As a result, animal models have been used to make biomedical research easier and more suited for disease investigations. The current study used zebrafish as an animal model to mimic a real-life scenario: acute exposure to an increased dose of pesticides, followed by prospective intervention-based therapy with vitamin B_{12} (vit. B_{12}). It is known that vit. B_{12} is involved in brain function nerve tissue, and red blood cell formation. Aside from this, the role of vit. B_{12} in the redox processes is recognized for its help against free radicals. To investigate the effect of vit. B_{12}, fish were divided into four different groups and exposed to a pesticide mixture (600 $\mu g\ L^{-1}$ fipronil + 600 $\mu g\ L^{-1}$ pyriproxyfen) and 0.24 $\mu g\ L^{-1}$ vit. B_{12} for 14 days. The impact of the compounds was assessed daily with EthoVision XT 11.5 software for behavioral observations, especially for sociability, quantified by the social interaction test. In addition, at the end of the study, the activities of superoxide dismutase (SOD), glutathione peroxidase (GPx), and malondialdehyde (MDA) were measured. The results showed significant improvements in locomotor activity parameters and a positive influence of the vitamin on sociability. Regarding the state of oxidative stress, high activity was found for SOD and GPx in the case of vit. B_{12}, while fish exposed to the mixture of pesticides and vit. B_{12} had a lower level of MDA. In conclusion, the study provides new data about the effect of vit. B_{12} in zebrafish, highlighting the potential use of vitamin supplementation to maintain and support the function of the organism.

Keywords: *Danio rerio*; behavior; autism spectrum disorder; pesticide; vitamin B_{12}; oxidative stress

1. Introduction

Being one of the eight vitamins of group B, vitamin B_{12} (vit. B_{12}), also called cobalamin due to the presence of the mineral cobalt in its structure, has often been mentioned as essential for cellular metabolism [1]. It is known to be involved in the synthesis of DNA molecules and myelin but also intervenes in the mediation of oxidative stress [2]. Its deficiency in the body has been linked to motor alterations, memory loss, irritability, poor balance, and cognitive impairment [1–3]. It has frequently been associated with increased anemia; alterations in the central or peripheral nervous system; and the onset of mechanisms prior to disorders such as autism spectrum disorder (ASD), schizophrenia, and epilepsy [3–5]. Despite the established recommended intake, which can vary across countries and continents, vit. B_{12} levels can be recorded at different values that indicate a deficiency. For instance, children, adolescents, women of childbearing age, and the elderly are considered vulnerable to vit. B_{12} deficiency, according to Vargas-Uricoechea et al. [6]. With an underrecognized capacity to be considered a serious disorder, this deficiency can be heightened by autoimmune conditions, alcohol consumption, malabsorption, or a dietary insufficiency (e.g., in vegetarians) [7]. Additionally, vit. B_{12} serves as a cofactor for two enzymes [8]. Methionine synthase in the cytoplasm requires vit. B_{12} in the form of methylcobalamin to catalyze the conversion of homocysteine to methionine. If the process is impaired due to a lack of vit. B_{12}, the intracellular homocysteine level increases, homocysteine being implicated in the mediation of ROS buildup, e.g., homocysteine auto-oxidation [9]. Vit. B_{12} is also essential for the mitochondrial enzyme methylmalonyl CoA mutase, which converts methylmalonyl CoA to succinyl CoA, a step in the oxidation of odd-chain fatty acids and the catabolism of ketogenic amino acids [1].

Mentioned for the first time in 1985, the concept of "oxidative stress" has been defined as an imbalance between oxidants and antioxidants, characterizing the capacity of an organism to maintain its physiological state [10–12]. Usually, increased levels of reactive oxygen species (ROS) are linked to important changes in cell functioning that lead to biomolecule damage and, in the end, can be a determining factor causing cell apoptosis [13,14]. It has been indicated that there is a strong correlation between ASD and oxidative stress [15].

Recognized through the presence of significant disruptions in speech and social skills and through repetitive behavior, ASD is a well-known neurodevelopmental illness that started to gain more attention due to its high incidence [16,17]. Recent data have highlighted the prevalence of ASD among US children, estimated at 1 in 36 [18]. The rate of prevalence depends on several variables. For instance, it has been shown that the frequency of ASD is greater for Asian children, non-Hispanic Black children, children with higher Social Vulnerability Index scores, and children who receive treatment in urban primary care locations [19]. Additionally, the sex-ratio difference is another concern among specialists. There are reports that present a much higher incidence for boys than girls in detecting ASD, and this is due to the complicated process needed to discover the specific features of autism in girls [20]. In real-world practice, according to the Diagnostic and Statistical Manual of Mental Disorders (DSM-V), ASD is diagnosed based on three main characteristics: difficulty in social communication; deficiencies in social relationships; and specific, repetitive patterns of behavior, activities or interests [21–23]. Although its etiology is not fully understood, ASD may be seen from a complex perspective that combines genetic and environmental components [17,24–26]. The most common cause is genetic susceptibility, although prenatal stress, infections, parental age, dysfunctional familial relationships, and exposure to neurotoxic chemicals are all believed to be risk factors [27–31].

For instance, the lack of a sufficient amount of cobalamin in the bodies of autistic people is mainly due to poor nutrition, specifically in terms of micronutrients, but this is not the only cause [4,32]. Data on the prevalence of clinical eating issues such as anorexia nervosa and bulimia nervosa in the population with autism are limited, but the latest results indicate that these conditions are more common in people with autism and/or attention-deficit/hyperactivity disorder (ADHD) than in the general population [33–36]. Moreover, screening for vit. B_{12} in children diagnosed with ASD showed lower vitamin levels in those children than in the control group, according to several studies [37–40]. Methylcobalamin supplementation has been proven to be effective for participants in several studies carried out, leading to a relief of autism-related symptoms [41–45]. Even though little research has been conducted on the effect of vit. B_{12} in ASD or its effectiveness in alleviating core or associated symptoms, it appears that the current evidence supports the vitamin's capacity to help and even to be regarded as a prospective treatment intervention [45].

The role of vit. B_{12} has long been recognized, starting with the preliminary data obtained from experimental research, whose outcomes contributed to new data acquisition. For instance, vitamin activity has been investigated in several studies that used animals as model organisms (zebrafish, mice, rats) for a specific disorder. Although an animal model cannot mimic 100% of human features, there are three rules for validating its suitability as a model; it should have similar causes or mechanisms of onset, similar symptoms, and similar responsiveness to treatment [46,47]. In this study, the zebrafish (*Danio rerio*) was chosen due to its multiple advantages, and it was considered to be eligible for development as an animal model for ASD, a fact highlighted by numerous reports [48–52]. In addition, it possesses the full complement of cobalamin metabolic enzymes, and a deficiency of this nutrient can be caused by mutations in mmachc, a gene responsible for vit. B_{12} activity regulation [8,53,54]. According to Sloan et al. [53], zebrafish with mmachc mutant alleles showed impaired growth and developmental delays but also responded to established therapies, suggesting that this may be a suitable model for studying cobalamin deficiency. A 2012 study evaluated the effect of various vit. B_{12} levels in zebrafish and demonstrated that 5 µg vit. B_{12} kg^{-1} was insufficient to support whole-body vitamin storage, but there were also no signs of deficiency [55]. When vit. B_{12} was administered in a mixture with 100 µg L^{-1} malathion, an organophosphate insecticide, it led to an arousal of the motor functions by modulating acetylcholinesterase activity. These results were further supported by the diminished oxidative-stress status [56].

Aside from the genetic component, the environment has recently attracted increased attention as a risk factor for ASD. Specialists started to point out the involvement of the environment in ASD and the negative impact [16,24,28,30]. An imbalance between excitatory and inhibitory neuronal activity in most cases of ASD has been hypothesized as a common underlying defect with many converging etiologies. For example, the impairment of gamma-aminobutyric acid (GABA) neurotransmission in autistic people is described by numerous reports [57–59]. These findings led to the choice of a mixture of pesticides (fipronil and pyriproxyfen), whose synergistic effect was correlated with the induction of GABA malfunction. Fipronil (FIP) is a compound from the phenylpyrazole class of insecticides that acts on the insect nervous system [60]. The main mechanism of action is the inhibition of GABA receptors and glutamate-gated chloride channels, and, depending of the dose, this can end in extreme neuronal excitation until the death of the organism [61,62]. Pyriproxyfen (PYR) is a compound that mimics the natural hormone for insect growth [63]. Both compounds, alone or in a mixture, are linked to developmental and histological abnormalities, behavioral disturbances, and elevated levels of oxidative stress [64–73].

Due to the increased role of the environment as a risk factor for ASD and the need for new therapeutic interventions for autistic people, the present study aimed to evaluate the effects of vit. of B_{12} and a mixture of pesticides administered individually or in combination in a zebrafish animal model, mimicking a real-life scenario. This objective was approached in the following steps: (1) evaluation of the effect of the compounds on locomotor activity, (2) characterization of sociability after exposure to the compounds, and (3) measurement of specific parameters of oxidative stress.

2. Materials and Methods

2.1. Animals

A total of 200 zebrafish juveniles (*Danio rerio*, WT AB, 2–3 months, ≈2 cm body length, 0.22 ± 0.05 g body weight, sex ratio 1:1) were obtained from an authorized local supplier and kept in the laboratory for three weeks as an acclimatization period. The water in the housing aquarium was replaced every 48 h with dechlorinated tap water, and the water in the experimental tanks was changed every single day. The water parameters were constantly measured and kept at normal values using filtration and an air pump (Table 1). The tanks were illuminated with LED bends (307.5 LUX) with a photoperiodic cycle of 14:10 h (light:dark). The fish were fed twice a day with TetraMin Tropical Flakes (5% of body weight in food per day, of which vit. B_{12} accounted for approximately 0.12 µg).

Table 1. Environmental conditions from the housing and experimental tanks observed during the experimental period.

Type of Tank	Temperature (°C)	pH	Conductivity (µS cm^{-1})	Salinity	Ammonia (mg L^{-1})	Dissolved Oxygen (%)
Housing tank	26 ± 0.5	7.6	551	0.26	0.05	90.8
Experimental tanks	25 ± 0.5	7.5	553	0.24	0.06	90.7

2.2. Chemicals

The pesticide mixture used in this study was purchased from a veterinary store in liquid form. The product purchased was mainly made up of the two pesticides (67.5 mg FIP and 67.5 mg PYR) but also contained other chemicals such as 0.3 mg of butylated hydroxyanisole, 60 mg of benzyl alcohol, and 0.15 mg of butylhydroxytoluene. The concentration of each pesticide compound was 600 µg L^{-1}, which was achieved by dissolving a certain quantity of the previously prepared stock solution into the medium. Vit. B_{12} was bought from a local pharmacy as tablets of a recommended product for dietary supplementation, and the formulation contained microcrystalline cellulose, dicalcium phosphate, hypromellose, cellulose powder, magnesium stearate, and stearic acid in addition to the vitamin. The concentration of the vitamin used was 0.24 µg L^{-1}. Each solution was prepared daily by grinding the tablets and dissolving the fragments in a 100 mL volumetric flask. Plastic vials with lids were filled with 40 mL of solution (prepared by dissolving a certain amount of the stock solution), and the fish were kept for 30 min according to Pena's protocol [74]. The chemicals used in this protocol (the pesticide mixture and the vitamin tablets) were commercial compounds, since it is more common to use them that way than in the pure state of the active ingredients (to avoid conflicts of interest, the brands of the products will not be mentioned). The oxidative stress analysis was performed using the Superoxide Dismutase Determination Kit (SOD, 19160-1KT-F,); Glutathione Peroxidase Cellular Activity Assay Kit (GPx, CGP1-1KT,); and Total Protein Kit, Micro Lowry, Peterson's Modification (TP0300-1KT) from Merck, Darmstadt, Germany. In addition, malondialdehyde (MDA) levels were assessed through the thiobarbituric acid-reactive substances assay according to the protocol of Balmus et al. [75].

2.3. Experimental Design

The fish were randomly transferred from the housing aquarium to the experimental tanks, with a capacity of 5 L each, and left to adjust to the new space. Four experimental groups were divided from each other as follows: untreated, 0.24 µg L^{-1} vit. B_{12}, 600 µg L^{-1} FIP + PYR, and 0.24 µg L^{-1} vit. B_{12} + 600 µg L^{-1} FIP + PYR. Zebrafish juveniles were exposed to a single dose of the pesticide mixture, while vit. B_{12} was administered for a period of two weeks in order to simulate a real-life situation.

Following the accommodation period, the initial behavior of each fish was evaluated through the locomotor activity and social interaction tests.

A newly prepared pesticide solution was dissolved directly into the experimental tanks for the mixture and mixture + vit. groups. As regards vitamin administration, this was performed by placing each fish in a plastic vial filled with vit. B_{12} solution and leaving it in for 30 min. The control and mixture groups simulated exposure to the vitamin. Each fish was tested in the T-maze to collect data on locomotor activity and sociability as in the initial assessment of behavior. These tests were repeated daily for two weeks. Data were acquired every day using a camera situated above the maze, connected to a computer with EthoVision XT 11.5 software (Noldus Information Technology, Wageningen, Holland), with which all the behavioral parameters were calculated. In the end, fish were killed by immersion in ice-cold water for a minimum of 5 min after opercular motion had stopped and then stored in the freezer at −80 °C for oxidative stress analysis. The study included two more replicates. A schematic representation of the entire study is presented in Figure 1.

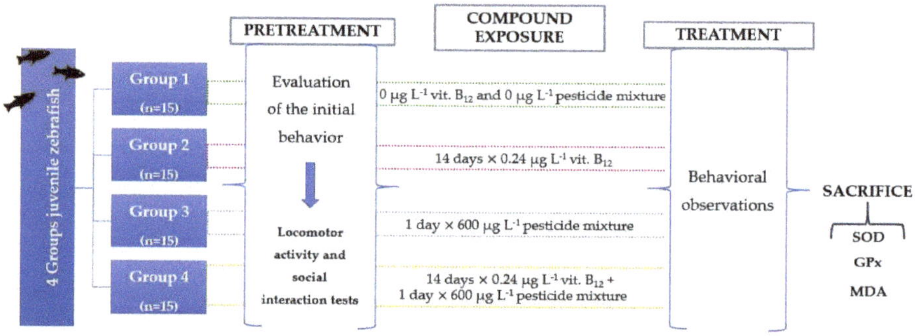

Figure 1. The experimental design of the study for evaluating the impact of vitamin B_{12} and pesticide mixture on zebrafish.

2.4. Behavioral Tests

2.4.1. Locomotor Activity Test

The specific locomotor activity parameters of the animals were measured before and after the treatment using a T-maze adapted for this test. The experimental apparatus is made from transparent Plexiglass (40 × 30 × 10 cm, length × height × width) and divided into three arms: left, right, and center (Figure 2). The starting point was established at the end of the center arm. To investigate the impact of the compounds on animals, a series of parameters were chosen to describe the locomotor activity. The total distance swum was the first one chosen; it represents the total distance travelled by fish in the T-maze (cm) during a trial. Secondly, the average velocity parameter refers to how fast the fish is moving (cm s^{-1}), while maximum acceleration is defined as the fish's maximum speed of reaction (cm s^{-2}). In addition, the time spent active or inactive describes the amount of time in which the fish was or was not moving (s). Each trial had a duration of 4 min, and an experimental session was carried out every day between 9 a.m. and 6 p.m.

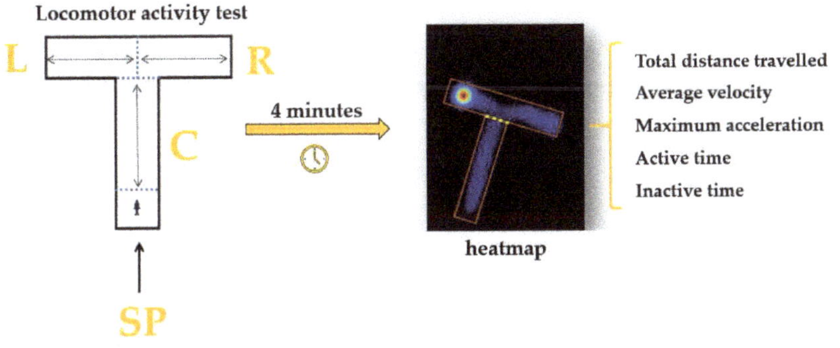

Figure 2. The T-maze adaptation for performing the locomotor activity test; C: center arm, L: left arm, R: right arm, and SP: start point.

2.4.2. Social Interaction Test

The social interaction test aims to assess the tendency of an individual to choose and/or spend time next to its conspecifics. This test used the same experimental apparatus described in the previous subsection, but with several adaptations. A transparent wall was added in the left arm to divide the area into two zones: the social stimulus and the tested zone (Figure 3). In the social stimulus zone was placed a group of three animals (from the same group tested and with a different sex ratio every day), while the tested zone corresponded to the experimental fish. Each fish was allowed to swim freely in all arms, except for the social stimulus zone, which was separated. Social behavior was quantified by recording the time spent by fish next to the social stimulus zone in a session of 4 min. Beside this, the time spent in the center and right arms was measured.

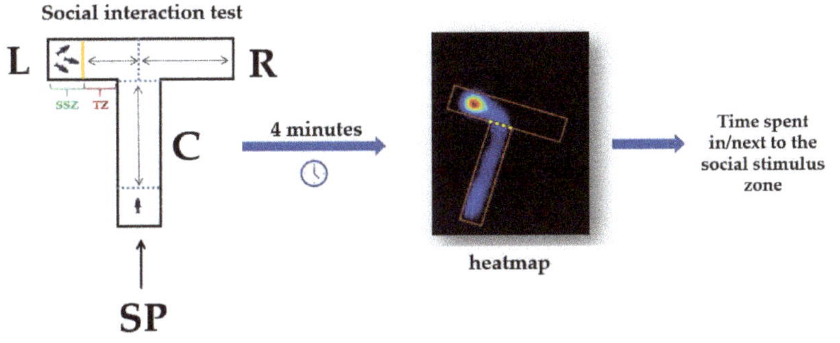

Figure 3. The T-maze adaptation for performing the social interaction test; C: center arm, L: left arm, R: right arm, SP: start point, SSZ: social stimulus zone, TZ: tested zone.

2.5. Oxidative Stress Measurement

At the end of the chronic exposure, all the experimental fish were killed by immersion in cold water (under 5 °C) and kept in the freezer for the oxidative stress analysis. To measure the oxidative stress markers, each fish was defrosted and homogenized in ice-cold saline (0.90% NaCl). Afterward, all the samples were centrifuged at 5500 rpm for 15 min following Jin's protocol [76]. The obtained supernatant was used to determine the SOD and GPx activity, MDA level, and protein concentrations. The enzyme activity was determined according to the suggested protocols from the kit packages and quantified with a Specord 210 Plus spectrophotometer from Analytik Jena, Jena, Germany, at the following specific wavelengths: 450 nm for SOD, 340 nm for GPx, and 532 nm for MDA. Protein was measured using the Bradford method and determined at 595 nm [77]. Each sample was tested in triplicate (Supplementary Materials), and values were presented as the average ± SEM.

2.6. Statistical Analysis

OriginPro v.9.8 software (OriginLab Corporation, Northampton, MA, USA, 2021) was used to realize the statistical analysis for both experimental tests. The first step in analyzing the data consisted of verifying of the normality of the data distribution through the Shapiro–Wilk test. When normality was confirmed, Tukey's post hoc test was applied to demonstrate the significant differences between group parameters before and after the treatment period. The α value was established at 0.05 to indicate the mean differences between the group, with the data being expressed as the average ± standard error of the mean (S.E.M.). The graphic presentation of the results for the locomotor activity and social interaction tests was generated using OriginPro software and Microsoft Package Excel files (Microsoft Office Professional Plus 2021) for oxidative stress results.

2.7. Ethical Note

The guidelines for the accommodation and care of animals used for experimental and other scientific purposes, Directive 2010/63/EU of the European Parliament, and the Council of 22 September 2010 on the protection of animals used for scientific purposes were strictly followed and maintained [78,79]. Additionally, this experiment was approved by the Ethical Commission of the Faculty of Veterinary Medicine, University of Agricultural Sciences and Veterinary Medicine Iasi, with registration number 750/04.07.2019.

3. Results

3.1. Short-Term Changes in Locomotor Activity Due to the Presence of Vitamin B_{12}

The total distance swum by the control group did not reveal any changes during the experimental period (initial behavior: 886.3 ± 206.1 cm vs. the average of the study period: 886.6 ± 181.3 cm, $p > 0.05$, Tukey, ANOVA). Compared to the control group's activity, the total distance for the 0.24 μg L^{-1} vit. B_{12} group registered increased values, with maximum peaks on D_5 (1518.3 ± 238.1 cm, $p = 0.03$, Tukey, ANOVA), D_7 (1333.4 ± 157.2 cm, $p = 0.04$, Tukey, ANOVA), and D_8 (1485.9 ± 152.8 cm, $p = 0.04$, Tukey, ANOVA) in contrast to the initial average: 755.1 ± 74.5 cm (Figure 4). A single exposure to the 600 μg L^{-1} FIP + PYR mixture triggered a decrease in the distance travelled in the first day (735.8 ± 166.4 cm, $p > 0.05$, Tukey, ANOVA) in comparison to the initial behavior (1090.1 ± 149.9 cm), but in the following days, the values of this parameter exhibited an upward trend—specifically, on D_2 (1638.5 ± 421.8 cm), D_5 (1592.6 ± 404.8 cm), and D_8 (1666.4 ± 294.5 cm)—without showing significant changes. Regarding the activity of the zebrafish exposed to the vitamin and pesticide mixture, the total distance value decreased on D_1 (707.2 ± 277.5 cm, $p > 0.05$, Tukey, ANOVA) vs. pretreatment (913.6 ± 53.8 cm), with ups and downs during the entire experimental period, ending at a greater value (1203.4 ± 323.8 cm) than was measured in the initial phase (Figure 4).

In regard to the parameter "swimming speed", it presented similar trends, as can be seen in Figure 5. Swimming speed registered high levels for the 0.24 μg L^{-1} (initial behavior: 3.14 ± 0.31 cm s^{-1} vs. end of the study: 5.07 ± 1.07 cm s^{-1}, $p > 0.05$, Tukey, ANOVA) and 600 μg L^{-1} FIP + PYR (initial behavior: 4.54 ± 0.62 cm s^{-1} vs. end of the study: 5.44 ± 0.81 cm s^{-1}, $p > 0.05$, Tukey, ANOVA) groups compared to the control (initial behavior: 4.09 ± 0.70 cm s^{-1} vs. end of the study: 4.50 ± 0.34 cm s^{-1}, $p > 0.05$, Tukey, ANOVA) and the remaining group (initial behavior: 3.78 ± 0.17 cm s^{-1} vs. end of the study: 5.01 ± 1.35 cm s^{-1} ($p > 0.05$, Tukey, ANOVA).

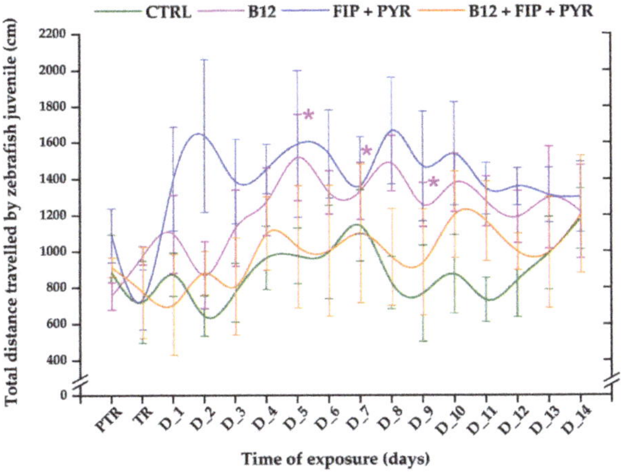

Figure 4. The total distance travelled by juveniles from experimental groups. D: day, PTR: pretreatment, TR: treatment, green: control, purple: 0.24 μg L^{-1} vit. B_{12}, blue: 600 μg L^{-1} FIP + PIR, and orange: 0.24 μg L^{-1} vit. B_{12} + 600 μg L^{-1} FIP + PIR. The data are expressed as average ± SEM (n = 15); * $p < 0.05$ (ANOVA, Tukey) is significant compared to the results from the PTR stage.

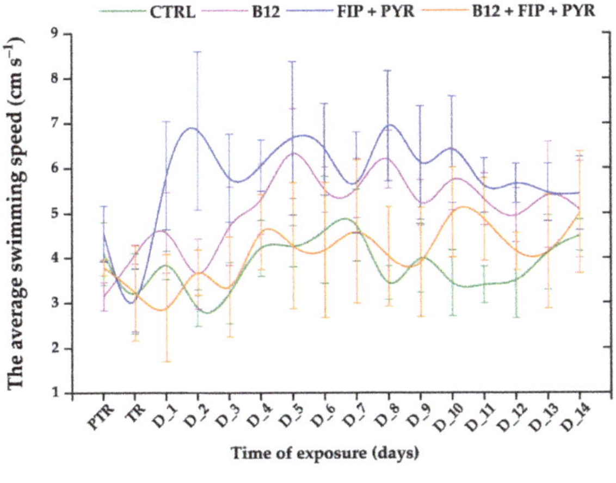

Figure 5. The average swimming speed of the experimental groups. D: day, PTR: pretreatment, TR: treatment, green: control, purple: 0.24 μg L^{-1} vit. B_{12}, blue: 600 μg L^{-1} FIP + PIR, and orange: 0.24 μg L^{-1} vit. B_{12} + 600 μg L^{-1} FIP + PIR. The data are expressed as average ± SEM (n = 15); $p < 0.05$ (ANOVA, Tukey) is significant compared to the results from the PTR stage.

Another quantified parameter for the locomotor activity characterization was "maximum acceleration". As can be seen in Figure 6, this parameter did not show important modifications in any group during the experimental period. In addition, the single exposure to the pesticide mixture triggered a slight increase in maximum acceleration on D_5: 235.8 ± 12.4 cm s^{-2} ($p > 0.05$, Tukey, ANOVA) compared to the pretreatment data: 211.9 ± 2.35 cm s^{-2}. On the other hand, when the vitamin was also present, the parameter of maximum acceleration was reduced on D_1 (192.6 ± 19.16 cm s^{-2}, $p > 0.05$, Tukey, ANOVA) and D_13 (191.1 ± 15.6 cm s^{-2}, $p > 0.05$, Tukey, ANOVA) versus the pretreatment value: 223.2 ± 11.06 cm s^{-2}.

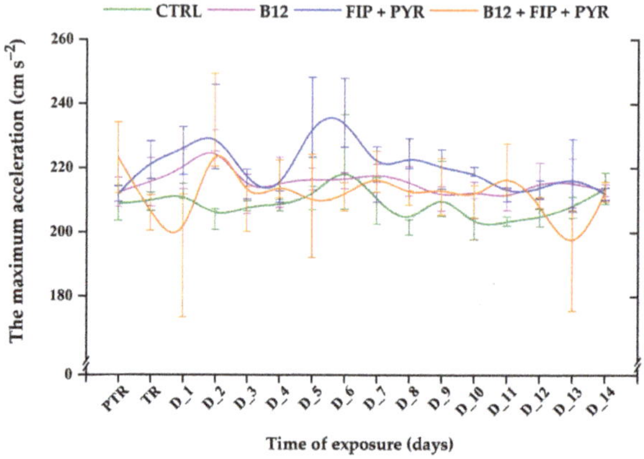

Figure 6. The maximum acceleration of the experimental groups. D: day, PTR: pretreatment, TR: treatment, green: control, purple: 0.24 µg L^{-1} vit. B_{12}, blue: 600 µg L^{-1} FIP + PIR, and orange: 0.24 µg L^{-1} vit. B_{12} + 600 µg L^{-1} FIP + PIR. The data are expressed as average ± SEM (n = 15); $p < 0.05$ (ANOVA, Tukey) is significant compared to the results from the PTR stage.

The "active swimming" parameter presented several changes in the activity of the fish. Although most zebrafish individuals did not exhibit important modifications in this parameter's values, a fluctuating trend was observed during the experimental period. The vit. B_{12} group was the only one with constant activity. Even though the 0.24 µg L^{-1} group showed constant activity, there was a decrease in it on D_2 (205.4 ± 8.54 s, $p > 0.05$, Tukey, ANOVA) in comparison to the pretreatment value: 217.6 ± 3.14 s (Figure 7). After the first week of exposure to the pesticide alone, fish were able to regain values close to the initial behavior (223.3 ± 7.43 s). Thus, the lowest values of this parameter were recorded on the treatment day (176.9 ± 41.1 s), D_2 (191.5 ± 31.7 s), and D_5 (199 ± 37.9 s). When fish were exposed to the vitamin and the pesticides, the active swimming parameter revealed unstable behavior. The highest value was recorded on D_12 (229.4 ± 3.91 s, $p > 0.05$, Tukey, ANOVA), and the lowest on D_1 (161.2 ± 32.7 s, $p > 0.05$, Tukey, ANOVA), compared to pretreatment (215.3 ± 10.2 s).

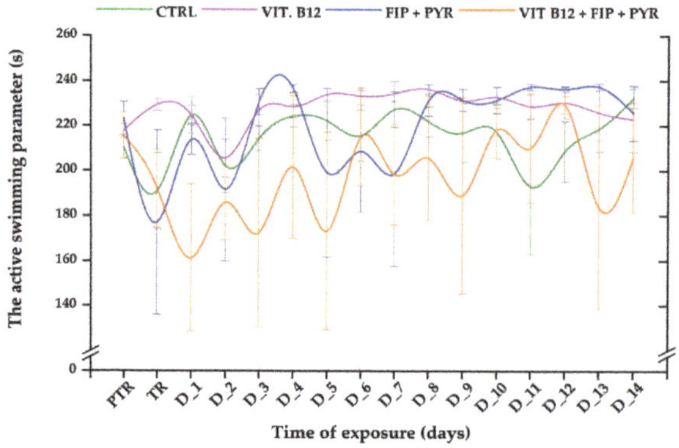

Figure 7. The active swimming parameter recorded for all the experimental groups. D: day, PTR: pretreatment, TR: treatment, green: control, purple: 0.24 µg L^{-1} vit. B_{12}, blue: 600 µg L^{-1} FIP + PIR, and orange: 0.24 µg L^{-1} vit. B_{12} + 600 µg L^{-1} FIP + PIR. The data are expressed as average ± SEM (n = 15); $p < 0.05$ (ANOVA, Tukey) is significant compared to the results from the PTR stage.

The "inactive status" parameter revealed short-term changes in the experimental groups during the tested period. In the first week of exposure, as can be seen from Figure 8, the group exposed to 0.24 μg L^{-1} vit. B_{12} + 600 μg L^{-1} FIP + PIR presented a more pronounced time spent in inactivity compared to the initial behavior (average of the week: 62.36 ± 35.10 s vs. initial behavior: 24.64 ± 10.29 s). When the compounds were given separately, this trend changed. For instance, the vitamin group exhibited the lowest values for this parameter, in contrast to the pesticide group, which had several elevated peaks recorded for the treatment day (63.01 ± 41.1 s), D_2 (48.44 ± 31.7 s), D_5 (40.9 ± 37.3 s), and D_7 (41.3 ± 41.1 s). The control group did not show any modifications to this parameter ($p > 0.05$, Tukey, ANOVA).

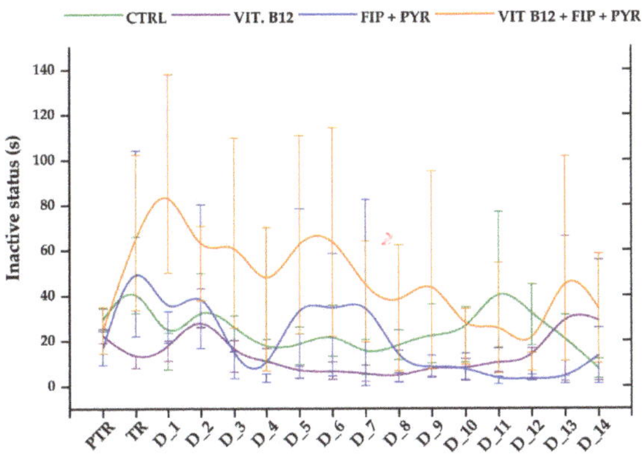

Figure 8. The inactive status recorded for all the experimental groups. D: day, PTR: pretreatment, TR: treatment; green: control, purple: 0.24 μg L^{-1} vit. B_{12}, blue: 600 μg L^{-1} FIP + PIR, and orange: 0.24 μg L^{-1} vit. B_{12} + 600 μg L^{-1} FIP + PIR. The data are expressed as average ± SEM (n = 15); $p < 0.05$ (ANOVA, Tukey) is significant compared to the results from the PTR stage.

3.2. Impact of the Presence of Vitamin B_{12} on Zebrafish Social Behavior

The sociability of zebrafish was evaluated through the social interaction test by measuring the time spent next to the stimulus zone. In Figure 9, the variations of this behavior during the experimental period are exhibited.

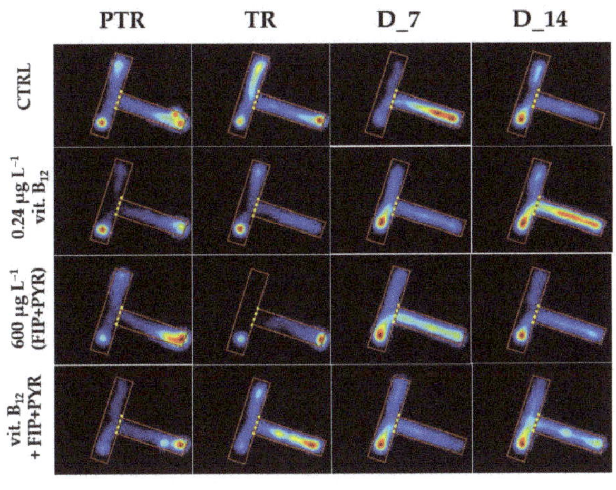

Figure 9. The time spent in the T-maze areas during the social interaction test, presented through heatmaps. D: day, PTR: pretreatment, TR: treatment.

The control group revealed a normal and natural behavior that is specific to this organism, with the most time spent next to the stimulus zone (124.5 ± 31.8 s), followed by the center arm (88.5 ± 27.3 s) and then the right arm (26.9 ± 15.7 s), with no significant difference between the experimental period and pretreatment (left: 135.04 ± 35.3 s vs. center: 92.4 ± 30.5 s, vs. right: 12.6 ± 8.84 s, $p > 0.05$, ANOVA) (Figure 10).

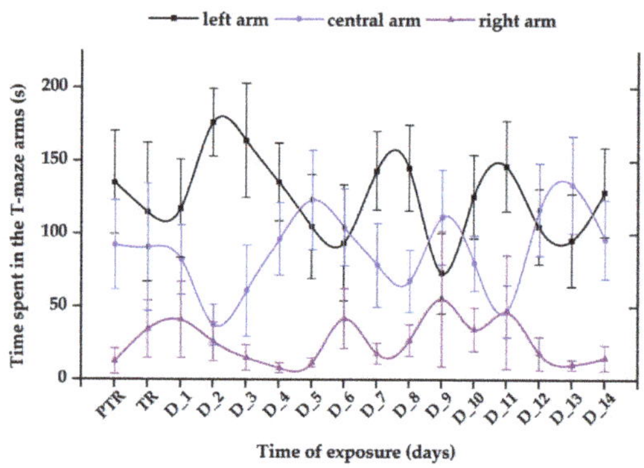

Figure 10. The time spent in the T-maze areas, recorded for the control group. D: day, PTR: pretreatment, TR: treatment. The data are expressed as average ± SEM (n = 15); $p < 0.05$ (ANOVA, Tukey_ is significant compared to the results from the PTR stage.

Regarding the 0.24 μg L^{-1} B_{12} group, the time spent in the maze arms reflected elevated values for the left and center arms (average of tested period: 111.3 ± 22.6 s vs. 106.1 ± 20.2 s) and a reduced value for the right arm (22.6 ± 9.71 s) compared to initial behavior (left: 157.9 ± 16.1 s vs. center arm: 41.5 ± 8.5 s vs. right arm: 34.6 ± 14.6 s) (Figure 11).

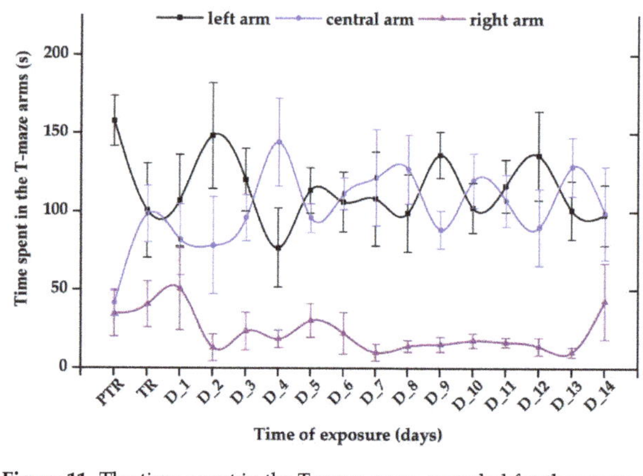

Figure 11. The time spent in the T-maze areas, recorded for the group exposed to 0.24 μg L^{-1} vit. B_{12}. D: day, PTR: pretreatment, TR: treatment. The data are expressed as average ± SEM (n = 15); $p < 0.05$ (ANOVA, Tukey) is significant compared to the results from the PTR stage.

Exposure to a single dose of 600 μg L^{-1} FIP + PIR did not trigger long-term effects on zebrafish sociability; however, this combination was able of disturbing this behavior after the first days of treatment. The time spent in the left arm decreased on D_1 (70.4 ± 43.1 s) and D_3 (96.7 ± 27.7 s) compared to the pretreatment period (124.1 ± 29.7 s). Thus, after these days, the fish started to regain their normal behavior, as can be observed in Figure 12. Additionally, the time spent in the right arm registered the lowest values (pretreatment:

20.2 ± 7.7 s vs. D_14: 14.1 ± 7.7 s), in contrast to the left arm (pretreatment: 95.7 ± 27.9 s vs. D_14: 75.1 ± 26.1 s) and center arm (pretreatment: 124.1 ± 29.7 s vs. D_14: 150.2 ± 33.1 s).

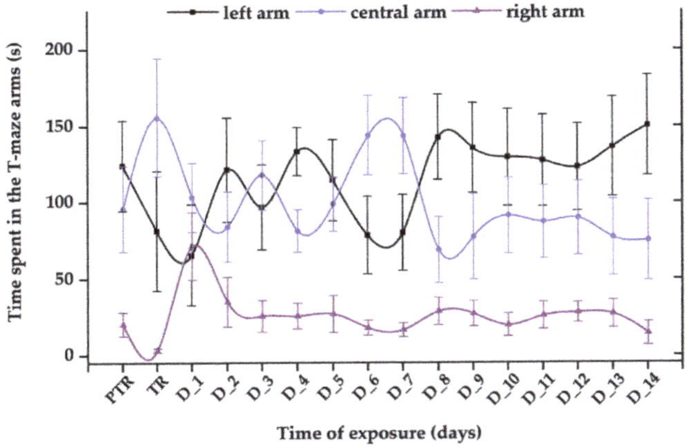

Figure 12. The time spent in the T-maze areas, recorded for the group exposed to 600 μg L^{-1} FIP + PIR mixture. D: day, PTR: pretreatment, TR: treatment. The data are expressed as average ± SEM (n = 15); $p < 0.05$ (ANOVA, Tukey) is significant compared to the results from the PTR stage.

The group treated with 0.24 μg L^{-1} vit. B_{12} and 600 μg L^{-1} FIP + PIR spent less time in the left arm on the treatment day (96.02 ± 42.1 s), D_1 (70.4 ± 43.1 s), and D_2 (108.1 ± 35.7 s) than during the pretreatment period (120.4 ± 23.2 s). Starting on D_3, the time spent in the stimulus zone gradually increased, registering an average of 128.6 ± 30.8 s, almost matching that from the initial period (Figure 13). Regarding the other areas of the maze, the time spent in the right and center arms by the fish presented ups and downs with no significant activity ($p > 0.05$, Tukey, ANOVA) (Figure 13).

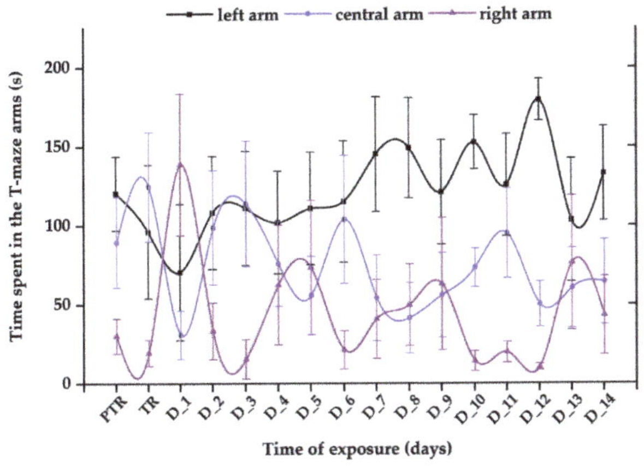

Figure 13. The time spent in the T-maze areas, recorded for the group exposed to 0.24 μg L^{-1} vit. B_{12} and 600 μg L^{-1} FIP + PIR mixture. D: day, PTR: pretreatment, TR: treatment. The data are expressed as average ± SEM (n = 15); $p < 0.05$ (ANOVA, Tukey) is significant compared to the results from the PTR stage.

3.3. Antioxidant Boost after Vitamin B_{12} Supplementation

The biochemical activity is represented in Figure 14. A single exposure to the pesticide mixture did not trigger significant changes in SOD activity; neither did exposure to the pesticides and vit. B_{12} ($p > 0.05$ Tukey, ANOVA). The same trend was observed for GPx activity ($p > 0.05$ Tukey, ANOVA). In contrast, 14 days of treatment with 0.24 μg L^{-1} vit. B_{12} resulted in increased activities for SOD ($p = 0.03$ Tukey, ANOVA) and GPx ($p = 0.02$ Tukey, ANOVA). Regarding the lipid peroxidation process, the MDA marker did not show important variations among the experimental groups except for the last group ($p = 0.03$ Tukey, ANOVA), exposed to the pesticide mixture and the vitamin.

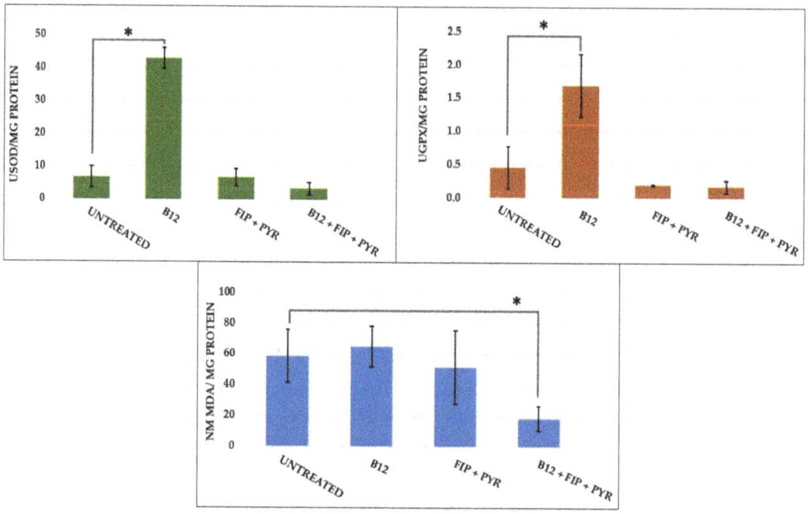

Figure 14. A graphical representation of the activity of superoxide dismutase (SOD), glutathione peroxidase (GPx), and malondialdehyde (MDA) for the experimental groups. The data are expressed as the average ± SEM; * $p < 0.05$ (Tukey) compared to the control.

4. Discussion

The purpose of this study was to determine whether vit. B_{12} can act as a therapeutic tool in an ASD animal model developed through environmental risk factor exposure. Modeling traits comparable to those reported in autistic people in another organism implies multiple phases. The first step in the construction of an animal model is the discovery of a suitable inductor, followed by the validation of the existence of ASD and the evaluation of an adequate response after trying a recognized therapeutic method. The effectiveness of vit. B_{12} in treating symptoms induced by exposure to FIP and PYR (already established to have the potential to produce ASD-like impairments) was assessed in this trial. To date, no animal studies have been performed to evaluate the effects of vit. B_{12} on locomotor activity, on social features, or in association with ASD. In this study, the first of its kind, the findings reveal that vit. B_{12} can assist in restoring normal behavior in zebrafish after exposure to a mixture of pesticides by interacting with enzymes of the antioxidant system. As shown in the study results section, supplementing the zebrafish diet with vit. B_{12} led to improved levels of movement parameters describing fish locomotor activity.

Hyperactivity was one of the main findings recorded for the pesticide group, which presented high values for distance, velocity, and maximum acceleration parameters in comparison to the other experimental groups. Even when no significant, differences could be seen between the pretreatment and treatment phases. Although there was only a single high exposure to the mixture of pesticides, the impact could be seen over the whole study period, particularly during the first week. This may be explained by the time required for pesticides to be metabolized in fish. Furthermore, excessive movement can also be a response to the interaction of fish with these two pesticides, which causes the appearance of stress and triggers an increase in cortisol secretion but also in ROS [80,81]. This observation has been made in many research studies after FIP and PYR exposure due to the pesticides' transformation into more toxic and lasting compounds. For example, the administration of a single oral dose of PYR (2 and 1000 mg kg^{-1}) to rats showed that this pesticide had not only a higher excretion rate but also a reduced depuration period when the presence of tissue residues was determined after 7 days [82]. A more recent work, in which zebrafish were exposed to 10 and 100 μg L^{-1} PYR for 30 days, demonstrated the ability of the pesticide to accumulate after only one day of exposure, while the depuration period of 14 days indicated different half-life values: 2.3 days and 92.5% on day 7 for the lowest dose compared to 1.2 days and 94.6% on day 7 for the highest. In addition, compared with the other metabolites, both doses of PYR inhibited the activity of CAT and SOD in the liver [83]. Similar results as well as elevated levels of lipid peroxidation in the brain and kidney were obtained after oral administration of 2.5, 5, and 10 mg kg^{-1} body weight FIP to mice for 28 days [67]. The same observations were made in zebrafish after 96 h of exposure to 0.5, 1, and 2 mg L^{-1} FIP [82]. Compared with the previous study, in the present work, no significant effects were recorded on the activity of SOD, GPx, or MDA after pesticide exposure. This may be explained by variations in dose, exposure time, and developmental stage that may trigger different consequences on zebrafish. Moreover, when this pesticide mixture was used in a 14-day treatment for zebrafish, it resulted in increased activities for SOD, GPx, and MDA [83]. Consequently, it can be concluded that there is a link between the transformation of pesticides and the occurrence of oxidative stress, especially through the overproduction of free radicals, which can overwhelm the antioxidant system.

Although an effect of vit. B12 on the social behavior of zebrafish was not evidenced, oscillations between the left and central arms were observed after two weeks of treatment. On the other hand, the group exposed to 0.24 μg L^{-1} vit. B_{12} and 600 μg L^{-1} FIP + PIR showed a clear preference for the region with social cues, suggesting that vit. B_{12} may participate in certain fish metabolic processes, allowing them to behave as prior to treatment. This observation could lead to the conclusion that the vitamin does not directly participate or act on social behavior, but its involvement in other metabolic processes could impact the behavior of individuals. For example, compared to the results of the previous group, a single dose of the pesticide mixture was capable to induce short- and medium-term changes in fish sociability in the first week of exposure. This behavioral alteration did not last until the end of experimental period, indicating that pesticides and their effects began to fade via the excretion process as soon as fish were transferred to system water. Even if the differences were not validated by a specific degree of significance, the graphical representations indicate certain trends for the behavioral parameters studied, which must be further investigated.

The potential antioxidant effect of vit. B_{12} has been mentioned several times, but it remains unclear, though its involvement as a broad-spectrum micronutrient is known [84]. A recently published study discovered associations between subclinical vit. B_{12} deficiency and serum metabolic markers linked to neuronal and mitochondrial function, along with increased oxidative stress [85]. Moreover, vit. B_{12} interacts with superoxide, a product of aerobic metabolism, at rates comparable to SOD, which highlights the mimetic behavior of the vitamin towards the enzyme. [86,87]. This may indicate a possible mechanism through which the vitamin protects against chronic inflammation and controls redox homeostasis. In this study, exposure to 0.24 μg L^{-1} vit. B_{12} for 14 days resulted in elevated activities for SOD and GPx, whereas, when the vitamin was given after the pesticide mixture, the activity was lower than for control group. Similar to these results, a 7-day treatment with 0.63 g kg^{-1} vit. B_{12} reduced the levels of hepatic enzymes (aminotransferase and aspartate aminotransferase), increased antioxidant activities, and diminished inflammatory cell infiltration and necrosis processes in a male rat study of acetaminophen hepatotoxicity [88].

A possible explanation for this finding could be the ability of the vitamin administered in a non-stressful environment to promote and enhance the activity of the enzymes of the antioxidant system. On the other hand, in a disturbed environment (exposure to a mixture of pesticides) the vitamin participated together with the antioxidant system in counteracting the effects induced by FIP and PYR even with a single exposure. At the same time, the rate of accumulation in the zebrafish body and the products resulting from the metabolism of FIP and PYR may cause variations in the response to contact with the compounds. The ability of FIP to accumulate and the rate of metabolite formation in rainbow trout (*Oncorhynchus mykiss*) was measured after 32 days of exposure followed by 96 days of depuration. That study concluded that FIP is rapidly converted to its metabolite, fipronil sulfone, known to have a longer half-life [89]. For instance, the elimination half-life of FIP was 8.5 h, compared to 208 h for fipronil sulfone, after administration of 4 mg kg^{-1} FIP in rats [62,90]. Additionally, the persistence of fipronil sulfone was confirmed after a 7-day depuration process in European sea bass (*Dicentrarchus labrax*) juveniles previously fed with 10 mg kg^{-1} FIP for 14 days [91].

Another parameter measured to identify the existence of oxidative stress was MDA, a popular marker for lipid peroxidation. Exposure to a single dose of pesticides followed by 14 days of vit. B_{12} led to a decrease in the MDA level compared to the other groups. This result indicates a possible intervention of the vitamin to regulate the balance between ROS products and antioxidants, which is also supported by the decreased activities of SOD and GPx. Dietary supplementation with vit. B_{12} had a positive influence on the methylation process, GSH activity, and oxidative stress in autistic children after an 8-week course of therapy [43]. Similar results were previously reported by Bertoglio et al. following a 3-month course of therapy with 0.06 mg kg^{-1} vit. B_{12} [42]. A substantially decreased level of vit. B_{12} was recently found by two studies that assessed the vitamin's activity in children with ASD [39,92]. Perturbation of vitamin activity can also occur due to genetic mutations, as demonstrated in zebrafish by mutations in the abcd4 gene, whose deficiency caused anemia, or the mmachc gene, responsible for processing the vitamin and transporting it to cells [53,93]. Vitamin deficiency was also proven in a mouse model of ischemic stroke, where both females and males had impaired balance and coordination as well as elevated homocysteine levels compared to the 0.025 mg kg^{-1} group [94]. Neurologic alterations such as anxiety, deficits in learning and memory, and changes in brain mass were obtained in a knockout mouse in which the transcobalamin receptor (TCblR) gene (CD320) was ablated [95].

Finally, the interaction among vit. B_{12}, antioxidants, and ROS should be further studied and developed using animal models in an environmental setting, especially due to the high incidence of side effects, but also in a neuropsychiatric context.

5. Conclusions

The usefulness of the vitamin will need to be examined by developing animal models with similar characteristics to ASD, considering the new research that has come to light indicating a lack of vitamin B_{12} in people with autism, whether it is genetic or environmental. Furthermore, the present findings revealed the vitamin's participation in an environment of oxidative stress, along with its contribution to zebrafish behavior. This study requires further attention to find out the optimal route of exposure, dose, and treatment duration; all of these are considered limitations of the current study.

Supplementary Materials: The following supporting information can be downloaded at: https://www.mdpi.com/article/10.3390/ani14030405/s1, Table S1: Superoxide dismutase results. Table S2: Glutathione peroxidase results. Table S3: Malondialdehyde results.

Author Contributions: Conceptualization, M.A.R.; methodology, M.A.R. and O.D.I.; software, M.A.R.; validation, A.C.; formal analysis, M.A.R. and O.D.I.; resources, M.N.N., L.E.R., D.U. and A.C.; data curation, M.A.R. and O.D.I.; writing—original draft preparation, M.A.R.; writing—review and editing, M.N.N., G.S. and A.C.; supervision, A.C.; project administration, M.N.N. and A.C.; funding acquisition, M.N.N. and D.U. All authors have read and agreed to the published version of the manuscript.

Funding: M.A.R. was supported by Project POCU/993/6/13/153322, project title "Educational and training support for PhD students and young researchers in preparation for insertion into the labour market", co-funded by the European Social Fund, through Operational Programme Human Capital 2014–2020. The other authors are thankful to the Romanian Ministry of Research, Innovation and Digitization, within Program 1—Development of the national RD system, Subprogram 1.2—Institutional Performance—RDI excellence funding projects, Contract no. 11PFE/30.12.2021, for financial support.

Institutional Review Board Statement: The animal study protocol was approved by the Ethical Commission of the Faculty of Veterinary Medicine, University of Agricultural Sciences and Veterinary Medicine Iasi, with registration number 750/04.07.2019.

Informed Consent Statement: Not applicable.

Data Availability Statement: Data supporting this study cannot be made available for ethical and commercial reasons.

Conflicts of Interest: The authors declare no conflict of interest.

References

1. Green, R.; Allen, L.H.; Bjorke-Monsen, A.-L.; Brito, A.; Gueant, J.-L.; Miller, J.W.; Molloy, A.M.; Nexo, E.; Stabler, S.; Toh, B.-H.; et al. Vitamin B12 deficiency. *Nat. Rev. Dis. Prim.* **2017**, *3*, 17040. [CrossRef]
2. Calderón-Ospina, C.A.; Nava-Mesa, M.O. B Vitamins in the nervous system: Current knowledge of the biochemical modes of action and synergies of thiamine, pyridoxine, and cobalamin. *CNS Neurosci. Ther.* **2020**, *26*, 5–13. [CrossRef] [PubMed]
3. Briani, C.; Dalla Torre, C.; Citton, V.; Manara, R.; Pompanin, S.; Binotto, G.; Adami, F. Cobalamin deficiency: Clinical picture and radiological findings. *Nutrients* **2013**, *5*, 4521–4539. [CrossRef] [PubMed]
4. Zhang, Y.; Hodgson, N.W.; Trivedi, M.S.; Abdolmaleky, H.M.; Fournier, M.; Cuenod, M.; Do, K.Q.; Deth, R.C. Decreased Brain Levels of Vitamin B12 in Aging, Autism and Schizophrenia. *PLoS ONE* **2016**, *11*, e0146797. [CrossRef]
5. Serin, H.M.; Arslan, E.A. Neurological symptoms of vitamin B12 deficiency: Analysis of pediatric patients. *Acta Clin. Croat.* **2019**, *58*, 295–302. [CrossRef]
6. Vargas-Uricoechea, H.; Nogueira, J.P.; Pinzón-Fernández, M.V.; Agredo-Delgado, V.; Vargas-Sierra, H.D. Population Status of Vitamin B12 Values in the General Population and in Individuals with Type 2 Diabetes, in Southwestern Colombia. *Nutrients* **2023**, *15*, 2357. [CrossRef] [PubMed]
7. Green, R.; Miller, J.W. Chapter Fifteen—Vitamin B12 deficiency. In *Vitamin B12*; Litwack, G., Ed.; Academic Press: Cambridge, MA, USA, 2022; Volume 119, pp. 405–439. ISBN 0083-6729.
8. Froese, D.S.; Kopec, J.; Fitzpatrick, F.; Schuller, M.; McCorvie, T.J.; Chalk, R.; Plessl, T.; Fettelschoss, V.; Fowler, B.; Baumgartner, M.R.; et al. Structural Insights into the MMACHC-MMADHC Protein Complex Involved in Vitamin B12 Trafficking. *J. Biol. Chem.* **2015**, *290*, 29167–29177. [CrossRef]
9. Hayden, M.R.; Tyagi, S.C. Homocysteine and reactive oxygen species in metabolic syndrome, type 2 diabetes mellitus, and atheroscleropathy: The pleiotropic effects of folate supplementation. *Nutr. J.* **2004**, *3*, 4. [CrossRef]
10. Sies, H.; Berndt, C.; Jones, D.P. Oxidative Stress. *Annu. Rev. Biochem.* **2017**, *86*, 715–748. [CrossRef]
11. Manivasagam, T.; Arunadevi, S.; Essa, M.M.; SaravanaBabu, C.; Borah, A.; Thenmozhi, A.J.; Qoronfleh, M.W. Role of Oxidative Stress and Antioxidants in Autism. *Adv. Neurobiol.* **2020**, *24*, 193–206. [CrossRef]
12. Liu, X.; Lin, J.; Zhang, H.; Khan, N.U.; Zhang, J.; Tang, X.; Cao, X.; Shen, L. Oxidative Stress in Autism Spectrum Disorder-Current Progress of Mechanisms and Biomarkers. *Front. Psychiatry* **2022**, *13*, 813304. [CrossRef]
13. Sies, H. Oxidative Stress: Concept and Some Practical Aspects. *Antioxidants* **2020**, *9*, 852. [CrossRef]
14. Jelinek, M.; Jurajda, M.; Duris, K. Oxidative Stress in the Brain: Basic Concepts and Treatment Strategies in Stroke. *Antioxidants* **2021**, *10*, 1886. [CrossRef]
15. Pangrazzi, L.; Balasco, L.; Bozzi, Y. Oxidative Stress and Immune System Dysfunction in Autism Spectrum Disorders. *Int. J. Mol. Sci.* **2020**, *21*, 3293. [CrossRef]
16. Fakhoury, M. Autistic spectrum disorders: A review of clinical features, theories and diagnosis. *Int. J. Dev. Neurosci.* **2015**, *43*, 70–77. [CrossRef] [PubMed]
17. Lord, C.; Elsabbagh, M.; Baird, G.; Veenstra-Vanderweele, J. Autism spectrum disorder. *Lancet* **2018**, *392*, 508–520. [CrossRef] [PubMed]
18. Wormwood, K.L.; Charette, L.; Ryan, J.P.; Darie, C.C.; Woods, A.G. A Proteomics Investigation of Salivary Profiles as Potential Biomarkers for Autism Spectrum Disorder (ASD). *Protein J.* **2023**, *42*, 607–620. [CrossRef] [PubMed]
19. Wallis, K.E.; Adebajo, T.; Bennett, A.E.; Drye, M.; Gerdes, M.; Miller, J.S.; Guthrie, W. Prevalence of autism spectrum disorder in a large pediatric primary care network. *Autism Int. J. Res. Pract.* **2023**, *27*, 1840–1846. [CrossRef] [PubMed]
20. Salari, N.; Rasoulpoor, S.; Rasoulpoor, S.; Shohaimi, S.; Jafarpour, S.; Abdoli, N.; Khaledi-Paveh, B.; Mohammadi, M. The global prevalence of autism spectrum disorder: A comprehensive systematic review and meta-analysis. *Ital. J. Pediatr.* **2022**, *48*, 112. [CrossRef]

21. Association, A.P. *Diagnostic and Statistical Manual of Mental Disorders*, 5th ed.; American Psychiatric Association: London, UK, 2013; ISBN 978-0-89042-554-1.
22. Zwaigenbaum, L.; Penner, M. Autism spectrum disorder: Advances in diagnosis and evaluation. *BMJ* **2018**, *361*, k1674. [CrossRef] [PubMed]
23. Al-Dewik, N.; Al-Jurf, R.; Styles, M.; Tahtamouni, S.; Alsharshani, D.; Alsharshani, M.; Ahmad, A.I.; Khattab, A.; Al Rifai, H.; Walid Qoronfleh, M. Overview and Introduction to Autism Spectrum Disorder (ASD). *Adv. Neurobiol.* **2020**, *24*, 3–42. [CrossRef]
24. Sealey, L.A.; Hughes, B.W.; Sriskanda, A.N.; Guest, J.R.; Gibson, A.D.; Johnson-Williams, L.; Pace, D.G.; Bagasra, O. Environmental factors in the development of autism spectrum disorders. *Environ. Int.* **2016**, *88*, 288–298. [CrossRef]
25. Lord, C.; Risi, S.; Lambrecht, L.; Cook, E.H.; Leventhal, B.L.; DiLavore, P.C.; Pickles, A.; Rutter, M. The Autism Diagnostic Observation Schedule—Generic: A Standard Measure of Social and Communication Deficits Associated with the Spectrum of Autism. *J. Autism Dev. Disord.* **2000**, *30*, 205–223. [CrossRef]
26. Scheffer, I.E.; Nabbout, R. SCN1A-related phenotypes: Epilepsy and beyond. *Epilepsia* **2019**, *60* (Suppl. S3), S17–S24. [CrossRef]
27. Moh, T.A.; Magiati, I. Factors associated with parental stress and satisfaction during the process of diagnosis of children with Autism Spectrum Disorders. *Res. Autism Spectr. Disord.* **2012**, *6*, 293–303. [CrossRef]
28. Modabbernia, A.; Velthorst, E.; Reichenberg, A. Environmental risk factors for autism: An evidence-based review of systematic reviews and meta-analyses. *Mol. Autism* **2017**, *8*, 13. [CrossRef] [PubMed]
29. Ramaswami, G.; Geschwind, D.H. Genetics of autism spectrum disorder. *Handb. Clin. Neurol.* **2018**, *147*, 321–329. [CrossRef] [PubMed]
30. Ongono, J.S.; Béranger, R.; Baghdadli, A.; Mortamais, M. Pesticides used in Europe and autism spectrum disorder risk: Can novel exposure hypotheses be formulated beyond organophosphates, organochlorines, pyrethroids and carbamates?—A systematic review. *Environ. Res.* **2020**, *187*, 109646. [CrossRef]
31. Wang, L.; Wang, B.; Wu, C.; Wang, J.; Sun, M. Autism Spectrum Disorder: Neurodevelopmental Risk Factors, Biological Mechanism, and Precision Therapy. *Int. J. Mol. Sci.* **2023**, *24*, 1819. [CrossRef]
32. Vissoker, R.E.; Latzer, Y.; Gal, E. Eating and feeding problems and gastrointestinal dysfunction in Autism Spectrum Disorders. *Res. Autism Spectr. Disord.* **2015**, *12*, 10–21. [CrossRef]
33. Schreck, K.A.; Williams, K. Food preferences and factors influencing food selectivity for children with autism spectrum disorders. *Res. Dev. Disabil.* **2006**, *27*, 353–363. [CrossRef] [PubMed]
34. Liu, X.; Liu, J.; Xiong, X.; Yang, T.; Hou, N.; Liang, X.; Chen, J.; Cheng, Q.; Li, T. Correlation between Nutrition and Symptoms: Nutritional Survey of Children with Autism Spectrum Disorder in Chongqing, China. *Nutrients* **2016**, *8*, 294. [CrossRef] [PubMed]
35. Sharp, W.G.; Postorino, V.; McCracken, C.E.; Berry, R.C.; Criado, K.K.; Burrell, T.L.; Scahill, L. Dietary Intake, Nutrient Status, and Growth Parameters in Children with Autism Spectrum Disorder and Severe Food Selectivity: An Electronic Medical Record Review. *J. Acad. Nutr. Diet.* **2018**, *118*, 1943–1950. [CrossRef] [PubMed]
36. Lundin Remnélius, K.; Neufeld, J.; Isaksson, J.; Bölte, S. Eating Problems in Autistic Females and Males: A Co-twin Control Study. *J. Autism Dev. Disord.* **2022**, *52*, 3153–3168. [CrossRef] [PubMed]
37. Al-Farsi, Y.M.; Waly, M.I.; Deth, R.C.; Al-Sharbati, M.M.; Al-Shafaee, M.; Al-Farsi, O.; Al-Khaduri, M.M.; Gupta, I.; Ali, A.; Al-Khalili, M.; et al. Low folate and vitamin B12 nourishment is common in Omani children with newly diagnosed autism. *Nutrition* **2013**, *29*, 537–541. [CrossRef] [PubMed]
38. Yektaş, Ç.; Alpay, M.; Tufan, A.E. Comparison of serum B12, folate and homocysteine concentrations in children with autism spectrum disorder or attention deficit hyperactivity disorder and healthy controls. *Neuropsychiatr. Dis. Treat.* **2019**, *15*, 2213–2219. [CrossRef] [PubMed]
39. Mahruba, S.; Begum, S.; Shahjadi, S.; Afroz, S.; Siddiqi, U.; Parvin, J. Serum vitamin B12 and folic acid status in Autism spectrum disorder children. *J. Bangladesh Soc. Physiol.* **2020**, *14*, 43–47. [CrossRef]
40. Li, B.; Xu, Y.; Pang, D.; Zhao, Q.; Zhang, L.; Li, M.; Li, W.; Duan, G.; Zhu, C. Interrelation between homocysteine metabolism and the development of autism spectrum disorder in children. *Front. Mol. Neurosci.* **2022**, *15*, 947513. [CrossRef]
41. Laud, R.B.; Girolami, P.A.; Boscoe, J.H.; Gulotta, C.S. Treatment outcomes for severe feeding problems in children with autism spectrum disorder. *Behav. Modif.* **2009**, *33*, 520–536. [CrossRef]
42. Bertoglio, K.; Jill James, S.; Deprey, L.; Brule, N.; Hendren, R.L. Pilot study of the effect of methyl B12 treatment on behavioral and biomarker measures in children with autism. *J. Altern. Complement. Med.* **2010**, *16*, 555–560. [CrossRef]
43. Hendren, R.L.; James, S.J.; Widjaja, F.; Lawton, B.; Rosenblatt, A.; Bent, S. Randomized, Placebo-Controlled Trial of Methyl B12 for Children with Autism. *J. Child Adolesc. Psychopharmacol.* **2016**, *26*, 774–783. [CrossRef]
44. Allen, L.H.; Miller, J.W.; de Groot, L.; Rosenberg, I.H.; Smith, A.D.; Refsum, H.; Raiten, D.J. Biomarkers of Nutrition for Development (BOND): Vitamin B-12 Review. *J. Nutr.* **2018**, *148*, 1995S–2027S. [CrossRef]
45. Rossignol, D.A.; Frye, R.E. The Effectiveness of Cobalamin (B12) Treatment for Autism Spectrum Disorder: A Systematic Review and Meta-Analysis. *J. Pers. Med.* **2021**, *11*, 784. [CrossRef]
46. Held, J.R. Appropriate animal models. *Ann. N. Y. Acad. Sci.* **1983**, *406*, 13–19. [CrossRef] [PubMed]
47. Davidson, M.K.; Lindsey, J.R.; Davis, J.K. Requirements and selection of an animal model. *Isr. J. Med. Sci.* **1987**, *23*, 551–555. [PubMed]
48. Kalueff, A.V.; Stewart, A.M.; Gerlai, R. Zebrafish as an emerging model for studying complex brain disorders. *Trends Pharmacol. Sci.* **2014**, *35*, 63–75. [CrossRef] [PubMed]

49. Stewart, A.M.; Nguyen, M.; Wong, K.; Poudel, M.K.; Kalueff, A. V Developing zebrafish models of autism spectrum disorder (ASD). *Prog. Neuro-Psychopharmacol. Biol. Psychiatry* **2014**, *50*, 27–36. [CrossRef] [PubMed]
50. Meshalkina, D.A.; Kizlyk, M.N.; Kysil, E.V.; Collier, A.D.; Echevarria, D.J.; Abreu, M.S.; Barcellos, L.J.; Song, C.; Warnick, J.E.; Kyzar, E.J.; et al. Zebrafish models of autism spectrum disorder. *Exp. Neurol.* **2018**, *299*, 207–216. [CrossRef]
51. Shams, S.; Rihel, J.; Ortiz, J.G.; Gerlai, R. The zebrafish as a promising tool for modeling human brain disorders: A review based upon an IBNS Symposium. *Neurosci. Biobehav. Rev.* **2018**, *85*, 176–190. [CrossRef] [PubMed]
52. Tayanloo-Beik, A.; Hamidpour, S.K.; Abedi, M.; Shojaei, H.; Tavirani, M.R.; Namazi, N.; Larijani, B.; Arjmand, B. Zebrafish Modeling of Autism Spectrum Disorders, Current Status and Future Prospective. *Front. Psychiatry* **2022**, *13*, 911770. [CrossRef] [PubMed]
53. Sloan, J.L.; Achilly, N.P.; Arnold, M.L.; Catlett, J.L.; Blake, T.; Bishop, K.; Jones, M.; Harper, U.; English, M.A.; Anderson, S.; et al. The vitamin B12 processing enzyme, mmachc, is essential for zebrafish survival, growth and retinal morphology. *Hum. Mol. Genet.* **2020**, *29*, 2109–2123. [CrossRef] [PubMed]
54. Hannibal, L.; Jacobsen, D.W. Intracellular processing of vitamin B(12) by MMACHC (CblC). *Vitam. Horm.* **2022**, *119*, 275–298. [CrossRef] [PubMed]
55. Hansen, A.-C.; Olsvik, P.A.; Hemre, G.-I. Effect of different dietary vitamin B12 levels on their retention in the body of zebrafish *Danio rerio* and on the gene expression of vitamin B12 binding proteins. *Aquac. Nutr.* **2013**, *19*, 413–420. [CrossRef]
56. Karmakar, S.; Sen Gupta, P.; Bhattacharya, S.; Sarkar, A.; Rahaman, A.; Mandal, D.P.; Bhattacharjee, S. Vitamin B12 alleviates malathion-induced toxicity in zebra fish by regulating cytochrome P450 and PgP expressions. *Toxicol. Mech. Methods* **2023**, *33*, 364–377. [CrossRef] [PubMed]
57. Coghlan, S.; Horder, J.; Inkster, B.; Mendez, M.A.; Murphy, D.G.; Nutt, D.J. GABA system dysfunction in autism and related disorders: From synapse to symptoms. *Neurosci. Biobehav. Rev.* **2012**, *36*, 2044–2055. [CrossRef] [PubMed]
58. Purkayastha, P.; Malapati, A.; Yogeeswari, P.; Sriram, D. A Review on GABA/Glutamate Pathway for Therapeutic Intervention of ASD and ADHD. *Curr. Med. Chem.* **2015**, *22*, 1850–1859. [CrossRef] [PubMed]
59. Umesawa, Y.; Matsushima, K.; Atsumi, T.; Kato, T.; Fukatsu, R.; Wada, M.; Ide, M. Altered GABA Concentration in Brain Motor Area Is Associated with the Severity of Motor Disabilities in Individuals with Autism Spectrum Disorder. *J. Autism Dev. Disord.* **2020**, *50*, 2710–2722. [CrossRef]
60. Gupta, R.C.; Miller Mukherjee, I.R.; Malik, J.K.; Doss, R.B.; Dettbarn, W.-D.; Milatovic, D. Chapter 26—Insecticides. In *Biomarkers in Toxicology*, 2nd ed.; Gupta, R.C., Ed.; Academic Press: Cambridge, MA, USA, 2019; pp. 455–475. ISBN 978-0-12-814655-2.
61. Gupta, R.C.; Anadón, A. Chapter 42—Fipronil. In *Veterinary Toxicology*, 3rd ed.; Gupta, R.C., Ed.; Academic Press: Cambridge, MA, USA, 2018; pp. 533–538. ISBN 978-0-12-811410-0.
62. Singh, N.S.; Sharma, R.; Singh, S.K.; Singh, D.K. A comprehensive review of environmental fate and degradation of fipronil and its toxic metabolites. *Environ. Res.* **2021**, *199*, 111316. [CrossRef]
63. Sullivan, J.J.; Goh, K.S. Environmental fate and properties of pyriproxyfen. *J. Pestic. Sci.* **2008**, *33*, 339–350. [CrossRef]
64. Bedient, P.; Horsak, R.; Schlenk, D.; Hovinga, R.; Pierson, J. Environmental Impact of Fipronil to the Louisiana Crawfish Industry. *Environ. Forensics* **2005**, *6*, 289–299. [CrossRef]
65. Mehrnoush, G.; Mehrdad, S.; Saeid, K.H.A. Effect of pyriproxyfen on function and tissue of testis in adult rat. *Int. J. Curr. Res. Rev.* **2013**, *5*, 66–74.
66. Wu, H.; Gao, C.; Guo, Y.; Zhang, Y.; Zhang, J.; Ma, E. Acute toxicity and sublethal effects of fipronil on detoxification enzymes in juvenile zebrafish (*Danio rerio*). *Pestic. Biochem. Physiol.* **2014**, *115*, 9–14. [CrossRef] [PubMed]
67. Badgujar, P.C.; Chandratre, G.A.; Pawar, N.N.; Telang, A.G.; Kurade, N.P. Fipronil induced oxidative stress involves alterations in SOD1 and catalase gene expression in male mice liver: Protection by vitamins E and C. *Environ. Toxicol.* **2016**, *31*, 1147–1158. [CrossRef] [PubMed]
68. Wang, X.; Martínez, M.A.; Wu, Q.; Ares, I.; Martínez-Larrañaga, M.R.; Anadón, A.; Yuan, Z. Fipronil insecticide toxicology: Oxidative stress and metabolism. *Crit. Rev. Toxicol.* **2016**, *46*, 876–899. [CrossRef] [PubMed]
69. Araújo, C.V.M.; Roque, D.; Blasco, J.; Ribeiro, R.; Moreira-Santos, M.; Toribio, A.; Aguirre, E.; Barro, S. Stress-driven emigration in complex field scenarios of habitat disturbance: The heterogeneous multi-habitat assay system (HeMHAS). *Sci. Total Environ.* **2018**, *644*, 31–36. [CrossRef] [PubMed]
70. Ghazanfar, M.; Shahid, S.; Qureshi, I.Z. Vitamin C attenuates biochemical and genotoxic damage in common carp (Cyprinus carpio) upon joint exposure to combined toxic doses of fipronil and buprofezin insecticides. *Aquat. Toxicol.* **2018**, *196*, 43–52. [CrossRef] [PubMed]
71. Gusso, D.; Reolon, G.K.; Gonzalez, J.B.; Altenhofen, S.; Kist, L.W.; Bogo, M.R.; Bonan, C.D. Pyriproxyfen Exposure Impairs Cognitive Parameters and Alters Cortisol Levels in Zebrafish. *Front. Behav. Neurosci.* **2020**, *14*, 103. [CrossRef]
72. Bownik, A.; Szabelak, A. Short-term effects of pesticide fipronil on behavioral and physiological endpoints of Daphnia magna. *Environ. Sci. Pollut. Res.* **2021**, *28*, 33254–33264. [CrossRef]
73. Staldoni de Oliveira, V.; Gomes Castro, A.J.; Marins, K.; Bittencourt Mendes, A.K.; Araújo Leite, G.A.; Zamoner, A.; Van Der Kraak, G.; Mena Barreto Silva, F.R. Pyriproxyfen induces intracellular calcium overload and alters antioxidant defenses in *Danio rerio* testis that may influence ongoing spermatogenesis. *Environ. Pollut.* **2021**, *270*, 116055. [CrossRef]

74. Pena, I.A.; Roussel, Y.; Daniel, K.; Mongeon, K.; Johnstone, D.; Weinschutz Mendes, H.; Bosma, M.; Saxena, V.; Lepage, N.; Chakraborty, P.; et al. Pyridoxine-Dependent Epilepsy in Zebrafish Caused by Aldh7a1 Deficiency. *Genetics* **2017**, *207*, 1501–1518. [CrossRef]
75. Balmus, I.-M.; Lefter, R.; Ciobica, A.; Cojocaru, S.; Guenne, S.; Timofte, D.; Stanciu, C.; Trifan, A.; Hritcu, L. Preliminary Biochemical Description of Brain Oxidative Stress Status in Irritable Bowel Syndrome Contention-Stress Rat Model. *Medicina* **2019**, *55*, 776. [CrossRef]
76. Jin, Y.; Liu, Z.; Liu, F.; Ye, Y.; Peng, T.; Fu, Z. Embryonic exposure to cadmium (II) and chromium (VI) induce behavioral alterations, oxidative stress and immunotoxicity in zebrafish (*Danio rerio*). *Neurotoxicol. Teratol.* **2015**, *48*, 9–17. [CrossRef]
77. Bradford, M.M. A rapid and sensitive method for the quantitation of microgram quantities of protein utilizing the principle of protein-dye binding. *Anal. Biochem.* **1976**, *72*, 248–254. [CrossRef]
78. The Commission of The European Communities. Commission Recommendation Guidelines for the accommodation and care of animals used for experimental and other scientific purposes (notified under document number C(2007) 2525). *Off. J. Eur. Union* **2007**, *50*, 90.
79. The European Parliament; The Council of The European Union. Directive 63 the protection of animals used for scientific purposes. *Off. J. Eur. Union* **2010**, *53*, 47.
80. Stehr, C.M.; Linbo, T.L.; Incardona, J.P.; Scholz, N.L. The developmental neurotoxicity of fipronil: Notochord degeneration and locomotor defects in zebrafish embryos and larvae. *Toxicol. Sci. Off. J. Soc. Toxicol.* **2006**, *92*, 270–278. [CrossRef]
81. Wang, C.; Qian, Y.; Zhang, X.; Chen, F.; Zhang, Q.; Li, Z.; Zhao, M. A metabolomic study of fipronil for the anxiety-like behavior in zebrafish larvae at environmentally relevant levels. *Environ. Pollut.* **2016**, *211*, 252–258. [CrossRef]
82. Matsunaga, H.; Yoshino, H.; Isobe, N.; Kaneko, H.; Nakatsuka, I.; Yamada, H. Metabolism of Pyriproxyfen in Rats. 1. Absorption, Disposition, Excretion, and Biotransformation Studies with [phenoxyphenyl-14C]Pyriproxyfen. *J. Agric. Food Chem.* **1995**, *43*, 235–240. [CrossRef]
83. Wei, Y.; Cui, J.; Zhai, W.; Liu, X.; Zhou, Z.; Wang, P.; Liu, D. Toxicity and fate of chiral insecticide pyriproxyfen and its metabolites in zebrafish (*Danio rerio*). *Environ. Pollut.* **2021**, *280*, 116894. [CrossRef] [PubMed]
84. Manzanares, W.; Hardy, G. Vitamin B12: The forgotten micronutrient for critical care. *Curr. Opin. Clin. Nutr. Metab. Care* **2010**, *13*, 662–668. [CrossRef] [PubMed]
85. Brito, A.; Grapov, D.; Fahrmann, J.; Harvey, D.; Green, R.; Miller, J.W.; Fedosov, S.N.; Shahab-Ferdows, S.; Hampel, D.; Pedersen, T.L.; et al. The Human Serum Metabolome of Vitamin B-12 Deficiency and Repletion, and Associations with Neurological Function in Elderly Adults. *J. Nutr.* **2017**, *147*, 1839–1849. [CrossRef] [PubMed]
86. Suarez-Moreira, E.; Yun, J.; Birch, C.S.; Williams, J.H.H.; McCaddon, A.; Brasch, N.E. Vitamin B(12) and redox homeostasis: Cob(II)alamin reacts with superoxide at rates approaching superoxide dismutase (SOD). *J. Am. Chem. Soc.* **2009**, *131*, 15078–15079. [CrossRef] [PubMed]
87. Ayesha, A.; Bahnson, E.M.; Kayashima, Y.; Wilder, J.; Huynh, P.K.; Hiller, S.; Maeda-Smithies, N.; Li, F. Vitamin B12 does not increase cell viability after hydrogen peroxide induced damage in mouse kidney proximal tubular cells and brain endothelial cells. *Adv. Redox Res.* **2022**, *4*, 100029. [CrossRef] [PubMed]
88. Ahmed Mohammed, R.; Fadheel, Q.J. Hepatoprotective Effect of Vitamin B12 in Acetaminophen Induce Hepatotoxicity in Male Rats. *Arch. Razi Inst.* **2023**, *78*, 419–425. [CrossRef] [PubMed]
89. Konwick, B.J.; Garrison, A.W.; Black, M.C.; Avants, J.K.; Fisk, A.T. Bioaccumulation, Biotransformation, and Metabolite Formation of Fipronil and Chiral Legacy Pesticides in Rainbow Trout. *Environ. Sci. Technol.* **2006**, *40*, 2930–2936. [CrossRef] [PubMed]
90. Mohamed, F.; Senarathna, L.; Percy, A.; Abeyewardene, M.; Eaglesham, G.; Cheng, R.; Azher, S.; Hittarage, A.; Dissanayake, W.; Sheriff, M.H.R.; et al. Acute Human Self-Poisoning with the N-Phenylpyrazole Insecticide Fipronil—A GABAA-Gated Chloride Channel Blocker. *J. Toxicol. Clin. Toxicol.* **2004**, *42*, 955–963. [CrossRef]
91. Dallarés, S.; Dourado, P.; Sanahuja, I.; Solovyev, M.; Gisbert, E.; Montemurro, N.; Torreblanca, A.; Blázquez, M.; Solé, M. Multibiomarker approach to fipronil exposure in the fish Dicentrarchus labrax under two temperature regimes. *Aquat. Toxicol.* **2020**, *219*, 105378. [CrossRef]
92. Metyas, M.M.; Abdelhakim, A.S.; Ghandour, H.H. Screening of vitamin B12 in children diagnosed as Autism Spectrum Disorder. *QJM Int. J. Med.* **2020**, *113*, hcaa063.006. [CrossRef]
93. Choi, Y.M.; Kim, Y.-I.; Choi, J.-H.; Bhandari, S.; Nam, I.-K.; Hong, K.; Kwak, S.; So, H.-S.; Park, D.-S.; Kim, C.-H.; et al. Loss of abcd4 in zebrafish leads to vitamin B12-deficiency anemia. *Biochem. Biophys. Res. Commun.* **2019**, *514*, 1264–1269. [CrossRef]
94. Yahn, G.; Wasek, B.; Bottiglieri, T.; Jadavji, N. A Dietary Vitamin B12 Deficiency Impairs Balance and Coordination After Ischemic Injury to the Sensorimotor Cortex in Adult Male and Female Mice. *Curr. Dev. Nutr.* **2021**, *5*, 932. [CrossRef]
95. Arora, K.; Sequeira, J.M.; Hernández, A.I.; Alarcon, J.M.; Quadros, E.V. Behavioral alterations are associated with vitamin B12 deficiency in the transcobalamin receptor/CD320 KO mouse. *PLoS ONE* **2017**, *12*, e0177156. [CrossRef] [PubMed]

animals

MDPI

Article

Tolerability of 2 and 4 mg/kg Dosing Every 12 Hour of a Cannabidiol- and Cannabidiolic Acid-Rich Hemp Extract on Mixed-Breed Dogs Utilized for Teaching in a Closed Colony

Trista Mills [1], Stephanie Myers [1], Daniel Hughes [2] and Joseph Wakshlag [3,*]

1 School of Veterinary Medicine, Texas Tech University, Amarillo, TX 79106, USA; trista.mills@ttu.edu (T.M.); stephanie.myers@ttu.edu (S.M.)
2 Ellevet Sciences, Portland, ME 04106, USA; daniel.hughes@ellevetsciences.com
3 Department of Clinical Sciences, College of Veterinary Medicine, Cornell University, Ithaca, NY 14850, USA
* Correspondence: jw37@cornell.edu

Simple Summary: Considering the increasing popularity of cannabinoid-rich hemp-based full-spectrum nutraceuticals, there is a need to better understand the tolerability and adverse events associated with their use. This study aimed to examine the effects on dogs when using a 2 mg/kg and 4 mg/kg dose of CBD/CBDA-rich hemp product every 12 h in an academic teaching colony of dogs when compared to the consumption of a placebo soft-gel capsule every 12 h for two weeks. The results indicated that although there were serum concentrations of CBD in the 30–100 ng/mL concentration and 100–200 ng/mL concentration of CBDA, there were no adverse effects or behavioral changes observed regardless of the treatment used, thus showing that in normal healthy dogs, 2–4 mg/kg every 12 h appears to a safe dosing regimen.

Abstract: With the increase in popularity of utilizing cannabidiol (CBD) for human ailments, owners are actively interested in the possible utilization of cannabinoid products for their pets. The evaluation of CBD-rich hemp as an anti-anxiolytic, anti-inflammatory, immunomodulator, and anti-epileptic supplement has been assessed in previous studies in dogs, with adverse events such as ataxia or lethargy noted. In this study, the utilization of CBD-rich hemp was assessed at two concentrations to ascertain the impact on behavior as well as the tolerability of the medication given in a typically recommended dose and then twice that dose. Eighteen dogs were utilized in a randomized, double-blinded, placebo-controlled, 3 × 3 designed study. Each group of six dogs was provided placebo, 2 mg/kg, and 4 mg/kg of a cannabidiol/cannabidiolic acid (CBD/CBDA)-rich hemp in two-week intervals with one-week washout periods between each treatment period. Throughout the 10-week treatment period, student evaluations were performed, simulating clients' subjective assessments. Improvements in anxiety-related behavior and adverse events related to lethargy and ataxia were not observed and may indicate that the utilization of CBD-rich hemp products for behavioral changes may require higher dosing to mitigate unwanted behaviors in normal, healthy dogs. Furthermore, serum chemistry and serum cortisol were evaluated after each treatment period showing only a mildly significant increase in serum alkaline phosphatase when dosing at 4 mg/kg every 12 h, which is consistent with previously reported CBD dosing at these higher concentrations. Adverse events associated with CBD/CBDA-rich hemp extract given at 2 and 4 mg/kg every 12 h for two weeks were not reported, suggesting that using CBD-rich hemp in young, healthy dogs was safe during two weeks of treatment.

Keywords: dog; cannabidiol; cannabidiolic acid; adverse events; tolerability

1. Introduction

The use of *Cannabis sativa* hemp strains for cannabinoid treatment has gained popularity among pet owners and veterinarians alike over the past 10 years [1,2]. Cannabis

Sativa in the United States that has less than 0.3% delta 9-tetrahydrocannabinol (THC) is considered hemp, and is federally legal, creating a burgeoning market of pet supplements made from these low THC cultivars [3]. Current research supports the potential use of cannabidiol (CBD) isolates and CBD/cannabidiolic acid-rich (CBDA) hemp extracts clinically in canine veterinary medicine for ailments including osteoarthritis, refractory idiopathic epilepsy and atopic dermatitis [4–10]. Currently, clinically relevant dosing has been established at approximately 2–2.5 mg/kg every 12 h generally for osteoarthritis and 2–4.5 mg/kg every 12 h for refractory seizure activity [4–10]. In general, these are considered safe doses based on 12–36 weeks safety studies [11–14], and older literature suggesting that even higher doses are potentially safe in dogs [15]. Though safe, there are still questions about adverse events with the continued use of CBD isolates or CBD-rich hemp extracts due to slightly higher doses causing potential lethargy, ataxia, somnolence or appetite changes at doses from 2 to 5 mg/kg either SID or BID [4–10]. Clinical veterinary assessments of CBD-rich hemp extract have reported physiological issues observed by veterinarians including mydriasis and mildly delayed hopping responses at doses 5–10 mg/kg as a single daily dose within 2 h of ingestion, yet there appears to be tolerance with chronic dosing of 5 mg/kg daily [16].

Behavioral issues or owner-perceived side effects have been observed in the 2–4.5 mg/kg every 12 h range, with some evidence that CBD-rich hemp can be anxietolytic or can possible hinder aggression [17–19]. A study assessing aggressive tendencies, using an approximate dose of 2–4 mg/kg daily, showed that over time there was a decrease in aggressive tendencies during 4 weeks of kenneling; however, when compared to placebo there were no significant differences [17]. Another study suggested that 1.4 mg/kg of CBD 4–6 h prior to a recorded thunderstorm event in shelter/teaching dogs at a University showed no behavioral changes related to this dose of CBD isolate after dosing [18]. In kenneled dog studies on separation and car ride anxiety models, utilizing 4 mg/kg of CBD isolate as a one-time dose, there was found to be minimal physiological alteration in parameters associated with anxiety within 2 h of dosing (i.e., cortisol, lip-licking or heart-rate variability), yet behaviorist video evaluations suggest a more relaxed demeanor [19]. To date, no clinical study in client-owned populations have been performed related to behavioral pathologies.

We hypothesized that increasing the dosage from 2 mg/kg every 12 h to 4 mg/kg every 12 h would elicit adverse effects, behavioral alterations resulting in tolerability issues. The aim of our study was to examine adverse events at two different doses of CBD/CBDA-rich hemp within the dosing range utilized in multiple studies using medical records and weekly veterinary examinations for adverse events; as well as student evaluations of the dogs in an "owner-like" unvalidated observation related to their kenneled lifestyle. A second objective was to determine the serum chemistry alteration that may be attributed to dosing of 2 mg/kg and 4 mg/kg every 12 h for two weeks in a randomized placebo blinded cross-over design to better understand tolerability.

2. Materials and Methods

2.1. Dogs

The study population included 20 dogs acquired from the local shelter chosen over a period of two days. Dogs that had "good temperament" and were considered "people friendly" were chosen. A 3-week acclimation period to the long-term teaching colony was observed for all dogs. During this time, unsterilized animals were spayed or neutered, screened for parasites and rickettsial diseases, and ancillary procedures necessary for optimal quality of life were performed. Dogs were allowed to undergo these procedures and were included in the study after these medical screens were deemed negative and/or treated appropriately. All dog's received a complete blood count and a serum biochemistry prior to enrollment and were deemed free of any clinically significant organ-related dysfunction with a physical examination showing all physiological parameters within normal limits. The study was performed with approval from the Texas Tech University School of Veterinary Medicine Institutional Care and Use Committee approval (protocol 2022-1272).

2.2. Randomization, Treatment and Physical Assessment

Twenty dogs were randomized, in a double-blinded, placebo-controlled, study design with one week washout periods between treatment periods (two week duration) and each dog was assigned to a sequence of treatment (i.e., ACB, BAC, or CBA). The cohort was randomized into two groups of 7 and one group of 6 dogs, each ranging in size from 10 to 40 kg, using a random number generator (randomizer app version 8.0). All resources for production including the hemp extract, sesame oil, and gelatin were food grade products made under certified and audited good manufacturing processes. Dogs were provided oral soft gel capsules (gelatin based) in groups A (2 mg/kg CBD/CBDA), B (placebo-sunflower oil), and C (4 mg/kg CBD/CBDA) using incremental dosing based on weight of the dog at the beginning of the study phase using capsules designed at 5 mg, 10 mg or 20 mg of total cannabinoid. Each ml of the oil utilized to fill the gel capsules was 29 mg/mL CBD, 30 mL CBDA, 1.2 mg of THC, 1.4 mg/mL tetrahydrocannabinolic acid (THCA), 0.9 mg/mL of cannabichromene (CBC), 1.0 mg/mL cannabichromenic acid (CBCA), 1.2 mg/mL cannabigerol (CBG), 1.2 mg/mL cannabigerolic acid (CBGA) and no other detectable cannabinoids based on third party analysis in a 17025 certified facility (Proverde Analytics, Milford, MA, USA). The hemp oil was also certified free of detectable nonpathogenic or pathogenic microbes, heavy metals, pesticides, extraction solvents and mycotoxins at the same certified facility. Treatment was provided every morning at approximately 7 am and in the evening at approximately 6 pm in a "pill pocket" with the dog's meals; dogs were weighed every 3 weeks and dose was adjusted appropriately. There was a 1-week washout period and then each group transitioned to the next treatment formulation based on the prior literature that behavioral effects are transient and that any residual cannabinoid in the serum would be negligible to final cannabinoid assessment after the 1-week washout and then two weeks of treatment [20]. To assess physiologic response to the treatments, blood was taken before and after each treatment period (6 samples total) on all dogs in the study to assess cannabinoid concentrations, cortisol, and serum biochemistry, with complete blood counts performed at the initiation and end of the 9-week study period. These samples were taken between 3 and 4 h after morning treatments to provide consistency for serum cannabinoid testing. Physical examinations were performed by the veterinary principle investigator (TM) every week where the dogs were examined and received neurological (i.e., cranial nerve, reflexes, ataxia assessment and proprioceptive testing) and orthopedic examinations (i.e., gait, lameness and proprioception).

2.3. Student Interaction Evaluations and Video Assessment

Two weeks before starting the study, students in their first year of the veterinary curriculum worked with their specifically assigned dog for teaching clinical skills examinations. Dogs were then started on the protocol as described and visualized in Figure 1, with both students and veterinarians blinded to treatments. Basic behavior evaluations assessing subjective anxiety, lethargy, ease of working with the dog, aggressive behaviors, jumping behavior, and vocalization/barking were tracked utilizing a Likert scale administered via online survey for the students. Students were asked to fill out evaluations at each interaction with the dog over the 9-week period (Supplemental Figure S1). Scaling was based on 0 suggesting no changes, scores of −1 being a little worse, −2 being a lot worse, 1 being a little better and 2 being a lot better.

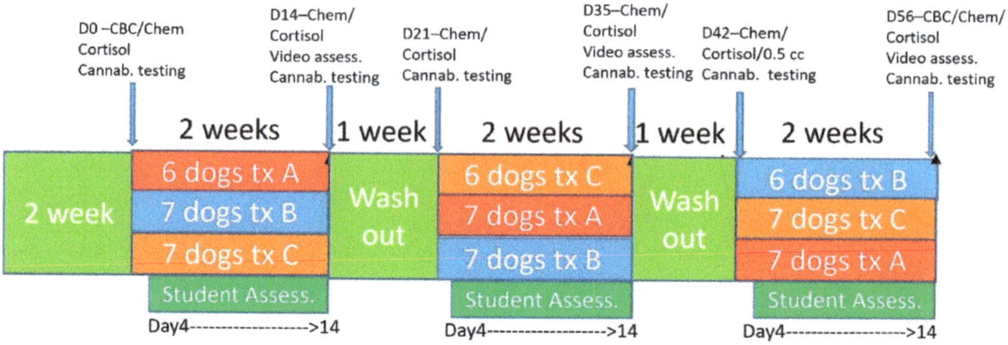

Figure 1. Timeline for treatment and procedures during the trial and treatment groups. Treatment A was 2 mg/kg BID, Treatment B was placebo, Treatment C was 4 mg/kg.

Evaluations were assessed as a change from baseline after interacting with the dogs for two weeks (week 0) for each student interacting with each dog only if they had an evaluation between days 4 and 14 of treatment in all three treatment periods. Typically, for each dog there were 4–6 complete student evaluations for each treatment period which were averaged across the students for each category of behavior/adverse event assessment and presented as a mean and standard deviation score for that specific dog during each treatment period.

A secondary behavior assessment was performed looking at panting, circling, self-mutilation/licking, posture in kennel, sleep habits, interest in enrichment, utilizing objective video recording performed once weekly between 6 and 7 pm for a 10 min duration approximately 1 h after evening dosing, which was recorded and assessed via remote observation. A running medical evaluation kept track of any illness experienced by the dogs through laboratory animal care attendants and veterinarians' observations for any illness including attitude changes, decreased appetite, vomiting, diarrhea, coughing, or other clinical signs related to illness or injury.

2.3.1. CBC, Serum Chemistry and Cannabinoid Analysis

Blood was drawn from each dog prior to and after the completion of each phase of treatment, the day before the treatment started and then again on day 14 of treatment. Two cc of blood was collected in a 4 mL EDTA tube (Beckton Dickenson, Franklin Lakes, NY, USA) while 4 cc was collected in a red top tube that was allowed to clot for 20–40 min before being spun at 3600 G for 10 min to collect serum with 1 cc allocated to clinical chemistry for serum biochemical and cortisol assessment. A 1 mL aliquot of serum was also frozen at −80 °C for eventual cannabinoid analysis. CBCs were performed at week 0 and week 9 of the study to assess any hemogram changes from initiation to study end (IDEXX Laboratories, Memphis, TN, USA). CBC parameters assessed were red blood cell count, hemoglobin, hematocrit, white blood cell count, neutrophils, lymphocytes, eosinophils, basophils and platelets. Serum biochemistry and cortisol assessment was performed prior to and at the completion of each phase of the experiment (IDEXX Laboratories, Memphis, TN, USA). Parameters assessed through serum chemistry included glucose, symmetric dimethyl arginine, serum urea nitrogen (SUN), creatinine, sodium, potassium, chloride, magnesium, calcium, phosphorus, total protein, globulin, albumin, alkaline phosphatase (ALP), alanine aminotransferase (ALT), aspartate aminotransferase (AST), bilirubin, cholesterol and cortisol concentrations.

At study end, all frozen samples were shipped on dry ice overnight to Cultivate Analytics (Portland, ME, USA) and were assessed utilizing liquid chromatography and mass spectroscopy (LC/MS/MS) for serum cannabinoids. Serum assessment included CBD, CBDA, THC, THCA, CBC, CBCA, CBGA, 6-hydroxy cannabidiol (6-OH-CBD), 7 hydroxy-cannabidiol (7-OH-CBD), 7 carboxy-cannabidiol (7-COOH-CBD), cannabinol (CBN) and glucoronidated-THC.

Analysis was performed with a fit-for-purpose LC/MS/MS method for measurement of seven cannabinoids and five of their metabolites at Cultivate (Portland, ME, USA). Matrix-matched calibration curves were generated for each compound using reference standards obtained from Cerilliant Corporation (Round Rock, TX, USA). An internal standard solution was generated in methanol at 1 μg/mL containing 7-OH-CBD-d3, 11-OH-delta-9-THC-d3, CBDA-d3, CBD-d3, delta 9-THC-d3, and THCA-A-d3. Dog serum samples were prepared for analysis by adding 100 μL of serum to 250 μL of methanol and 50 μL of internal standard solution. Samples were vortexed for at least 1 min and centrifuged at 10,000 rpm (9300× *g*) at 4 °C. The supernatant was transferred to autosampler vials for analysis via LC-MS/MS (Agilent 1260 Infinity II HPLC coupled to an Agilent 6490 Triple Quadrupole; Santa Clara, CA, USA). A volume of 10 μL of each sample was injected onto an Agilent column (Poroshell 120 EC-C18 2.7 μm 3.0 × 100 mm). The columns were equilibrated with 50% mobile phase A (0.1% formic acid in water) and 50% mobile phase B (0.1% formic acid in acetonitrile). The column compartment was held at 50 °C. The compounds were eluted by a starting gradient of 50% B held for 0.5 min, ramped to 100% B over 7 min, and held at 100% B for 1 min. The column was re-equilibrated to the initial mobile phase composition for 1.5 min. The flow rate was 0.8 mL/min for the entire analysis. The compounds were detected in electrospray ionization positive and/or negative mode as described in Supplemental Table S1. The gas temperature and sheath gas temperature were set to 120 °C and 400 °C, respectively. The gas flow and sheath gas flow were set to 11 L/min and 12 L/min, respectively. The nebulizer was set to 30 psi. The capillary and nozzle voltage were set to 3000 V and 2000 V, respectively. Concentrations were calculated using Agilent Mass Hunter Quantitative Analysis version 10.0 using a linear regression with 1/c weighing based on relative response for each compound. The lower limit of detection and quantitation in dog serum is provided in Supplemental Table S2.

2.3.2. Statistical Analysis

Student Adverse Event/Behavioral Evaluations

The means from student evaluations from each treatment phase as changes from baseline were assessed for normality utilizing Shapiro–Wilk test, and residual plots were examined. If normality was rejected, the data were log transformed and visually inspected for normal distribution before analysis, utilizing repeated measures mixed-model analysis on JMP 16 (Wittington House, UK). Variables included in the model as fixed effects were gender, treatment, time, sequence, and trazodone use. Random effects were period and dog nested within period. Tukey's post hoc tests were performed for multiple comparison correction of *p*-values for all pairwise least square means (LSM) comparisons found to be significant, with a value of 0.05 or less being deemed a significant finding.

2.3.3. CBC and Serum Chemistry

All CBC and serum chemistry data were assessed utilizing Shapiro–Wilk test for normality, and residual plots were examined. When normality was rejected, the data was log transformed and visually inspected for normal distribution before analysis utilizing repeated measures mixed-model analysis on JMP 16 (Wittington House, UK). Different covariance structures were tested for each model and the data was then back transformed for reporting if logarithmic analysis was utilized. For the serum chemistry, the variables included in the model as fixed effects were gender, sequence of treatment, time, treatment, and the interaction term treatment × time. Random effects were period and dog nested within period. For CBC pre- and post-trial results, the variables included in the model were gender, sequence of treatment, time with the random effects of period and dog nested within period. Tukey's post hoc tests were performed for multiple comparison correction of *p*-values for all pairwise LSM comparisons found to be significant, with a value of 0.05 or less being deemed a statistically significant finding.

2.3.4. Serum Cannabinoids

Serum cannabinoids that were detectable within the LLOQ of detection were assessed using descriptive statistics to provide serum concentrations found during each treatment phase. Serum was collected prior to the initiation of each phase and then again between 3 and 4 h after treatment on day 14 of each group. Descriptive statistics including means (medians and ranges) for the two treatments are reported to examine relative cannabinoids and cannabinoid metabolites observed in this population of dogs.

3. Results

3.1. Physical Examinations

During the 9-week protocol, there were two dogs that were returned to the shelter due to inability to control inter-dog aggression at week 4 of the protocol, leaving 16 dogs for complete data assessment. Demographics including presumed predominant breed, age, gender and weights over the trial are reported in Table 1. Each weekly physical examination of each dog revealed no abnormalities including physical examination, neurologic (deficits in cranial nerves, reflexes, ataxia, or proprioception/hopping responses) or orthopedic examination (gait or lameness evaluations) at any time point. All dogs showed normal appetite throughout the protocol with the average weight of the dogs being 23.7 ± 6.7 kg prior to the trial and 24.1 ± 6.6 kg at the end of the trial. During the protocol, there were two incidences of diarrhea which were treated with metronidazole and probiotic for a 5-day duration; one being during the treatment with 2 mg/kg twice daily and another dog during the treatment with placebo. No other adverse events were noted during the treatment or washout periods that could be attributed to the treatments provided.

Table 1. Canine demographics of the cohort that completed the 10-week trial with assumed ages and weights during the trial.

Breed	Est. Age	Sex	Weight D0 (kg)	Weight D20 (kg)	Weight D41 (kg)
Pit mix	2 y	MN	33.2	34.0	33.6
Pit mix	2 y	FS	20.5	20.9	20
Lab Mix	2 y	FS	19.5	19.5	19.5
GSD Mix	2 y	MN	34.1	34.5	34.5
Border Collie Mix	7 m	FS	13.6	13.6	15
Great Dane mix	4 y	MN	21.8	27.3	32.7
German Shepherd Mix	2 y	MN	29.1	30.5	30
Shar pei mix	6 y	MN	26.4	26.4	25.9
Great Dane Mix	1 y	FS	28.6	29.5	30.4
Pit bull mix	2 y	FS	23.2	22.7	22.7
Pit bull mix	2 y	FS	22.7	22.7	22.7
Pit bull mix	2 y	MN	22.7	22.7	22.7
Lab Mix	1 y	FS	20.9	20.5	20.5
Terrier	2 y	FS	21.4	21.8	21.8
Coonhound	2 y	FS	33.2	33.6	33.6
Boxer mix	2 y	MN	25.9	25.9	25
Papillon	6 m	MN	9.1	10.5	11.4
Pit mix	2 y	FS	20.5	20.5	20.5
Border Collie Mix	1 y	MN	14.5	15.0	15

Note: These animals were acquired from the local shelter with minimal to nonexistent historical information. The ages were estimated and may not reflect true age.

Due to kennel management issues, some dogs were placed on trazadone treatment at 5 mg/kg body weight due to clinical assessments by handlers in managing dogs through the recommendation of the clinical vets from the laboratory animal veterinary care services. There were 6 dogs treated with approximately 5 mg/kg every q 12 h trazodone during the placebo treatment, 4 dogs during the 2 mg/kg CBD-rich hemp treatment, and 6 dogs during the 4 mg/kg CBD-rich hemp treatment. Treatment was deemed necessary for exuberant behavior and easier handling of the dogs by students who were performing required enrichment and for teaching purposes related to physical examination as part of their training.

3.2. Student Adverse Event/Behavioral Evaluations

At the beginning of the trial, there were 7–8 students assigned to each dog to partake in evaluations during each phase of the trial. After examining all students that responded during each phase of the trial periods, there were between 4 and 6 evaluations from students that had an evaluation for each phase of the study for their respective dog. The average response score from each student over the three phases was averaged for each treatment period and reported as the mean and standard deviation (Table 2). All data collected were normally distributed, so no transformations of the data were required before statistical analysis. Across all the evaluations, there were no differences found in treatment, gender, sequence or trazodone treatment for lethargy, anxiety, jumping, mouthing/biting, or vocalization. A significance was found for handling and treatment effects ($p = 0.008$), whereby post hoc assessment showed improved handling between the 2 mg/kg and 4 mg/kg treatment groups ($p = 0.004$), but not with the placebo. Additionally, the sequence was significantly different for handling ($p = 0.04$) with this difference being between the sequence of 2 mg/kg–4 mg/kg–placebo vs. 4 mg/kg–placebo–2 mg/kg for biting/mouthing behaviors. It was found that there was a significant increase in vocalization during period 2 when compared to period 3 ($p = 0.02$).

Table 2. Change from baseline scoring of dogs during students' weekly evaluations during protocol based on 5-point Likert scaling: −2—much worse, −1—a little worse, 0—no change, 1—a little better, 2—a lot better.

Δ From Baseline	Placebo	2 mg/kg	4 mg/kg	Period	Tx	Seq	Gender	Traz
Anxiety	0.53 ± 0.58	0.48 ± 0.26	0.66 ± 0.56	0.47	0.27	0.10	0.36	0.81
Lethargy	0.46 ± 0.34	0.38 ± 0.37	0.50 ± 0.39	0.66	0.48	0.93	0.84	0.96
Handling	0.73 ± 0.58	0.63 ± 0.44	0.77 ± 0.59 *	0.70	0.008	0.04	0.3	0.89
Jumping	0.28 ± 0.48	0.14 ± 0.28	0.28 ± 0.34	0.47	0.41	0.96	0.76	0.14
Biting/mouthing	0.35 ± 0.52	0.20 ± 0.44	0.54 ± 0.52	0.20	0.08	0.57	0.79	0.14
Vocalizing	0.22 ± 0.42	0.16 ± 0.44	0.50 ± 0.49	0.02	0.19	0.18	0.43	0.07

* Asterisk indicates a significant difference between 4 mg/kg and 2 mg/kg treatment.

3.3. Video Evaluation

Ten-minute evaluations of each dog were recorded to assess kennel behaviors including pacing, cage biting, kennel positioning, and vocalization as markers of stress and anxiety in the kenneled environment between 7 p.m. and 7:30 p.m. on day 7 of treatment and at the end of each phase of testing on day 14. Video recordings of all 16 dogs that remained in the study for the duration showed that 15 of the 16 dogs were all recumbent on their sides or in a curled posture primarily sleeping for the duration of each video assessment. There was one dog that was observed to be vocalizing during each evaluation recording, regardless of the treatment period and was persistently vocalizing at the front of the cage for the entire 10 min time period.

3.4. Complete Blood Count

Of the CBC results analyzed, all the data was found to be normally distributed. Blood counts assessed at week 0 and week 9 of the study revealed time-related differences in a few parameters (Table 3). There was a significant decrease in reticulocyte across the population of dogs, yet all remained within the reference range ($p < 0.001$). Hematocrit and hemoglobin concentrations were also significantly higher at the end of the study ($p = 0.004$ and $p = 0.003$, respectively). Overall, white blood cell and neutrophil counts were significantly lower at the end of the study as well, ($p = 0.02$ and $p = 0.015$ respectively) with only one dog being above the reference range for white blood cells and neutrophils at the beginning of the study period which normalized at the end of the study. The basophil counts were also significantly decreased from baseline by the end of the study, with all dogs being within reference range at each time point ($p = 0.015$).

Table 3. Means and standard deviations of CBC parameters ($n = 16$) at the beginning and end of the study period. Time, gender, and sequence significances are reported with $p < 0.05$ being significant and bolded.

Analyte (Ref. Range)	Pre Trial	Post Trial	Time	Gender	Tx Seq
Red blood cells (5.39–8.70 M/µL)	6.88 ± 0.79	7.14 ± 0.52	0.06	0.21	0.41
Hematocrit (38.3–56.6%)	46.8 ± 5.2	49.7 ± 5.1	**0.004**	0.08	0.5
Hemoglobin (13.4–20.7 g/dL)	15.7 ± 1.9	16.6 ± 1.5	**0.003**	0.08	0.47
Reticulocyte (10–110 K/µL)	70 ± 22	43 ± 15	**<0.001**	0.54	0.32
White blood cells (4.9–17.6 thous/µL)	14.1 ± 4.6	11.4 ± 3.6	**0.02**	0.78	0.43
Neutrophil (2.94–1270 thous/µL)	9.4 ± 4.0	6.7 ± 2.2	**0.015**	0.55	0.46
Lymphocytes (1.06–4.95 thous/µL)	3.28 ± 1.36	3.21 ± 1.49	0.99	0.22	0.83
Monocytes (0.13–1.15 thous/µL)	0.63 ± 0.23	0.55 ± 0.45	0.48	0.82	0.3
Eosinophils (0.07–1.49 thous/µL)	0.74 ± 0.45	0.93 ± 0.48	0.09	0.37	0.4
Basophils (0–0.1 thous/µL)	0.05 ± 0.03	0.02 ± 0.02	**0.015**	0.31	0.63
Platelets (143–448 thous/µL)	270 ± 114	230 ± 78	0.17	0.18	0.54

3.5. Serum Biochemistry and Cortisol

Of the serum biochemistry evaluated, only ALP and cortisol were found to be non-normally distributed and log transformation was performed before evaluation and back transformed for reporting purposes (Table 4). Serum mineral and electrolyte changes were not observed as treatment effects; however, there was a time effect on both serum potassium and serum calcium concentrations. Calcium was typically higher pretreatment for each group than post-treatment ($p < 0.001$), while serum potassium was slightly higher in the post-treatment intervals than prior to treatments ($p < 0.001$). Additionally, serum glucose showed mild significant differences over time ($p < 0.001$), with pretreatment samples being slightly higher than post-treatment samples. Serum proteins including total protein and albumin were significantly higher in males than in females, yet all parameters fell within normal reference ranges ($p = 0.02$ and 0.01, respectively). All serum hepatic enzymes and renal parameters showed no differences regardless of time or treatment except ALP values which showed a treatment*time effect ($p = 0.001$), with post hoc analysis showing the 4 mg/kg every 12 h ALP was higher with 3 of 16 values above the reference range at the end of the treatment period (Figure 2). Serum cortisol showed no significant differences over the treatment period or between treatment groups. Both bilirubin and ALT were elevated in the group designated to the CBA series of treatment compared to the other two randomization sequences ($p = 0.002$ and $p = 0.01$, respectively).

Table 4. Mean and standard deviations of serum chemistry parameters ($n = 16$) at the beginning and end of the study period. Time, treatment (Tx), Tx*time, gender and sequence significances are reported, with $p < 0.05$ being significant.

Analyte (Ref. Range)	Time	Placebo	2 mg/kg	4 mg/kg	Tx	Time	Tx*Time	Gender	seq
Glucose	Pre	83 ± 11	79 ± 12	82 ± 8	0.37	<0.001	0.14	0.69	0.58
(53–114 mg/dL)	Post	76 ± 13	76 ± 11	70 ± 15					
SDMA	Pre	11 ± 1	12 ± 3	11 ± 2	0.91	0.15	0.82	0.2	0.14
(0–14 ug/dL)	Post	10 ± 3	11 ± 2	11 ± 2					
Creatinine	Pre	1.1 ± 0.2	1.0 ± 0.3	1.0 ± 0.2	0.79	0.1	0.43	0.94	0.06
(0.5–1.5 mg/dL)	Post	1.1 ± 0.3	1.1 ± 0.2	1.0 ± 0.1					
SUN	Pre	22 ± 7	22 ± 7	19 ± 6	0.25	0.24	0.86	0.75	0.06
(9–31 mg/dL)	Post	23 ± 9	22 ± 5	23 ± 5					
Phosphorus	Pre	6 ± 2	5.8 ± 1.3	5.9 ± 1.5	0.21	0.02	0.08	0.57	0.57
(2.5–6.1 mg/dL)	Post	5.2 ± 1	5.6 ± 1.4	5.9 ± 1.3					
Calcium	Pre	10.0 ± 0.4	9.9 ± 0.8	9.9 ± 0.5	0.34	<0.001	0.65	0.62	0.91
(8.4–11.8 mg/dL)	Post	9.4 ± 0.5	9.4 ± 0.6	9.7 ± 0.6					
Sodium	Pre	147 ± 4	144 ± 6	147 ± 2	0.14	0.76	0.41	0.23	0.75
(142–152 mmol/L)	Post	144 ± 9	146 ± 3	148 ± 3					
Potassium	Pre	4.6 ± 0.4	4.5 ± 0.3	4.6 ± 0.3	0.1	<0.001	0.43	0.09	0.89
(4.0–5.4 mmol/L)	Post	4.7 ± 0.4	4.7 ± 0.4	4.9 ± 0.5					
Chloride	Pre	110 ± 3	107 ± 5	110 ± 2	0.06	0.11	0.06	0.76	0.58
(108–119 mmol/L)	Post	110 ± 2	110 ± 2	110 ± 2					
Total protein	Pre	6.1 ± 0.5	6.0 ± 0.4	6.0 ± 0.5	0.77	0.18	0.3	0.02	0.27
(5.5–7.5 g/L)	Post	6.0 ± 0.4	5.9 ± 0.4	6.1 ± 0.5					
Albumin	Pre	3.0 ± 0.3	3.0 ± 0.3	3.0 ± 0.3	0.88	0.96	0.76	0.01	0.73
(2.7–3.9 g/L)	Post	3.0 ± 0.3	3.0 ± 0.3	3.1 ± 0.4					
Globulin	Pre	3.1 ± 0.4	3.0 ± 0.4	3.0 ± 0.4	0.73	0.07	0.12	0.55	0.4
(2.4–4.0 g/L)	Post	3.0 ± 0.4	2.9 ± 0.3	3.0 ± 0.4					
ALT	Pre	38 ± 11	40 ± 14	39 ± 9	0.66	0.95	0.49	0.19	0.01
(18–121 U/L)	Post	40 ± 10	42 ± 11	39 ± 8					
AST	Pre	29 ± 6	31 ± 8	31 ± 7	0.4	0.74	0.42	0.02	0.68
(16–55 U/L)	Post	30 ± 7	32 ± 9	30 ± 5					
ALP	Pre	116 ± 111	75 ± 40	94 ± 79	0.92	<0.001	<0.001	0.29	0.27
(5–160 U/L)	Post	92 ± 79	105 ± 88	155 ± 187 *					
Bilirubin	Pre	0.1 ± 0.1	0.1 ± 0.1	0.1 ± 0.1	0.98	0.29	0.07	0.37	0.002
(0–0.2 U/L)	Post	0.1 ± 0.1	0.1 ± 0.1	0.0 ± 0.0					
Cholesterol	Pre	232 ± 60	214 ± 52	228 ± 57	0.91	0.38	0.06	0.37	0.14
(131–345 mg/dL)	Post	221 ± 47	227 ± 47	227 ± 46					
Cortisol	Pre	1.3 ± 0.6	1.6 ± 1.1	1.9 ± 1.1	0.23	0.98	0.44	0.27	0.61
(0.6–3.4 µg/dL)	Post	1.4 ± 0.8	1.3 ± 0.6	2.2 ± 2.1					

* Asterisk indicates a significant difference between 4 mg/kg treatment from both placebo and 2 mg/kg treatment.

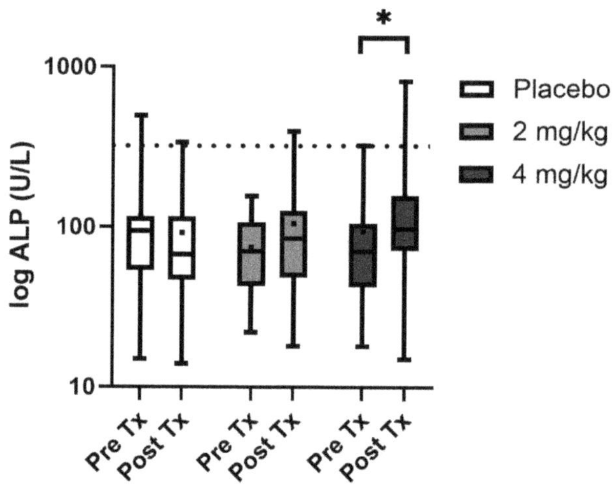

Figure 2. Serum ALP box and whisker plot with boxes showing the 25th and 75th median quartiles and whiskers indicating the minimum and maximum concentrations (dot within the box is mean) before treatment (day 0) and post-treatment (day 14) for each phase. Dotted line depicts the upper reference range. * Depicts a significant difference between the groups pre- and post-treatment.

3.6. Cannabinoid and CBD Metabolite Concentrations

Detectable cannabinoids and metabolites in the serum were CBD, CBDA, 9-THC, THCA, CBCA, 6-hydroxy cannabidiol (6 OH-CBD), and 7 carboxy cannabidiol (7 COOH-CBD) above their lower limits of quantitation in the 2 mg/kg and 4 mg/kg treatment groups (Table 5). All other cannabinoids were non-detectable in the serum of the dogs. Serum samples collected after each one-week wash out showed no residual cannabinoids above the LLOQ for any of the cannabinoids or metabolites. The analysis of the CBD concentrations on the last day of each treatment period, performed 3–4 h after the morning dose, had the expected results for Group A (placebo) with no detectable cannabinoids for all animals involved. Group B's (2 mg/kg) post-treatment analysis can be found in Table 5. For metabolites 6-OH-CBD and 7-COOH-CBD at 2 mg/kg, nearly all dogs (>12) had values below the LLOQ and are thus not reported. At 4 mg/kg dosing, four dogs were in between the LLOQ and LLOD; therefore, the values utilized for calculation were half of the LLOQ at 2.5 ng/mL for 6OH-CBD. The 7-COOH-CBD concentrations at 4 mg/kg revealed eight dogs with values between the LLOD and LLOQ; therefore, half of the LLOQ being 0.5 mg/mL was entered as data points for those eight dogs to provide the mean, median and range for this metabolite.

Table 5. Mean (median; range) serum concentration of cannabinoids and CBD-related metabolites (n = 16) 3–4 h after morning dose on day 14 of 2 and 4 mg/kg BID dosing of CBD/CBDA-rich hemp extract.

Analyte	LLOD	LLOQ	2 mg/kg	4 mg/kg
CBD	5	10	37.9 (37.4; 10.5–82.8)	80.4 (80.7; 17.0–119.8)
CBDA	1	2.5	101.5 (90; 33.1–221.0)	189.7 (154.4; 35.6–674.6)
THC	1	2.5	1.5 (1.3; 0–5.0)	4.8 (5.3; 1.3–8.2)
THCA	1	2.5	6.3 (6.0; 1.3–13.6)	8.6 (7.8; 3.1–14.7)
CBCA	1	2.5	16 (25.6; 4.3–30.2)	24.3 (20.2; 7.3–51.7)
6-OH CBD	1	5	LLOQ	4.2 (3.9; 2.5–6.9)
7-COOH-CBD	0.5	1	LLOQ	1.1 (1.2; 0.5–2.3)

LLOQ indicates values were below the lower limit of quantification.

4. Discussion

The use of CBD-rich hemp has been observed to induce transient clinical signs of a delayed hopping response and mydriasis in one clinical study at 5 mg/kg, which, when dosed over 5 days diminished with repeated 5 mg/kg daily dosing. Based on veterinary examinations weekly, this was not observed at the end of week one or week two of our study period, suggesting that acclimation to the dose may be occurring or that this unique hemp blend did not induce these physical examination changes. No other clinical signs or observations by veterinarians or students suggested any adverse events related to every 12 h treatment with 2 or 4 mg/kg. In clinical studies utilizing CBD/CBDA-rich hemp extract to determine effect on pruritis, Loewinger reported a portion of the study participants (5/17 dogs) experienced lethargy or calmness attributed to the treatment with no other clinically notable adverse effects when utilizing 2 mg/kg q 12 h [7]. While studies utilizing CBD concurrently with traditional seizure medication (singular or combination use of phenobarbital, zonisamide, levetiracetam and potassium bromide), McGrath and colleagues noted adverse effects including somnolence and ataxia with the addition of 2.5 mg/kg to every 12 h dosing of a CBD product to established treatment protocols for epilepsy [9]. This agrees with the findings reported by Garcia et al. as 3/14 dogs utilized in their study developed transient ataxia during the course of treatment with 2 mg/kg twice daily dosing of CBD/CBDA-rich hemp added to an established treatment protocol of 2 or more anti-seizure medications [8]. Both of these studies note that anti-seizure medications and CBD undergo metabolism via hepatic and gastrointestinal cytochrome p450 and hepatic conjugation activities which could alter the serum concentrations of typical anti-epileptic drugs; however, in the Garcia study, no serum alterations of phenobarbital or zonisamide were observed [8,9,21]. In a later study by Donovan et al., the interactions of CBD and phenobarbital were elegantly examined showing no influence of CBD on phenobarbital serum concentrations in normal healthy beagles at similar or higher dosing [22].

In our study, we did not see any notable alterations in CBC parameters that were related to a treatment effect; however, CBCs were not performed at each stage of the study. Repeated CBCs at each phase were not performed due to prior studies showing no alterations in any CBC parameters using doses between 5 and 10 mg/kg per day in studies examining mixed cannabinoids or CBD-rich hemp products, to date [11,21]. All of the changes over time surrounded primarily red blood cell alterations and reticulocytosis which could be related to environment change as feral dogs and treatment of GI parasitism. More importantly, these changes were not clinically significant as all dogs fell within the normal ranges for RBC and HCT.

Serum chemistry was followed for each phase of treatment as multiple studies utilizing between 2 and 10 mg/kg total daily dose of various CBD products have shown alterations in ALP, with hints towards ALT rises when providing 10 mg/kg as a single daily dose in dogs [4,9,10,12–14]. An ALP increase is attributed to the upregulation of cytochrome P450 enzymatic activity, while ALT rises can be attributed to hepatocellular damage [10,12]. In the current study, only dogs given 4 mg/kg CBD/CBDA-rich hemp every 12 h showed significant alterations in ALP with 3/16 dogs showing elevations above the reference range. All other serum chemistry alterations were related to the time or sequence of treatment which may be related to the new environment or differences in feeding from their prior shelter or feral status. These rises in ALP appear to be innocuous as they are not accompanied by other serum hepatic enzyme alterations and prior investigations have shown that these rises are reversable when treatment is discontinued [14]. While several of the dogs were on concurrent trazodone for ease of handling for teaching purposes, it should be noted there was no evidence of neurologic deficits during co-administration of these treatments. Nor were there any adverse events or behavioral alteration noted by the student evaluation during co-treatment or even single-agent delivery of trazodone. Similarly, a report on the behavioral alterations in dogs when specifically co-administered trazodone at 10 mg/kg along with 1.4 mg/kg of CBD isolate as a single dose showed no behavioral alterations during co-administration or with each as single-agent therapy [17].

The lack of any behavioral or adverse events with the 2 mg/kg and 4 mg/kg every 12 h dosing regimen was surprising; however, the dogs used in this study were all under the estimated age of six years old and healthy with no comorbidities unlike clinical studies for epilepsy, arthritis and atopic dermatitis where there were concomitant treatments ongoing in dogs with a wider age range [4,7,8]. It must be noted that the veterinary evaluations were performed between 7:30 a.m. and video at 7 p.m. generally 30–60 min after morning dosing at 7 a.m. and 6 p.m. in the evening. Any anxiolytic or adverse events may peak at 1–2 h after dosing; therefore, our evaluations were not carried out just prior to peak serum exposure, similar to Hunt and colleagues [18]. Student assessments were typically performed throughout the day between 10 a.m. and 4 p.m., presenting a major limitation in our study being the lack of a standard timing for these evaluations, which was not possible due to the varied student activities throughout the day during this study. It must also be noted that this was not a validated survey and the variability in each student's assessment could be related to timing; however, there were no real adverse events related to lethargy or somnolence and globally the dogs did not show any significant behavior changes during this chronic exposure. Though speculative, we might consider the student observations to be similar to what owners might report. Based on this information of no perceived differences between the treatment groups of placebo, 2 mg/kg and 4 mg/kg, it could be suggested that the administration of up to 4 mg/kg of this full-spectrum hemp product should not cause any significant adverse events or positive/negative behavioral effects in normal healthy dogs.

The management of stress and stress-related co-morbidities in canines has a limited number of viable pharmaceutical treatment options. In human psycho-therapeutic medicine, CBD has been purported to benefit users who suffer from anxiety, depression, and PTSD [23]. Veterinary medicine has begun to examine the behavioral effect of CBD in areas such as aggression and anxiety. Recent studies by Hunt and colleagues have examined a single car ride as well as repeated car rides and separation anxiety in kenneled dogs given a single oral dose of 4 mg/kg CBD isolate showing a lack of traditional measures such as lip licking, cortisol or heart rate variability changes globally [18,24]. However, behaviorist video assessment using qualitative behavioral ratings suggested lower stress, sad, tense and uncomfortable behaviors during vehicle travel [18]. This proved to be inconsistent in a follow-up study when examining multiple car rides at a single 4 mg/kg dose 1–2 h before three different car rides over 3 months [24]. The inconsistency and lack of definitive effects globally suggest that a CBD isolate may only have mild effects on anxiety and dosing may need to be higher. As noted by Hunt et al., studies on clinically affected dogs rather than kenneled dogs with no known anxiety disorders are needed to evaluate efficacy with owner surveys and board-certified veterinary behaviorist evaluation in a clinical population [18,24].

Blood was drawn from each dog three to four hours after the morning dose of the last day of each treatment period to assess cannabinoids found in the serum after dosing to assess relative steady state. It was evident that CBDA was absorbed and retained approximately two-fold better than CBD with 2 mg/kg every 12 h, with serum concentrations being approximately half of what was found of both cannabinoids when dosed at 4 mg/kg every 12 h, as expected. Interestingly, of the other minor cannabinoids in the product, the acidic THCA and CBCA appear to be absorbed and retained at some level suggesting that acidic cannabinoids may be absorbed better and preferable to the neutral cannabinoids such as THC and CBD. This has been shown in multiple species including parrots, humans, horses, primates and rabbits [20,24–28]. As expected, low concentrations of THC were found in the bloodstream, being a potential psychotropic cannabinoid, with the highest concentration observed being 8.3 ng/mL in the serum. With no psychotropic effects observed at the 4 mg/kg every 12 h in any dog, this suggests that this is a safe dose free of adverse events for normal healthy dogs.

As with any study, there were limitations to this study and in the interpretation of the data. The cohort utilized here were relatively young dogs and therefore may have different metabolic capacity than older dogs. Future studies utilizing these higher doses and potentially even higher doses in geriatric dogs (the typical cohort utilizing such products) is needed to fully assess the safety. This study only examined a short 2-week dosing regimen which may not be long enough to fully evaluate safety, similar to other studies showing safety in chronic dosing [11–14]; therefore, we cannot say what longer dosing regimens may reveal at 4 mg/kg. Lastly, as healthy dogs without any other significant medications on board, we cannot suggest that the use of this higher dose would necessarily be safe with other concomitant medications, although CBD and CBD-rich hemp products appeared to be safe when given with lower doses alongside non-steroidal anti-inflammatories and anti-epileptic drugs in 1–3 month clinical studies [4,6,8–10].

5. Conclusions

In this cohort of apparently healthy, young dogs, no adverse events were reported with the utilization of CBD/CBDA-rich hemp at 2 mg/kg and 4 mg/kg every 12 h. Additionally, at 2 mg/kg every 12 h, serum chemistry results had no significant findings and at 4 mg/kg every 12 h, a small portion of the dogs (3/16) had an elevation in ALP above the reference range, with no corresponding ALT elevation. Furthermore, even with concurrent use of trazodone in some dogs, hepatic injury was not apparent in the serum chemistry results. These findings, no adverse reactions/events and an innocuous rise in ALP, indicate that there is an adequate margin of safety in the use of CBD/CBDA-rich hemp extract for sub-acute use in dogs, though the use of a larger population of apparently healthy dogs with a wider range of ages would be prudent in future long-term studies utilizing CBD/CBDA-rich hemp at the higher dose. Regarding anxiety behavior, this study suggests minimal to no effect on behavior as observed by non-experts. Further evaluation utilizing board-certified behaviorists and possibly higher concentrations of cannabinoid could further define the necessary dose for anxiolytic effect.

Supplementary Materials: The following supporting information can be downloaded at: https://www.mdpi.com/article/10.3390/ani14131863/s1, Figure S1: Student Survey for adverse events and behavioral changes figure of questions asked; Table S1: LC-MS/MS parameters for cannabinoid detection; Table S2: Percent Accuracy and percent coefficient of variation of assay. Analysis was done in triplicate on three days.

Author Contributions: Conceptualization, T.M.; methodology, T.M. and D.H.; formal analysis, T.M., S.M., D.H. and J.W.; investigation, T.M., S.M. and D.H.; data curation, T.M. and S.M.; writing—original draft, T.M.; writing—review and editing, T.M., S.M., D.H. and J.W.; supervision, T.M.; funding acquisition, J.W. All authors have read and agreed to the published version of the manuscript.

Funding: Please add: This research was funded by Ellevet Sciences, grant number TTU 2315.

Institutional Review Board Statement: This study was approved under the guidance of the Texas Tech University Institutional Animal Care and Use Committee—Approval # 2022-1272.

Informed Consent Statement: The shelter from which these dogs were acquired approved the use of these dogs for teaching and non-invasive research in accordance with procedures outlined and approved by the Texas Tech University Animal Care and Use Committee.

Data Availability Statement: The original contributions presented in the study are included in the Article/Supplementary Materials; further inquiries can be directed to the corresponding author/s.

Acknowledgments: Authors would like to thank Joshua Cabello for his technical support during this project All authors have read and agreed to the published version of this manuscript.

Conflicts of Interest: T.M. and S.M. have no conflicts of interest to declare. J.W. and D.H. are paid consultants for Ellevet Sciences.

References

1. Kogan, L.; Schoenfeld-Tacher, R.; Hellyer, P.; Rishniw, M. US Veterinarians' Knowledge, Experience, and Perception Regarding the Use of Cannabidiol for Canine Medical Conditions. *Front. Vet. Sci.* **2019**, *5*, 338. [CrossRef] [PubMed]
2. Corsato Alvarenga, I.; MacQuiddy, B.; Duerr, F.; Elam, L.H.; McGrath, S. Assessment of cannabidiol use in pets according to a national survey in the USA. *J. Small Anim. Pract.* **2023**, *64*, 513–521. [CrossRef] [PubMed]
3. Wakshlag, J.J.; Cital, S.; Eaton, S.J.; Prussin, R.; Hudalla, C. Cannabinoid, Terpene, and Heavy Metal Analysis of 29 Over-the-Counter Commercial Veterinary Hemp Supplements. *Vet. Med. Res. Rep.* **2020**, *11*, 45–55. [CrossRef] [PubMed]
4. Gamble, L.J.; Boesch, J.M.; Frye, C.W.; Schwark, W.S.; Mann, S.; Wolfe, L.; Brown, H.; Berthelsen, E.S.; Wakshlag, J.J. Pharmacokinetics, Safety, and Clinical Efficacy of Cannabidiol Treatment in Osteoarthritic Dogs. *Front. Vet. Sci.* **2018**, *5*, 165. [CrossRef] [PubMed]
5. Verrico, C.D.; Wesson, S.; Konduri, V. A randomized, double-blind, placebo-controlled study of daily cannabidiol for the treatment of canine osteoarthritis pain. *Pain* **2020**, *161*, 2191–2202. [CrossRef] [PubMed]
6. Brioschi, F.A.; Di Cesare, F.; Gioeni, D. Oral Transmucosal Cannabidiol Oil Formulation as Part of a Multimodal Analgesic Regimen: Effects on Pain Relief and Quality of Life Improvement in Dogs Affected by Spontaneous Osteoarthritis. *Animals* **2020**, *10*, 1505. [CrossRef] [PubMed]
7. Loewinger, M.; Wakshlag, J.J.; Bowden, D.; Peters-Kennedy, J.; Rosenberg, A. The effect of a mixed cannabidiol and cannabidiolic acid based oil on client-owned dogs with atopic dermatitis. *Vet. Dermatol.* **2022**, *33*, 329. [CrossRef] [PubMed]
8. Garcia, G.A.; Kube, S.; Carrera-Justiz, S.; Tittle, D.; Wakshlag, J.J. Safety and efficacy of cannabidiol-cannabidiolic acid rich hemp extract in the treatment of refractory epileptic seizures in dogs. *Front. Vet. Sci.* **2022**, *9*, 939966. [CrossRef] [PubMed]
9. McGrath, S.; Bartner, L.R.; Rao, S.; Packer, R.A.; Gustafson, D.L. Randomized blinded controlled clinical trial to assess the effect of oral cannabidiol administration in addition to conventional antiepileptic treatment on seizure frequency in dogs with intractable idiopathic epilepsy. *J. Am. Vet. Med. Assoc.* **2019**, *254*, 1301–1308. [CrossRef]
10. Rozental, A.J.; Weisbeck, B.G.; Corsato Alvarenga, I.; Gustafson, D.L.; Kusick, B.R.; Rao, S.; Bartner, L.R.; McGrath, S. The efficacy and safety of cannabidiol as adjunct treatment for drug-resistant idiopathic epilepsy in 51 dogs: A double-blinded crossover study. *J. Vet. Intern. Med.* **2023**, *37*, 2291–2300. [CrossRef]
11. Deabold, K.A.; Schwark, W.S.; Wolf, L.; Wakshlag, J.J. Single-dose pharmacokinetics and preliminary safety assessment with use of CBD-rich hemp nutraceutical in healthy dogs and cats. *Animals* **2019**, *9*, 832. [CrossRef] [PubMed]
12. Corsato Alvarenga, I.; Wilson, K.M.; McGrath, S. Tolerability of long-term cannabidiol supplementation to healthy adult dogs. *J. Vet. Intern. Med.* **2024**, *38*, 326–335. [CrossRef] [PubMed]
13. Bookout, W.; Dziwenka, M.; Valm, K.; Kovacs-Nolan, J. Safety study of cannabidiol products in healthy dogs. *Front. Vet. Sci.* **2024**, *11*, 1349590. [CrossRef] [PubMed]
14. Bradley, S.; Young, S.; Bakke, A.M.; Holcombe, L.; Waller, D.; Hunt, A.; Pinfold, K.; Watson, P.; Logan, D.W. Long-term daily feeding of cannabidiol is well-tolerated by healthy dogs. *Front. Vet. Sci.* **2022**, *9*, 977457. [CrossRef] [PubMed]
15. Whalley, B.J.; Lin, H.; Bell, L.; Hill, T.; Patel, A.; Gray, R.A.; Elizabeth Roberts, C.; Devinsky, O.; Bazelot, M.; Williams, C.M.; et al. Species-specific susceptibility to cannabis-induced convulsions. *Br. J. Pharmacol.* **2019**, *176*, 1506–1523. [CrossRef] [PubMed]
16. Corsetti, S.; Borruso, S.; Malandrucco, L.; Spallucci, V.; Maragliano, L.; Perino, R.; D'Agostino, P.; Natoli, E. *Cannabis sativa* L. may reduce aggressive behaviour towards humans in shelter dogs. *Sci. Rep.* **2021**, *11*, 2773. [CrossRef]
17. Morris, E.M.; Kitts-Morgan, S.E.; Spangler, D.M.; McLeod, K.R.; Costa, J.H.C.; Harmon, D.L. The Impact of Feeding Cannabidiol (CBD) Containing Treats on Canine Response to a Noise-Induced Fear Response Test. *Front. Vet. Sci.* **2020**, *7*, 569565. [CrossRef]
18. Hunt, A.B.G.; Flint, H.E.; Logan, D.W.; King, T. A single dose of cannabidiol (CBD) positively influences measures of stress in dogs during separation and car travel. *Front. Vet. Sci.* **2023**, *10*, 1112604. [CrossRef]
19. Chicoine, A.; Illing, K.; Vuong, S.; Pinto, K.R.; Alcorn, J.; Cosford, K. Pharmacokinetic and Safety Evaluation of Various Oral Doses of a Novel 1:20 THC:CBD Cannabis Herbal Extract in Dogs. *Front. Vet. Sci.* **2020**, *7*, 583404. [CrossRef]
20. Wakshlag, J.J.; Schwark, W.S.; Deabold, K.A.; Talsma, B.N.; Cital, S.; Lyubimov, A.; Iqbal, A.; Zakharov, A. Pharmacokinetics of Cannabidiol, Cannabidiolic Acid, Δ9-Tetrahydrocannabinol, Tetrahydrocannabinolic Acid and Related Metabolites in Canine Serum after Dosing with Three Oral Forms of Hemp Extract. *Front. Vet. Sci.* **2020**, *7*, 505. [CrossRef]
21. Court, M.H.; Mealey, K.L.; Burke, N.S.; Jimenez, T.P.; Zhu, Z.; Wakshlag, J.J. Cannabidiol and cannabidiolic acid: Preliminary in vitro evaluation of metabolism and drug-drug interactions involving canine cytochrome P-450, UDP-glucuronosyltransferase, and P-glycoprotein. *J. Vet. Pharmacol. Ther.* **2024**, *47*, 1–13. [CrossRef] [PubMed]
22. Doran, C.E.; McGrath, S.; Bartner, L.R.; Thomas, B.; Cribb, A.E.; Gustafson, D.L. Drug-drug interaction between cannabidiol and phenobarbital in healthy dogs. *Am. J. Vet. Res.* **2021**, *83*, 86–94. [CrossRef]
23. Sholler, D.J.; Schoene, L.; Spindle, T.R. Therapeutic Efficacy of Cannabidiol (CBD): A Review of the Evidence from Clinical Trials and Human Laboratory Studies. *Curr. Addict. Rep.* **2020**, *7*, 405–412. [CrossRef] [PubMed]
24. Flint, H.E.; Hunt, A.B.G.; Logan, D.W.; King, T. Daily dosing of cannabidiol (CBD) demonstrates a positive effect on measures of stress in dogs during repeated exposure to car travel. *J. Anim. Sci.* **2024**, *102*, skad414. [CrossRef] [PubMed]
25. Rooney, T.A.; Carpenter, J.W.; KuKanich, B.; Gardhouse, S.M.; Magnin, G.C.; Tully, T.N. Feeding decreases the oral bioavailability of cannabidiol and cannabidiolic acid in hemp oil in New Zealand White rabbits (*Oryctolagus cuniculus*). *Am. J. Vet. Res.* **2022**, *83*, 1–7. [CrossRef] [PubMed]

26. Wang, T.; Zakharov, A.; Gomez, B.; Lyubimov, A.; Trottier, N.L.; Schwark, W.S.; Wakshlag, J.J. Serum Cannabinoid 24 h and 1 Week Steady State Pharmacokinetic Assessment in Cats Using a CBD/CBDA Rich Hemp Paste. *Front. Vet. Sci.* **2022**, *9*, 895368. [CrossRef] [PubMed]
27. Johns, T.N.; Wakshlag, J.J.; Lyubimov, A.V.; Zakharov, A.; Burnside, W.M. Pharmacokinetics of cannabidiol-/cannabidiolic acid-rich hemp oil in juvenile cynomolgus macaques (*Macaca fascicularis*). *Front. Vet. Sci.* **2023**, *10*, 1286158. [CrossRef]
28. Sosa-Higareda, M.; Guzman, D.S.; Knych, H.; Lyubimov, A.; Zakharov, A.; Gomez, B.; Beaufrère, H. Twice-daily oral administration of a cannabidiol and cannabidiolic acid-rich hemp extract was well tolerated in orange-winged Amazon parrots (*Amazona amazonica*) and has a favorable pharmacokinetic profile. *Am. J. Vet. Res.* **2023**, *84*, 1–11. [CrossRef]

animals

MDPI

Review

An Overview of the Health Effects of Bisphenol A from a One Health Perspective

Ana M. Molina-López [1,*], Francisca Bujalance-Reyes [2], Nahúm Ayala-Soldado [2,*], Rafael Mora-Medina [2], Antonio Lora-Benítez [2,†] and Rosario Moyano-Salvago [1,†]

[1] Departamento Anatomía y Anatomía Patológica Comparadas y Toxicología, Unidad de Investigación Competitiva Zoonosis y Enfermedades Emergentes desde la Perspectiva de Una Salud ENZOEM, Universidad de Córdoba, Campus de Rabanales, Edificio Darwin, E-14071 Córdoba, Spain; r.moyano@uco.es

[2] Departamento Anatomía y Anatomía Patológica Comparadas y Toxicología, Universidad de Córdoba, Campus de Rabanales, Edificio Darwin, E-14071 Córdoba, Spain; v02buref@uco.es (F.B.-R.); v02momer@uco.es (R.M.-M.); v12lobea@uco.es (A.L.-B.)

* Correspondence: ft2moloa@uco.es (A.M.M.-L.); v22ayson@uco.es (N.A.-S.)

† These authors contributed equally to this work.

Simple Summary: Endocrine disruptors are substances with a capacity to alter the endocrine system, one of the best known being bisphenol A. Bisphenol A is employed in the manufacture of a multitude of utensils used daily, and it is constantly being found polluting the environment and food. It is also an important aquatic pollutant, and its presence has been detected in coastal areas, rivers, and streams, among others. Due to its ubiquity, human and animal populations are frequently exposed to this compound. This work has compiled the effects on health of this substance, which are highly varied and are relevant in affecting reproduction and causing metabolic or immune system alterations, among others, as well as related to an increase in hormone-dependent pathologies, obesity, or type 2 diabetes. Monitoring the populations at risk and establishing a safe exposure level are proposed as being fundamental points in the control of exposure to this compound.

Abstract: Bisphenol A (BPA) is a chemical compound, considered as an "emerging pollutant", that appears ubiquitously, contaminating the environment and food. It is an endocrine disruptor, found in a multitude of consumer products, as it is a constituent of polycarbonate used in the manufacture of plastics and epoxy resins. Many studies have evaluated the effects of BPA, using a wide range of doses and animal models. In this work, we carried out a review of relevant research related to the effects of BPA on health, through studies performed at different doses, in different animal models, and in human monitoring studies. Numerous effects of BPA on health have been described; in different animal species, it has been reported that it interferes with fertility in both females and males and causes alterations in their offspring, as well as being associated with an increase in hormone-dependent pathologies. Similarly, exposure to BPA has been related to other diseases of great relevance in public health such as obesity, hypertension, diabetes, or neurodevelopmental disorders. Its ubiquity and nonmonotonic behavior, triggering effects at exposure levels considered "safe", make it especially relevant when both animal and human populations are constantly and inadvertently exposed to this compound. Its effects at low exposure levels make it essential to establish safe exposure levels, and research into the effects of BPA must continue and be focused from a "One Health" perspective to take into account all the factors that could intervene in the development of a disease in any exposed organism.

Keywords: bisphenol A; One Health; transgenerational; reproductive effects; metabolic disorder

1. Introduction

Bisphenol A (BPA) is an endocrine disruptor (EDC), whose use is authorized in materials entering into contact with food in the European Union (EU), in accordance with

Regulation (EU) no. 10/2011 [1] on material and plastic objects destined for that purpose. In January 2011, the European Commission banned the use of BPA in the manufacture of polycarbonate feeding bottles for infants. In February 2018, the EU introduced stricter limits for BPA in materials associated with food conservation, derived from the temporary tolerable daily intake (TDI) established by the European Food Safety Agency (EFSA) in 2015. Since September 2018, BPA has been prohibited in bottles and plastic containers of food for infants, and for children under 3 years of age [2]. Its use was also constrained in thermal paper as from January 2020, in the European Union [3]. Regarding toys manufactured with BPA-based polymers, and given that the final users comprise a population group at great risk, in the EU, there is currently a limit on the amount of BPA that can become detached from toys for children of up to three, which has been fixed at 0.04 mg/L since 26 November 2018. This order was adopted in accordance with Directive 2017/898 of 24 May 2017 [4]. The two main uses of BPA, accounting for approximately 95% of its production, are in the manufacture of polycarbonate plastic and of epoxy resins [5]. About 70% of the BPA produced in the industry is used to make the former, and approximately 25% is found in the latter. The remaining 5% is found in a wide variety of products, including phenolic resins, unsaturated polyester resins, can coatings, as an antioxidant and end-polymerization inhibitor in the manufacture of polyvinyl (vinyl chloride) plastics, as an intermediate in the manufacture of thermal paper, and in car tires or flame retardants [6]. The emission of BPA into the atmosphere occurs mainly because of industrial activity. In a study in which the atmospheric levels of BPA in samples collected on five continents were evaluated, pg/m^3 was detected in coastal areas, the highest levels being reported on the east coast of Asia. The areas of large agglomerations in Asia, New Zealand, and the United States presented levels of 170–880 pg/m^3, detecting mean concentrations of 4.55 ng/m^3 in urban areas of India [7]. Regarding water and effluents, BPA usually appears in surface waters in low concentrations. The occurrence of various EDCs, including BPA, was studied in 14 rivers in Portugal. Analyses of the samples revealed widespread contamination by BPA, with the highest concentration reaching 98.4 ng/L. Investigations conducted in 16 large rivers in Taiwan determined BPA concentrations ranging from 0.01 to 44.65 g/dm^3, whereas, in the sediments, they were 0.37–491.54 g/kg. In a similar context, in an analysis of surface, river, and spring water in Poland, BPA was found in all the samples tested at concentrations ranging from 6–427 ng/L in surface water to 629 ng/L in stream water [8,9].

As a consequence of the enormous production of BPA, and the multiple uses of this compound, it is found everywhere in the environment and in food, with both the human and the animal populations being continuously and inadvertently exposed to this endocrine disruptor. Due to its significant effects on health, attempts have been made to find alternatives to its use, although there is currently no safe option for this compound, despite a large number of studies focusing on the search for safe exposure levels [10–12]. BPA is considered to be an "emerging pollutant" to which we are constantly being exposed, and the environment, animals, and people can be affected by its possible harmful effects [13,14]. The effects on reproduction of BPA, at which most of the studies have initially been aimed, are well known. However, for some years, research has gone deeper into the effects of BPA at other levels, since it has been possible to verify how certain levels of exposure would not produce harmful effects on the reproductive system, whereas they could be observed at other levels, such as on the immune system [6,15,16].

It is, therefore, very important to find out the effects of BPA on health at different levels and systems, thus avoiding their underestimation at certain levels of exposure. In this sense, the EFSA experts, in their latest 2023 report, concluded that people of all age groups with medium and high exposure to BPA would exceed the new TDI, which is a reason for concern in terms of health.

In investigating the effects of BPA, the "One Health" perspective acquires special relevance. Studying them on different biomodels, as well as monitoring the exposure of certain animal species, could serve to understand their possible impact on the human population, in addition to evaluating the likely incidence of inadvertent exposure to BPA in the conservation of biodiversity. The objective of this work was to carry out a review highlighting appropriate studies on the relationships between BPA and its important adverse effects on health. For this purpose, we took studies published during the last 10 years, in which a wide range of doses was used in different animal models and human monitoring studies, from different bibliographic databases (Scopus, Pubmed, WoS and Science Direct). In addition, we consulted EFSA reports and pages from the Official Journal of the European Union, as well as official legislation websites.

2. Health Effects of Bisphenol A

Exposure to BPA through different routes has demonstrated its impact on both human and animal health, describing effects on different systems and organic levels. Prominent effects described are (1) those on reproduction, (2) those on development, (3) transgenerational and multigenerational effects (4) those on the metabolism, (5) immunological effects, (6) those on the thyroid function, and (7) those on oxidative stress and inflammation, among others (Figure 1) [11,17,18].

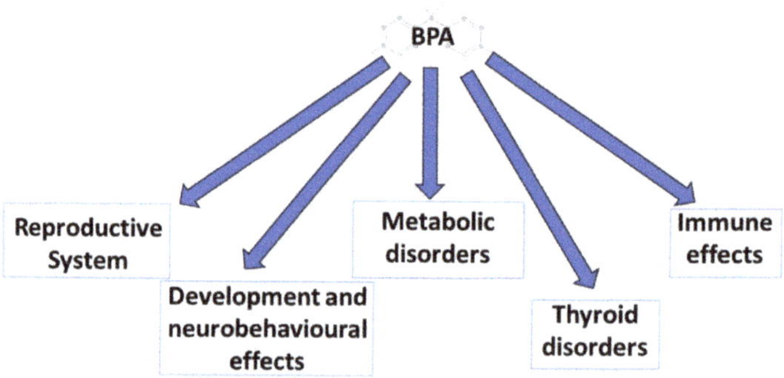

Figure 1. BPA multisystem toxicity.

2.1. *Effects on the Reproductive System*

Many studies have shown that the reproductive system is affected by BPA [19–23]. Figure 2 depicts a reproduction toxicity study in two generations. In studies on humans, the most outstanding effects are its disruption of sex hormone activity, and its influence on the development and function of the reproductive system. In this context, it has been proposed that BPA could increase serum estradiol (E2), progesterone, luteinizing hormone (LH), and testosterone (T) levels, as well as decrease cortisol concentrations [20]. Other studies, however, revealed that BPA would reduce serum T concentration and increase E2 concentration [24].

Furthermore, it is important to mention that estrogens are largely responsible for the development of the sexually dimorphic anatomical, functional, and behavioral characteristics that are essential for reproduction in vertebrates. For instance, a key enzyme in estrogen synthesis is cytochrome P450 aromatase [25]. Aromatase converts androstenedione to estrone (E1) or testosterone (T) to 17β-estradiol (E2), the major estrogens in mammals. Aromatase activity is found in invertebrate brain and gonadal tissue; however, in mammals, including humans, this enzyme is also active in the placenta, adipose tissue, and fetal liver [25]. In healthy human breast tissue, aromatase expression is regulated by promoter regions via the protein kinase A (PKA) phosphorylation pathway. In addition, the bioactive lipid prostaglandin E2 (PGE2) has been shown to regulate the activity of the aromatase enzyme [26]. PGE2 is generated by the activity of cyclooxygenase-2 (COX-2), the rate-limiting enzyme that catalyzes the conversion of arachidonic acid to proteinoids [27]. COX-2 inhibition negatively regulates aromatase activity and decreases tumor Leydig cell proliferation [28], which suggests that COX-2 would play an important role in aromatase synthesis and steroidogenesis.

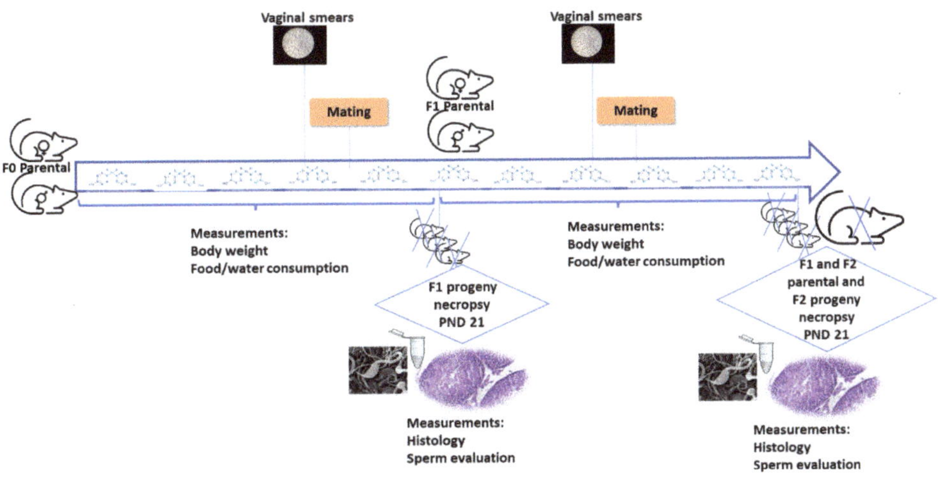

Figure 2. Diagram of a study on reproduction toxicity in two generations (see OCDE 416 "Two-Generation Reproduction Toxicity" [29]).

In animal experiments, exposure to BPA has been shown to have adverse effects on the reproductive system [10]. In female reproduction, neonatal or perinatal exposure to BPA has been reported as causing significant histological changes in the reproductive tract [30,31], alteration in the cyclicity of heat [32], decreased reproductive capacity [33], and changes in hormone levels in adult life [34]. In the ovary, interruption of follicular development and reduction in the number of primordial follicles [35,36] have been noted. In the case of males, an increase in the weight of the prostate, a decrease in the weight of the epididymis, a reduction in the production of spermatozoa, and a decrease in the concentrations of LH and testosterone in the blood serum have been found [37,38].

2.1.1. Effects on the Ovary

Experimental animal studies indicate that prenatal and postnatal exposure to BPA would cause decreased ovarian weight, follicle number, and primordial follicle recruitment, as well as an increased corpus luteum number, even at low doses [39–41]. In different mammalian species, BPA decreases the number of primordial follicles and induces atresia; in both mice and lambs, this effect has been related to the acceleration of follicular recruitment. In addition, exposure to very high doses of BPA (300 mg/kg) in rats would cause an increase in cystic follicles and a decrease in corpora lutea and antral follicles [42]. In addition, BPA has been seen to reduce the number of primary and secondary follicles, as well as increase DNA damage biomarkers, suggesting that this could be an ovarian toxicity effect [43]; in fact, some studies affirm that these impacts on the ovary could be transgenerational. Thus, a study on BPA exposure in the ovaries of F1 generation mice found effects on the ovary in the F3 generation [30]. Numerous studies have concluded that BPA affects follicular growth and increases the number of atretic follicles [23,35,44,45].

Another of the associations most studied is the correlation between the highest levels of BPA in serum with the appearance of the polycystic ovarian syndrome (PCOS). PCOS is a highly prevalent disorder that affects women of a reproductive age, and it is clinically characterized by hyperandrogenism, ovulatory dysfunction, and polycystic ovary morphology, together with dysfunctions related to metabolism such as hyperinsulinemia, obesity, and insulin resistance. BPA mimics the activity of 17-βestradiol, and it has been observed to have the ability to interrupt steroid feedback at the hypothalamic–pituitary level and steroid action at the ovarian level, which would suppress the pituitary–ovarian axis functions [46]. This includes hypersecretion of circulating LH and increased follicle-stimulating hormone

(FSH) levels, which would cause altered LH:FSH ratios [47]. In addition, BPA contributes to the metabolomic profile seen in PCOS, which includes insulin resistance, association with obesity, and chronic inflammation. BPA can affect ovarian steroidogenesis in the case of there being exposure during the periods known as "critical exposure windows", which would lead to irreversible effects, as demonstrated by Fernández et al. [17], who investigated the effects of neonatal exposure to BPA in female Sprague-Dawley rats, which exhibited a PCOS-like syndrome during adulthood. This suggests a possible relationship between the development of a PCOS-like syndrome and early exposure to BPA.

In relation to oocytes, some studies have demonstrated that BPA alters their meiotic division [48]. Along the same lines, Nakano et al. [49] analyzed the effects of exposure to BPA on mice oocyte maturation in vitro. The oocytes were cultured in the presence of BPA (2, 20, 50, or 100 μg/mL) for 18 h. At concentrations of 50 and 100 μg/mL, BPA inhibited oocyte maturation and caused cell-cycle delay under these conditions. In animal studies, BPA has also been known to disrupt the transition from prophase I to MII in oocytes, with this adverse effect being related primarily to altered microtubule organization [48–51].

2.1.2. Effects on the Uterus

A large number of experimental animal studies have shown that exposure to BPA produces adverse effects on the uterus. Neff et al. [52] demonstrated that exposure to environmentally relevant doses of BPA (60 μg/kg/day) had an uterotrophic effect in mice that showed increased proliferation in the uterine glandular epithelium, which is the site of origin of endometrial hyperplasia and cancer. This finding has been backed up by studies using low- and high-dose exposure in rodents (0.004 and 40 mg/kg/day) [53]. In studies conducted in CD-1 mice, exposure to low doses (60–600 μg/kg/day) of BPA increased glandular density, peri glandular collagen accumulation, and abnormal functions of the endometrial epithelium and stroma [54], indicating that BPA could have an inducing role in endometrial cancer [55].

2.1.3. Effects on the Placenta

BPA exposure has been linked to certain obstetric complications associated with the placenta, including preeclampsia, decreased fetal growth, miscarriage, and preterm birth. The current findings suggest that BPA would cause pathological changes in the placenta by interrupting its metabolic activities. Depending on the exposure concentrations, BPA could trigger apoptotic or antiapoptotic signals in trophoblasts, potentially interfering with pregnancy [56].

In the last decade, several studies have examined the effects of BPA on mouse placenta [57–61]. Many investigations showed that BPA interferes with the placental epigenome of mammals. Strakovsky et al. [62] found that BPA affected placental imprinting loss and decreased DNA methylation. In the placental IGF2/H19 domain, loss of imprinting and decreased methylation led to disrupted nutrient allocation and impaired fetal growth. Likewise, in that study, in placentas of the same age, without fetal malformations, they found that there were miR-146a alterations after exposure to BPA.

Other female reproductive abnormalities due to perinatal BPA exposure include early-onset vaginal opening and puberty, as well as alterations in estrous cyclicity, plasma LH levels, vaginal and uterine histology, and mammary gland, uterus, and ovarian morphology [63,64].

2.1.4. Effects on the Fetus

Birth Weight

Multiple studies in women have shown a negative correlation between BPA concentrations in amniotic fluid and urine and birth weight [65,66]. On the contrary, in some works, no association has been reported between BPA concentrations in maternal serum and urine at the beginning of gestation and at birth, with a lower weight than expected for gestational age [67,68].

Hu et al. [69] observed a significant dose–response curve for reduced birth weight after BPA exposure during gestation. In this study, a total of 452 mother–child pairs were selected in the city of Wuhan, China during 2012–2014. Mothers with low-birth-weight infants had significantly higher urinary BPA levels (4.70 μg/L) compared to mothers in the control group (2.25 μg/L). That association was more pronounced among female infants than among male ones, evidencing the relationship between the highest levels of BPA in urine and the sex of the offspring with a lower weight. Scientific research in this regard has been focused on determining the concentration of BPA in the placenta. In their study, Troisi et al. [70] analyzed placenta samples from 200 individuals, with BPA levels being measured by gas chromatography/mass spectrometry (GC–MS). Additional data on the mother and infant were collected from medical records and correlated with BPA levels in the placenta. The results of this study gave a significant negative correlation between the calculated birth weight percentile and placental BPA levels. Low-birth-weight infants and those small for their gestational age also had significantly higher placental BPA concentrations compared with infants of a normal weight or average/large for their gestational age.

In animal studies, it has been found that early exposure to BPA probably influences several important mechanisms for body weight regulation, including adipocyte deposition, glucose uptake, and homeostasis. Susiarjo et al. [71] demonstrated that BPA exposure during gestation and lactation affected postnatal growth of offspring of C57BL/6 mice. In that study, F1 males exposed to the lowest doses (10 μg/kg/day) of BPA exhibited accelerated weight gain after weaning, with no difference observed in food intake of F1 male mice in the different exposure groups. This effect appears to be sex-dependent, as no significant differences in body weight, body fat content, or bone mineral content and density were detected in females.

Premature Labor

There are few data on the correlation between preterm birth and BPA levels in pregnant mothers [72–74]. However, Smarr et al. [74] showed that this weak correlation is stronger for newborn girls than for boys.

In a similar context Behnia et al. [75] evaluated plasma and amniotic fluid in a sample of pregnant mothers, showing that mothers with higher plasma concentrations of BPA had a risk of a shorter gestation or premature rupture of membranes. Furthermore, some studies such as that of Cantonwine et al. [72] and Weinberger et al. [73] described an inverse correlation between the concentration of BPA in maternal urine and the length of gestation. However, the results of some research with animals indicate that, in females exposed to high concentrations of BPA, there was a lengthening of the gestation period, although this fact could not be directly attributed to exposure to BPA [11].

Fetal Malformation

Several studies have observed BPA-related fetal malformations, which would suggest that this endocrine disruptor is transferred trans-placentally to the embryo–fetal compartment [76]. Guida et al. [77] investigated total, free, and conjugated BPA measured in the blood of 151 pregnant women divided into two groups: one with an established diagnosis of the developmental defect, and the other with the normally developing fetus. The results showed that free BPA was higher in the blood of women pregnant with a fetus with chromosomal malformations and those of the central and peripheral nervous system, compared to women in the control group. This suggests a greater susceptibility to abnormalities among "poor metabolizers", which could be due to the free fraction being the active one, i.e., the one capable of binding to its sites of action and producing its adverse effects. Having a higher free proportion implies that a larger amount of BPA is able to reach its action sites. In addition, BPA possibly interferes with the progression of meiotic maturation (as demonstrated in vitro) and causes alterations in spindle organization and chromosome alignment.

On another note, the effect of BPA on male genital malformations has been demonstrated in rats and humans [78,79]. In human male studies, Fernández et al. [80] observed an increased risk of genital malformations due to high placental concentrations of BPA. Furthermore, Mammadov et al. [81] correlated decreased anogenital distance (AGD) in male offspring with high parental exposure to BPA. Cryptorchidism and hypospadias are among the most frequent neonatal malformations associated with multiple exogenous factors although they could not be significantly correlated with BPA exposure. Dobrzyńska et al. [82] demonstrated, in a study with mice, the parents (males) of which were exposed for 8 weeks to 5, 10, and 20 mg/kg bw of BPA, that the frequency of abnormal skeletons in the F1 offspring increased dose-dependently, observing malformations such as the concavity of the parietal bones and the presence of extra ribs.

2.1.5. Effects on Male Reproduction

Various in vivo and in vitro studies suggest that BPA and its analogs have deleterious effects on the male reproductive function and sperm quality. In this sense, it is known that BPA antagonizes endogenous hormones and interferes with steroid-mediated processes that affect male reproduction. Chianese et al. [83] demonstrated the existence of alterations in the testes in male rats after exposure to BPA from the fetal period to sexual maturation, demonstrating an alteration in the cytoarchitecture of the seminiferous epithelium. The oxidative stress mechanisms and a massive production of reactive oxygen species (ROS) would explain the interruption of functional communications between Sertoli and germ cells, as well as the alteration of spermatogenesis and cell damage in post-meiotic stages. Zhang et al. [84] demonstrated that BPA would increase the number of germ cells entering meiosis, causing an abnormal state of proliferation. The production of ROS in the testes and the DNA damage in post meiotic spermatids would justify the fact that BPA can induce the formation of poor-quality sperm, with possible transgenerational effects on the offspring.

Regarding Leydig cells, the main effects of BPA exposure on their activity are the alteration of the hormonal microenvironment in the testes, and the upregulation of key steroidogenic enzymes. In addition to Sertoli and germ cells, Leydig cells are also targets for BPA. The main effects of the latter's exposure on Leydig cell activity are the alteration of the hormonal microenvironment in the testes and the upregulation of steroidogenic enzymes, with an increase in estrogen production. In this sense, Lan et al. [85] demonstrated that the ratio of sex hormones (testosterone/estradiol) decreased in male rats administered for 5 days with BPA doses of 0.5 μg/kg/day. In their study, they observed that the ratio of sex hormones (T/E) was dramatically reduced in the BPA group compared to the control.

In humans, BPA has been known to reduce sperm quality, decrease sexual function, and reduce fertility. The correlation between BPA exposure and decreased semen quality, assessed as sperm count, motility, and vitality, has been seen to impact capacity and acrosomal reaction [86]. In particular, BPA modulates the motility of human spermatozoa in vitro, affecting their mitochondrial potential in a pathway that involves free Ca^{2+} as a second messenger [87]. Ji et al. [88] conducted a cross-sectional study in the Chinese city of Sandu with a sample of 774 men between the ages of 18 and 55, who underwent a semen analysis, and their BPA levels were associated with linearity, oscillation, amplitude of lateral displacement of head, mean angular displacement, and sperm concentration. This is consistent with many other studies showing that infertile men had higher levels of BPA in urine and plasma [89]. In general, BPA could affect the normal reproductive function by altering the activity of sex hormones, even triggering the onset of infertility. Similarly, Manfo et al. [90] found that men exposed to BPA had reduced libido levels, increased erection and ejaculation difficulties, and decreased satisfaction with their sex life.

2.2. *Developmental and Neurobehavioral Effects*

Maternal exposure to BPA and its level in umbilical cord blood have been reported to have a sex-specific effect on shortened AGD in children [91]. Barrett et al. [92] found that girls who had been exposed to higher levels of BPA during the first trimester of pregnancy had a shorter AGD. In rodents, Liu et al. [93] demonstrated that, in knockout mice exposed to BPA at a dose of 100 mg/L/day per gavage, the anogenital distance was shortened, and both the male testicular weights and the testosterone levels were reduced. The development of puberty has also been linked to the levels of exposure to BPA. Chen et al. [94] found that BPA levels were associated with idiopathic central precocious puberty (PPCI) in school-age girls. However, the study by Berger et al. [95], found that higher BPA concentrations could induce delayed puberty in girls and earlier puberty in boys, demonstrating a sex-dependent effect.

In addition, the neuroendocrine regulation inhibition induced by BPA could cause a series of mental and behavioral alterations in offspring. Chen et al. [94] investigated the effects of gestational exposure to BPA related to mental and behavioral problems in preschool children. They found that increased maternal exposure to BPA could be a potential risk factor for unusual conduct in children, especially boys, of preschool age. Perera et al. [96] found that prenatal BPA exposure was significantly associated with depression and anxiety in children, whereas postnatal BPA exposure was not related to these illnesses. Therefore, exposure to BPA during gestation, the critical exposure window, could interfere with brain development in offspring and increase the risk of behavioral problems. In addition, it was suggested that BPA could be associated with hyperactivity disorder, antisocial behavior, problems related to sleep, and language development [94,97,98].

Animal studies have reported that exposure to BPA during the prenatal, postnatal, and juvenile periods causes neurotoxic effects on the brain, and behavioral changes. Zhang et al. [99] in a multigenerational study with mice observed that even a low dose of maternal exposure to BPA (0.5 μg/kg/day) could significantly affect, depending on sex, the learning and memory capacity of male F1 mice, but not of the F2 generation. They also observed a decrease in the number of neurons in the hippocampus of the F1 and F2 generations after maternal exposure to BPA, and DNA damage to brain cells, but only in the F1 offspring. In addition, according to these authors, maternal exposure to BPA could lead to variations in hippocampal neurotransmitter levels, indicated by a decrease in the glutamic acid/gamma aminobutyric acid (Glu/GABA) ratio in F1 offspring. Bi et al. [100] exposed transgenic mice orally to BPA (0.05 mg/kg/day) from postnatal day (PND) 0 to PND 60, subsequently subjecting them to behavioral tests. Their results suggest potentially detrimental effects after BPA exposure on the excitatory neuronal circuitry in spatial memory formation.

Neurobehavioral and adult brain effects are mostly due to BPA exposure during critical life stages; they are subsequently transmitted to their offspring and can persist or further develop in adulthood. In this regard, Wang et al. [101] demonstrated that intrauterine exposure to BPA in adult CD-1 mice induced permanent changes in the gene expression in the brain, including a significant diminution in motor activity, in learning capacities, in long-term memory, and an increase in anxiety in young mice evaluated at 18 months of age. Fetal exposure, and that in the first years of life, permanently affected neurobehavioral functions, which deteriorated with age. They, therefore, revealed that BPA exposure could worsen aging effects, long-term memory, and an increase in anxiety.

In addition, it has been demonstrated that, after exposure during adult life, similar effects are produced. For example, Ni et al. [102] exposed adult, male and female, C57BL/6J mice at 8 weeks of age to 0.05, 0.5, 5, and 50 mg/kg of BPA during 22 weeks, and observed that exposure impaired the memory and learning capacity of the male mice, which was associated with an increase in neuroinflammation and a harmed hemato-encephalic barrier.

In studies with fish, authors such as Heredia-García et al. [103] evaluated the neurotoxic effects of acute exposure to BPA (96 h) at environmentally relevant concentrations (220, 1180, and 1500 ng/L) in adult zebrafish (*Danio rerio*), subsequently performing swimming behavior assessment tests (novel tank). Their results indicated that exposure to 1500 ng/L of BPA reduces the total distance traveled and increases the stopping time of the fish, concluding that environmentally relevant BPA concentrations could cause anxiety-like behavior and neurotoxic effects in adult zebrafish.

On the same lines of the study on the effects on the brain in the adult animal, Schirmer et al. [104] studied the effects, in the goldfish (*Carassius auratus*), after 1 month's exposure to environmentally relevant concentrations of BPA (1 and 10 $\mu g \cdot L^{-1}$) on the Mauthner neurone, an essential one in vertebrates to trigger "flight from predators" behavior. Their findings demonstrated that this exposure for 1 month strongly affected visual and acoustic processes occurring in those neurons, thus generating an impact on the essential communication functions in the brain of adult vertebrates. These effects, nevertheless, were not produced after acute exposure (1 h) in those same vertebrates.

2.3. Transgenerational and Multigenerational Effects

The multigenerational and transgenerational inheritance mechanisms of abnormal developmental phenotypes include epigenetic misregulation in germ cells. Multigenerational effects involve direct exposure of the factor influencing in the development of the disease, in contrast to transgenerational effects, in which transmission between generations does not imply direct exposure. Very many studies support the theory that BPA could alter epigenetic marks in rodents and humans. These epigenetic marks include DNA methylation, histone post-translational modifications, and noncoding RNAs [105,106]. The transgenerational effects of BPA have been demonstrated in mammals and nonmammals [107,108]. There is also evidence of multigenerational and transgenerational inheritance of abnormal developmental changes in offspring after exposure to this endocrine disruptor. BPA exposure is related to the transgenerational inheritance of reproductive, metabolic, or neurological phenotypes [22,63,109,110].

In rodents, developmental BPA exposure has been associated with social recognition and behavioral differences in three-generation studies [107]. In that study, after exposing the mothers to concentrations of 20 μg/day during mating and gestation, it was observed that, in subsequent generations of animals, juvenile mice exposed to BPA showed more active exploratory behavior than controls, without finding any sex differences in the performance of any of the behavioral tests carried out. These results demonstrated that exposure to BPA during pregnancy has lasting transgenerational effects on social recognition and activity in mice.

Various studies have shown that intrauterine exposure to BPA affects the reproductive function in developing mice, and that function can be altered for up to three generations [111,112]. Mahalingam et al. [111] exposed FVB mice to BPA at low concentrations (0.5, 20, and 50 μg/kg/day orally) to investigate the multigenerational effects of BPA on the F1, F2, and F3 generations. The results revealed that intrauterine BPA exposure decreased cytochrome P450 aromatase and estradiol mRNA levels in the F1 generation. Likewise, it was found that this exposure decreased testosterone levels and altered the mRNA levels of several steroidogenic factors in the F2 generation, producing multigenerational effects on the ovary and steroidogenesis in mice up to the F2 generation. In adulthood, effects were observed on the reproduction indices in generations F2 and F3, such as a decrease in fertility. Of note is that some of the most pronounced effects were measured in mice whose parents received the lowest dose of BPA. This would be related to the results that back up the theory that BPA shows a nonmonotonic dose–response curve. A monotonic response is characterized by a slope that does not change its sign. In contrast, a nonmonotonic dose–response curve (NMDRC) is characterized by a slope that changes its sign within the tested dose range. Some curves are U-shaped, some are inverted U-shaped, and, in others, the sign of the curve may change at multiple points throughout the range of doses studied. One of the characteristics of endocrine disruptors, specifically BPA, is that they produce nonmonotonic dose–response curves (Figure 3).

Furthermore, Shi et al. [115] examined the transgenerational effects of BPA on male reproductive functions using CD-1 mice as a model, and exposing them orally to BPA and other analogs, at concentrations of 0.5 and 50 μg/kg/day and using mice of F1 and F2 offspring to generate F3 males. Prenatal exposure to BPA was found to decrease sperm count and motility, and interrupt the progression of germ cell development in F3 males.

Deregulated serum levels of 17β-estradiol and testosterone were also observed, as well as steroidogenic enzyme expression in adult testes in F3. The results of this study suggest that prenatal exposure to BPA would originate transgenerational effects on male reproductive functions due to an altered epigenetic modification in neonatal and adult testes.

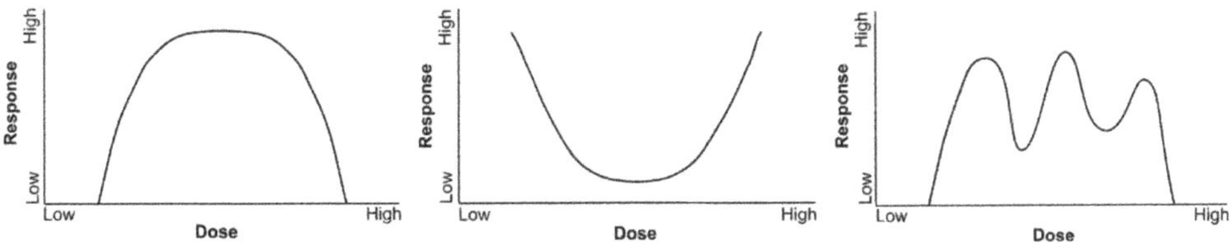

Figure 3. Example of nonmonotonic behavior dose–response curves (see [11,113,114]).

Rahman et al. [112] investigated the histological changes in the testes, together with the functional, biochemical, and epigenetic (DNA methylation) properties of spermatozoa from male CD-1 mice exposed to BPA (4 and 50 mg/kg/day) for 6 weeks and crossed with untreated females to produce up to a third generation (F3). The results showed that paternal exposure to BPA disrupted spermatogenesis, leading to a decrease in the total sperm count of the F0–F2 offspring. In addition, they demonstrated that a dose of 50 mg/kg/day decreased sperm motility in F0–F2 males by mediating the overproduction of ROS. BPA was also shown to compromise sperm fertility in F0–F2 generation mice in both dose groups, but in F3 only in the high-dose group.

In this context, Bansal et al. [110] used C57BL/6J (F0) mice that were exposed to BPA doses of 10 μg/kg/day (LowerB) and 10 mg/kg/day (UpperB), to study the effects on the pancreatic islets of offspring in the first (F1), second (F2), and third generations (F3). Male F1 and F2 offspring exposed to the low dose of BPA had reduced β-cell mass and smaller islets, which was associated with increased glucose-stimulated insulin secretion. The same did not occur in the case of females, which exhibited comparable results with controls.

The transgenerational effects of BPA in relation to neurobehavioral actions have also been described in many studies. In this line, Wolstenholme et al. [116] examined social recognition behaviors in third-generation mice after gestational exposure to BPA. In their study, they demonstrated that transgenerational exposure to BPA interrupted social interactions in mice and deregulated the normal expression of genes involved in excitatory postsynaptic density (PSD), closely related to neurobehavioral disorders during neuronal development.

2.4. Metabolic Effects

Experimental studies have shown that exposure to BPA generates weight gain, changes in blood glucose levels, and insulin resistance, as well as the development of dyslipidemia and alterations in lipid metabolism [117–119]. Epidemiological evidence found positive associations between BPA exposure and the onset of metabolic diseases such as obesity and type 2 diabetes. Likewise, numerous animal studies indicated that BPA exposure resulted in glucose intolerance, insulin resistance, and modifications in glucose homeostasis [120,121]. The alteration of different biochemical parameters could likewise be observed throughout different generations and be considered an indirect indicator of effects derived from chronic exposure to BPA. In this respect, Bujalance et al. [11], in a study of several generations of mice exposed to different concentrations of BPA (0.5, 2, 4, 50 and 100 μg/kg/day), reported that alterations were produced in the biochemical parameters throughout the generations exposed, modifying glucose, albumin, and total protein levels. Regarding glucose levels, it could be said that exposure to BPA causes a hyperglycemic effect, possibly due to an alteration in glucose metabolism in the pancreas. In addition, the variations in the levels of total proteins and albumin could be explained by the action of BPA, which would give rise to an alteration in the liver, resulting in a modification mainly in protein synthesis.

Exposure to BPA produces obesogenic effects, which not only occur in exposed subjects, but could also cause transgenerational outcomes. A direct interruption of endocrine regulation, of neuroimmune and signaling pathways, as well as of the intestinal microbiota, has been identified as being due to exposure to BPA, which would lead to overweight or obesity creating, in these cases, cardiovascular complications, one of the main consequences derived from obesity [122].

As a consequence of these obesogenic effects, there is an alteration in energy homeostasis, the lipid composition of the liver, and insulin signaling in insulin-sensitive organs such as the liver, muscle, and adipose tissues [123]. Furthermore, the link between energy homeostasis and reproduction has been demonstrated, in both animal and human models, with leptin, a peptide hormone produced in white adipose tissue, which is the main peripheral biomarker of metabolic status. Leptin (adipokine involved in the control of food intake through appetite suppression) can also stimulate oxidative stress, inflammation, thrombosis, arterial stiffness, angiogenesis, and atherogenesis. These leptin-induced effects could lead to a predisposition to suffer from cardiovascular diseases. Leptin levels have been positively associated with the presence, severity, extent, and complexity of coronary atherosclerosis lesion, as well as the presence and severity of ischemic and hemorrhagic strokes. In addition, leptin has been shown to independently predict common carotid intima–media thickness and carotid plaque instability. Elevated leptin levels have also been linked to the incidence and progression of chronic kidney disease, as well as insulin resistance, type 2 diabetes, and microvascular and macrovascular diabetic complications.

BPA directly affects food intake by modulating the activity of metabolic sensors produced in the arcuate hypothalamic nucleus (ARC), thus interfering in the interaction between the gonadotropin-releasing hormone (GnRH) and neural networks involved in the metabolic control of reproduction [124,125].

In studies on humans, BPA has been confirmed as being closely related to some metabolic diseases by altering the neuroendocrine function, potentially representing an important factor leading to the development of chronic diseases. Aktag et al. [126] found that urinary BPA levels in children during their prepubertal stage were positively associated with metabolic syndrome (MetS). Shu et al. [127], for their part, demonstrated that the serum concentration of BPA was positively associated with the increase in fasting plasma glucose levels. This study suggested that BPA might contribute to obesity and the development of type 2 diabetes with insulin resistance.

In animal studies, Moon et al. [120] demonstrated that oral exposure to BPA in mice produced glucose intolerance and insulin resistance. Yang et al. [128], observed that BPA promoted adiposity in 5 week old mice exposed to doses of 5–5000 μg/kg/day of BPA with a low-calorie diet in a nonmonotonic dose–response manner. Shu et al. [129] demonstrated that prenatal exposure in mice to BPA doses of 5 mg/kg/day by oral gavage caused transcriptomic and methylomic alterations in the liver, adipose tissue, and hypothalamus of the male offspring, with inter-tissue alterations in the metabolism of the lipids, and tissue-specific alterations in glucose metabolism, histone proteins, and the extracellular matrix.

Regarding the different metabolic alterations associated with exposure to BPA, high concentrations of this endocrine disruptor in urine were correlated with higher levels of blood pressure, indicating that it could possibly contribute to the development of cardiovascular diseases [130]. Therefore, the peripheral arterial disease (PAD) would be positively associated with urinary BPA levels, which could be used as a subclinical measure of atherosclerotic vascular disease, since there are positive associations, demonstrated in epidemiological studies, between urinary or blood levels of BPA and the development of coronary artery stenosis, carotid atherosclerosis, and peripheral kidney disease. Recent epidemiological studies have also verified that urine or serum BPA levels were positively associated with coronary artery stenosis, carotid atherosclerosis, and peripheral artery disease, suggesting that BPA exposure might be an emerging risk factor for the development of atherosclerosis [131].

Lastly, it should be noted that bone metabolism could also be affected by BPA through the interruption of calcium phosphate metabolism and the consequent reduction in bone mineral density [89]. It is known that BPA interferes with bone modeling and remodeling by altering hormonal regulation and causing the epigenetic alteration of target genes, which would cause osteoporotic lesions [132]. In particular, BPA has been shown to exert an estrogen-like action via estrogen receptors α and β (ERα and ERβ) and ER-related γ (ERRγ); however, unlike estrogens, it harms concomitant bone development with the inhibition of osteogenic gene expression levels [133,134], which would indicate that, after exposure to BPA, the agonist effects induced on the ER could inhibit osteogenesis, increasing bone loss.

2.5. Immunological Effects on Oxidative Stress and Inflammation

BPA is closely linked to immune function, inflammation, and oxidative stress [15,135]. It can also induce mitochondrial damage and cell apoptosis [136]. Xu et al. [137] found that immune cell populations and innate and adaptive immune system functions were altered upon exposure to BPA during development, including decreased regulatory T cells and upregulated proinflammatory and anti-inflammatory cytokines and chemokines. In 2019, this same research group found that BPA modulated immune function and the gut microbiome, which would be closely associated with a higher incidence of type 1 diabetes. In their study on animals, they demonstrated that BPA exposure caused a change in proinflammatory factors in females, while, in men, the same exposure caused elevated levels of anti-inflammatory immune factors and a decrease in the proinflammatory gut microbiome [138].

In this respect, taking into account the evidence from animal data and observational studies in humans, the immune system has been identified as being the one most sensitive to BPA exposure. One effect on T helper 17 lymphocytes (Th17 cells) in mice was identified as being critical; these cells are vital in cellular immune mechanisms and are involved in the development of inflammatory conditions, including autoimmunity and lung inflammation. On the basis of all this scientific evidence, the EFSA experts have established a TDI of 0.2 ng/kg/day, replacing the previous temporary level of 4 µg/kg/day, establishing in April 2023 a TDI approximately 20,000 times lower than that previously established [6].

Oxidative stress is another BPA toxicity mechanism. As a metabolic and endocrine disruptor, BPA alters redox homeostasis by increasing oxidative mediators and reducing antioxidant enzymes, leading to mitochondrial dysfunction, disruption of cell signaling pathways, and induction of apoptosis. Antioxidant enzymes are a class of essential enzymes that can protect against oxidative damage. BPA could reduce these antioxidant enzymes and increase free-radical generation and lipid peroxidation, leading to oxidative stress damage [135,139]. BPA can disrupt the balance of the antioxidant system and cause adverse effects by inhibiting antioxidant enzyme activity, downregulating antioxidant gene expression, and lipid peroxidation (LPO) formation.

Kaur et al. [140] observed that BPA could be an environmental risk factor for autism by inducing oxidative stress and mitochondrial dysfunction. Kazemi et al. [141] showed that BPA could promote the generation of ROS and increase the expression levels of the antioxidant gene in liver tissue, causing hepatotoxicity. In the study by Yuan et al. [142], BPA was found to cause oxidative stress in the testis and to reduce hydrogen peroxide (H_2O_2) primarily through the stimulation of catalase (CAT) activity. In animal models, it has been observed that chronic exposure to BPA could increase the levels of malondialdehyde (MDA) and IL-18, as well as reduce the levels of superoxide dismutase (SOD) in the lung tissue of adult male rats, which could result in inflammatory lung diseases [143]. BPA may also increase glutathione (GSH) content, CAT activity, and the formation of mitochondrial reactive oxygen species (ROS) and LPO in the kidney of adult male Wistar rats, leading to impaired renal function [144].

2.6. Effects on Thyroid Function

The thyroid hormone is essential for development, growth, and metabolism, and it plays an especially important role in neurodevelopment. Therefore, the alterations that may exist in the function of the thyroid hormone could hamper these vital functions. BPA can interfere with thyroid function through several mechanisms. It can inhibit thyroid hormone synthesis by altering thyroid hormone regulation through its interference at the pituitary and hypothalamic levels [145]. Less likely, it can also interfere with thyroid hormone transport and metabolism, although it is thought that the T_3 nuclear receptor (TR) antagonist effect of BPA may be the primary mechanism through which it disrupts the thyroid function.

In some animal studies, Da Silva et al. [146] administered BPA to Wistar rats, subsequently measuring their thyroid hormone levels. Exposure to BPA (40 mg/kg, 15 days, orally) in adult rats increased T_4 levels. Furthermore, Fernández et al. [17] investigated neonatal exposure to BPA (2.5–6.2 mg/kg, 10 days, subcutaneously), observing decreased T_4 levels and increased thyrotropin (TSH) levels in adulthood.

Likewise, maternal exposure to BPA in rats can affect thyroid hormone levels in their offspring. In a study with rats, Silva et al. [147] observed that maternal exposure to BPA during pregnancy and lactation (10 and 50 µg/kg/day, orally) decreased T_3 and T_4 levels in the offspring (postnatal day [PND] 15). For their part, Xu et al. [148] observed that maternal exposure to BPA induced a transient increase in T_4 (PND7) levels, followed by a decrease in T_4 (PND21) in the male offspring. However, other investigators showed that perinatal exposure to BPA (0.0025–40 mg/kg, orally or subcutaneously) did not alter TSH and T_4 levels in the offspring [110,149].

In humans, studies such as the one by Sanlidag et al. [150] evaluated dose-dependent maternal exposure to BPA effects on thyroid functions in neonates. The levels of BPA, TSH, and free T_4 were measured in the umbilical cord blood, not detecting any significant effect on thyroid hormones.

For their part, Li et al. [151], conducted an epidemiological study in China to examine the association between urinary BPA and thyroid nodules (TN) in women. A higher concentration of BPA in urine was associated with a higher risk of TN only in those with positive thyroid autoantibodies. Furthermore, this association was dose-dependent, which would indicate that any increase in BPA exposure was related to an increased risk of TN.

3. Conclusions

BPA is an environmental and food contaminant, which is found ubiquitously in different sources, whereby both the animal and the human populations remain continuously and inadvertently exposed to it. Numerous monitoring studies have concluded that exposure to BPA is constant; thus, the potential health effects of exposed organisms cannot be underestimated. The effects of BPA follow a nonmonotonic behavior, typical of endocrine disruptors, which do not behave dose-dependently. Among other reasons, the evaluation of the risk of exposure to this compound is more complex, and harmful effects may appear at lower doses. There are multiple effects on health at different levels and systems from this endocrine disruptor. The initial studies on it focused on evaluating its impact on reproduction, demonstrating that it interfered with fertility, and that it was related to the increase in hormone-dependent pathologies, among others. Similarly, a multitude of studies have shown that BPA exerts important effects, which could cause serious pathologies that would compromise the long-term life of exposed organisms, by triggering effects at different levels, such as metabolic, immune system, or neurodevelopmental ones, or those related to obesity, hypertension, diabetes, or diseases such as depression or anxiety, among others. The variety of pathologies with which long-term exposure to BPA is associated is so wide, acting or not at certain stages of development (critical exposure windows); hence, it is a real challenge to identify safe exposure limits, since that which may be innocuous for a certain system may not be so for another, and exposed organisms may suffer from subclinical diseases. At present, it is not known how its long-term effect will evolve in free-living animals, and research on its direct impact on the conservation of biodiversity has focused on the evaluation of toxicity in laboratory animals, or on monitoring in the human population, demonstrating its adverse effects on multiple systems. However, BPA is an "emerging contaminant", whose action affects all exposed organisms; hence, the monitoring of these species has acquired a special relevance, making it essential to focus the studies according to the "One Health" concept. It is urgent to establish new lines of research that evaluate the effects at an environmental, animal, or human level, as well as to establish measures to prevent environmental and food contamination and foster an essential restriction of its use and the maintenance of exposure surveillance, as being conducted by regulatory agencies, while continuing to search for a safe alternative to the use of BPA.

Author Contributions: Conceptualization, A.M.M.-L., F.B.-R. and R.M.-S.; investigation, A.M.M.-L., F.B.-R., N.A.-S., R.M.-M., A.L.-B. and R.M.-S.; resources, A.M.M.-L., F.B.-R., N.A.-S., R.M.-M., A.L.-B. and R.M.-S.; writing—original draft preparation, A.M.M.-L., F.B.-R., N.A.-S., A.L.-B. and R.M.-S.; writing—review and editing, A.M.M.-L., F.B.-R. and R.M.-S.; supervision, A.M.M.-L. and R.M.-S.; project administration, A.M.M.-L. and R.M.-S.; funding acquisition, A.M.M.-L. and R.M.-S. All authors have read and agreed to the published version of the manuscript.

Funding: This research was funded by Junta de Andalucía, Proyectos I + D + I Programa Operativo FEDER Andalucía (1381098-R).

Institutional Review Board Statement: Not applicable.

Informed Consent Statement: Not applicable.

Data Availability Statement: Not applicable.

Conflicts of Interest: The authors declare no conflict of interest. The funders had no role in the design of the study; in the collection, analyses, or interpretation of data; in the writing of the manuscript, or in the decision to publish the results.

References

1. Commission Regulation (EU) No 10/2011 of 14 January 2011 on Plastic Materials and Articles Intended to Come into Contact with Food. Available online: https://eur-lex.europa.eu/legal-content/EN/TXT/?uri=celex%3A32011R0010 (accessed on 12 July 2023).
2. Commission Regulation (EU) 2018/213 of 12 February 2018 on the Use of Bisphenol A in Varnishes and Coatings Intended to Come into Contact with Food and Amending Regulation (EU) No 10/2011 as Regards the Use of that Substance in Plastic Food Contact Materials. Available online: https://eur-lex.europa.eu/eli/reg/2018/213/oj (accessed on 12 July 2023).
3. Commission Regulation (EU) 2016/2235 of 12 December 2016 Amending Annex XVII to Regulation (EC) No 1907/2006 of the European Parliament and of the Council Concerning the Registration, Evaluation, Authorisation and Restriction of Chemicals (REACH) as Regards Bisphenol A. Available online: https://eur-lex.europa.eu/legal-content/EN/TXT/?uri=CELEX%3A32016R2235 (accessed on 12 July 2023).
4. Commission Directive (EU) 2017/898 of 24 May 2017 Amending, for the Purpose of Adopting Specific Limit Values for Chemicals Used in Toys, Appendix C to Annex II to Directive 2009/48/EC of the European Parliament and of the Council on the Safety of Toys, as Regards Bisphenol A. Available online: https://eur-lex.europa.eu/legal-content/EN/TXT/PDF/?uri=CELEX:32017L0898 (accessed on 12 July 2023).
5. Scientific Committee on Consumer Safety (SCCS). 2020. Available online: https://health.ec.europa.eu/other-pages/health-sc-basic-page/final-opinion-bpa-clothing-articles_en (accessed on 12 July 2023).
6. EFSA CEP Panel (EFSA Panel on Food Contact Materials, Enzymes and Processing Aids). Scientific Opinion on the re-evaluation of the risks to public health related to the presence of bisphenol A (BPA) in foodstuffs. *EFSA J.* **2023**, *21*, e6857. [CrossRef]
7. Fu, P.; Kawamura, K. Ubiquity of bisphenol A in the atmosphere. *Environ. Pollut.* **2010**, *158*, 3138–3143. [CrossRef]
8. Rocha, S.; Domingues, V.F.; Pinho, C.; Fernandes, V.C.; Delerue-Matos, C.; Gameiro, P.; Mansilha, C. Occurrence of bisphenol A, estrone, 17β-estradiol and 17α-ethinylestradiol in Portuguese rivers. *Bull. Environ. Contam. Toxicol.* **2013**, *90*, 73–78. [CrossRef]
9. Lee, C.C.; Jiang, L.Y.; Kuo, Y.; Hsieh, C.Y.; Chen, C.S.; Tien, C.J. The potential role of water quality parameters on occurrence of nonylphenol and bisphenol A and identification of their discharge sources in the river ecosystems. *Chemosphere* **2013**, *91*, 904–911. [CrossRef]
10. Vom Saal, F.S.; Vandenberg, L.N. Update on the Health Effects of Bisphenol A: Overwhelming Evidence of Harm. *Endocrinology* **2021**, *162*, bqaa171. [CrossRef]
11. Bujalance-Reyes, F.; Molina-López, A.M.; Ayala-Soldado, N.; Lora-Benitez, A.; Mora-Medina, R.; Moyano-Salvago, R. Analysis of Indirect Biomarkers of Effect after Exposure to Low Doses of Bisphenol A in a Study of Successive Generations of Mice. *Animals* **2022**, *12*, 300. [CrossRef] [PubMed]

12. Trullemans, L.; Koelewijn, S.F.; Scodeller, I.; Hendrickx, T.; Van Puyvelde, P.; Sels, B. A guide towards safe, functional and renewable BPA alternatives by rational molecular design: Structure-property and structure-toxicity relationships. *Polym. Chem.* **2021**, *12*, 5870–5901. [CrossRef]
13. Kim, J.-J.; Kumar, S.; Kumar, V.; Lee, Y.-M.; Kim, Y.-S. Bisphenols as a legacy pollutant, and their effects on organ vulnerability. *Int. J. Environ. Res. Public Health* **2020**, *17*, 112. [CrossRef]
14. Chen, D.; Kannan, K.; Tan, H.; Zheng, Z.; Feng, Y.; Wu, Y.; Widelka, M. Bisphenol Analogues Other Than BPA: Environmental Occurrence, Human Exposure, and Toxicity—A Review. *Environ. Sci. Technol.* **2016**, *50*, 5438–5453. [CrossRef]
15. Cho, Y.J.; Park, S.B.; Park, J.W.; Oh, S.R.; Han, M. Bisphenol A modulates inflammation and proliferation pathway in human endometrial stromal cells by inducing oxidative stress. *Reprod. Toxicol.* **2018**, *81*, 41–49. [CrossRef]
16. Di Paola, D.; Capparucci, F.; Lanteri, G.; Cordaro, M.; Crupi, R.; Siracusa, R.; D'Amico, R.; Fusco, R.; Impellizzeri, D.; Cuzzocrea, S.; et al. Combined Toxicity of Xenobiotics Bisphenol A and Heavy Metals on Zebrafish Embryos (*Danio rerio*). *Toxics* **2021**, *9*, 344. [CrossRef]
17. Fernandez, M.O.; Bourguignon, N.S.; Arocena, P.; Rosa, M.; Libertun, C.; Lux-Lantos, V. Neonatal exposure to bisphenol A alters the hypothalamic-pituitary-thyroid axis in female rats. *Toxicol. Lett.* **2018**, *285*, 81–86. [CrossRef]
18. Ma, Y.; Liu, H.; Wu, J.; Yuan, L.; Wang, Y.; Du, X.; Wang, R.; Marwa, P.W.; Petlulu, P.; Chen, X.; et al. The adverse health effects of bisphenol A and related toxicity mechanisms. *Environ. Res.* **2019**, *176*, 108575. [CrossRef]
19. Rochester, J.R. Bisphenol A and human health: A review of the literature. *Reprod. Toxicol.* **2013**, *42*, 132–155. [CrossRef] [PubMed]
20. Wisniewski, P.; Romano, R.M.; Kizys, M.M.; Oliveira, K.C.; Kasamatsu, T.; Giannocco, G.; Chiamolera, M.I.; Dias-da-Silva, M.R.; Romano, M.A. Adult exposure to bisphenol A (BPA) in Wistar rats reduces sperm quality with disruption of the hypothalamic-pituitary-testicular axis. *Toxicology* **2015**, *329*, 1–9. [CrossRef]
21. Lora, A.J.; Molina, A.M.; Bellido, C.; Blanco, A.; Monterde, J.G.; Moyano, M.R. Adverse effects of bisphenol A on the testicular parenchyma of zebrafish revealed using histomorphological methods. *Vet. Med.* **2016**, *61*, 577–589. [CrossRef]
22. Santangeli, S.; Consales, C.; Pacchierotti, F.; Habibi, H.R.; Carnevali, O. Transgenerational effects of BPA on female reproduction. *Sci. Total. Environ.* **2019**, *685*, 1294–1305. [CrossRef]
23. Molina, A.M.; Abril, N.; Morales-Prieto, N.; Monterde, J.G.; Lora, A.J.; Ayala, N.; Moyano, R. Evaluation of toxicological endpoints in female zebrafish after bisphenol A exposure. *Food Chem. Toxicol.* **2018**, *112*, 19–25. [CrossRef]
24. Zeng, J.Y.; Chen, P.P.; Liu, C.; Deng, Y.; Miao, Y.; Zhang, M.; Cui, F.P.; Lu, T.T.; Shi, T.; Yang, K.D.; et al. Bisphenol A analogues in associations with serum hormone levels among reproductive-aged Chinese men. *Environ. Int.* **2022**, *167*, 107446. [CrossRef]
25. Di Nardo, G.; Zhang, C.; Marcelli, A.G.; Gilardi, G. Molecular and Structural Evolution of Cytochrome P450 Aromatase. *Int. J. Mol. Sci.* **2021**, *22*, 631. [CrossRef]
26. Subbaramaiah, K.; Iyengar, N.M.; Morrow, M.; Elemento, O.; Zhou, X.K.; Dannenberg, A.J. Prostaglandin E_2 down-regulates sirtuin 1 (SIRT1), leading to elevated levels of aromatase, providing insights into the obesity-breast cancer connection. *J. Biol. Chem.* **2019**, *294*, 361–371. [CrossRef]
27. Donnini, S.; Bazzani, L.; Ziche, M.; Terzuoli, E. Nitric Oxide and PGE-2 Cross-Talk in EGFR-Driven Epithelial Tumor Cells. *Crit. Rev. Oncog.* **2016**, *21*, 325–331. [CrossRef]
28. Duliban, M.; Gorowska-Wojtowicz, E.; Tworzydlo, W.; Rak, A.; Brzoskwinia, M.; Krakowska, I.; Wolski, J.K.; Kotula-Balak, M.; Płachno, B.J.; Bilinska, B. Interstitial Leydig Cell Tumorigenesis-Leptin and Adiponectin Signaling in Relation to Aromatase Expression in the Human Testis. *Int. J. Mol. Sci.* **2020**, *21*, 3649. [CrossRef]
29. OECD. Test No. 416: Two-Generation Reproduction Toxicity. In *OECD Guidelines for the Testing of Chemicals, Section 4*; OECD: Paris, France, 2001. [CrossRef]
30. Berger, A.; Ziv-Gal, A.; Cudiamat, J.; Wang, W.; Zhou, C.; Flaws, J.A. The effects of in utero bisphenol A exposure on the ovaries in multiple generations of mice. *Reprod. Toxicol.* **2016**, *60*, 39–52. [CrossRef]
31. Liang, M.; Zhou, J.; Sun, X.; He, C.; Zhang, K.; Hu, K. Effects of bisphenol A on apoptosis of ovarian preantral follicular granulosa cells and ovarian development in mice. *J. South. Med. Univ.* **2021**, *41*, 93–99. [CrossRef]
32. Wang, W.; Hafner, K.S.; Flaws, J.A. In utero bisphenol A exposure disrupts germ cell nest breakdown and reduces fertility with age in the mouse. *Toxicol. Appl. Pharmacol.* **2014**, *276*, 157–164. [CrossRef]
33. Meng, Y.; Lin, R.; Wu, F.; Sun, Q.; Jia, L. Decreased Capacity for Sperm Production Induced by Perinatal Bisphenol A Exposure Is Associated with an Increased Inflammatory Response in the Offspring of C57BL/6 Male Mice. *Int. J. Environ. Res. Public Health* **2018**, *15*, 2158. [CrossRef]
34. Ma, S.; Shi, W.; Wang, X.; Song, P.; Zhong, X. Bisphenol A Exposure during Pregnancy Alters the Mortality and Levels of Reproductive Hormones and Genes in Offspring Mice. *Biomed Res. Int.* **2017**, *2017*, 3585809. [CrossRef]
35. Zhu, X.; Tian, G.G.; Yu, B.; Yang, Y.; Wu, J. Effects of bisphenol A on ovarian follicular development and female germline stem cells. *Arch. Toxicol.* **2018**, *92*, 1581–1591. [CrossRef]
36. Hu, Y.; Wen, S.; Yuan, D.; Peng, L.; Zeng, R.; Yang, Z.; Liu, Q.; Xu, L.; Kang, D. The association between the environmental endocrine disruptor bisphenol A and polycystic ovary syndrome: A systematic review and meta-analysis. *Gynecol. Endocrinol.* **2018**, *34*, 370–377. [CrossRef]
37. Liu, X.; Wang, Z.; Liu, F. Chronic exposure of BPA impairs male germ cell proliferation and induces lower sperm quality in male mice. *Chemosphere* **2021**, *262*, 127880. [CrossRef]

38. Nguyen, J.L.; Ricke, E.A.; Liu, T.T.; Gerona, R.; MacGillivray, L.; Wang, Z.; Timms, B.G.; Bjorling, D.E.; Vom Saal, F.S.; Ricke, W.A. Bisphenol-A analogs induce lower urinary tract dysfunction in male mice. *Biochem. Pharmacol.* **2022**, *197*, 114889. [CrossRef]
39. Li, Y.; Zhang, W.; Liu, J.; Wang, W.; Li, H.; Zhu, J.; Weng, S.; Xiao, S.; Wu, T. Prepubertal bisphenol A exposure interferes with ovarian follicle development and its relevant gene expression. *Reprod. Toxicol.* **2014**, *44*, 33–40. [CrossRef]
40. Patisaul, H.B.; Mabrey, N.; Adewale, H.B.; Sullivan, A.W. Soy but not bisphenol A (BPA) induces hallmarks of polycystic ovary syndrome (PCOS) and related metabolic co-morbidities in rats. *Reprod. Toxicol.* **2014**, *49*, 209–218. [CrossRef]
41. Santamaría, C.; Durando, M.; Muñoz de Toro, M.; Luque, E.H.; Rodriguez, H.A. Ovarian dysfunctions in adult female rat offspring born to mothers perinatally exposed to low doses of bisphenol A. *J. Steroid. Biochem. Mol. Biol.* **2016**, *158*, 220–230. [CrossRef]
42. Delclos, K.B.; Camacho, L.; Lewis, S.M.; Vanlandingham, M.M.; Latendresse, J.R.; Olson, G.R.; Davis, K.J.; Patton, R.E.; Gamboa da Costa, G.; Woodling, K.A.; et al. Toxicity evaluation of bisphenol A administered by gavage to Sprague Dawley rats from gestation day 6 through postnatal day 90. *Toxicol. Sci.* **2014**, *139*, 174–197, Erratum in: *Toxicol. Sci.* **2016**, *153*, 212. [CrossRef]
43. Ganesan, S.; Keating, A.F. Bisphenol A-Induced Ovotoxicity Involves DNA Damage Induction to Which the Ovary Mounts a Protective Response Indicated by Increased Expression of Proteins Involved in DNA Repair and Xenobiotic Biotransformation. *Toxicol. Sci.* **2016**, *152*, 169–180. [CrossRef]
44. Migliaccio, M.; Chioccarelli, T.; Ambrosino, C.; Suglia, A.; Manfrevola, F.; Carnevali, O.; Fasano, S.; Pierantoni, R.; Cobellis, G. Characterization of Follicular Atresia Responsive to BPA in Zebrafish by Morphometric Analysis of Follicular Stage Progression. *Int. J. Endocrinol.* **2018**, *2018*, 4298195. [CrossRef]
45. Ruiz, T.F.R.; Grigio, V.; Ferrato, L.J.; de Souza, L.G.; Colleta, S.J.; Amaro, G.M.; Góes, R.M.; Vilamaior, P.S.L.; Leonel, E.C.R.; Taboga, S.R. Impairment of steroidogenesis and follicle development after bisphenol A exposure during pregnancy and lactation in the ovaries of Mongolian gerbils aged females. *Mol. Cell. Endocrinol.* **2023**, *566–567*, 111892. [CrossRef]
46. Wang, C.; Zhang, J.; Li, Q.; Zhang, T.; Deng, Z.; Lian, J.; Jia, D.; Li, R.; Zheng, T.; Ding, X.; et al. Low concentration of BPA induces mice spermatocytes apoptosis via GPR30. *Oncotarget* **2017**, *8*, 49005–49015. [CrossRef]
47. Vahedi, M.; Saeedi, A.; Poorbaghi, S.L.; Sepehrimanesh, M.; Fattahi, M. Metabolic and endocrine effects of bisphenol A exposure in market seller women with polycystic ovary syndrome. *Environ. Sci. Pollut. Res. Int.* **2016**, *23*, 23546–23550. [CrossRef]
48. Acuña-Hernández, D.G.; Arreola-Mendoza, L.; Santacruz-Márquez, R.; García-Zepeda, S.P.; Parra-Forero, L.Y.; Olivares-Reyes, J.A.; Hernández-Ochoa, I. Bisphenol A alters oocyte maturation by prematurely closing gap junctions in the cumulus cell-oocyte complex. *Toxicol. Appl. Pharmacol.* **2018**, *344*, 13–22. [CrossRef] [PubMed]
49. Nakano, K.; Nishio, M.; Kobayashi, N.; Hiradate, Y.; Hoshino, Y.; Sato, E.; Tanemura, K. Comparison of the effects of BPA and BPAF on oocyte spindle assembly and polar body release in mice. *Zygote* **2016**, *24*, 172–180. [CrossRef] [PubMed]
50. Machtinger, R.; Orvieto, R. Bisphenol A, oocyte maturation, implantation, and IVF outcome: Review of animal and human data. *Reprod. Biomed. Online* **2014**, *29*, 404–410. [CrossRef]
51. Loup, B.; Poumerol, E.; Jouneau, L.; Fowler, P.A.; Cotinot, C.; Mandon-Pépin, B. BPA disrupts meiosis I in oogonia by acting on pathways including cell cycle regulation, meiosis initiation and spindle assembly. *Reprod. Toxicol.* **2022**, *111*, 166–177. [CrossRef]
52. Neff, A.M.; Blanco, S.C.; Flaws, J.A.; Bagchi, I.C.; Bagchi, M.K. Chronic Exposure of Mice to Bisphenol-A Alters Uterine Fibroblast Growth Factor Signaling and Leads to Aberrant Epithelial Proliferation. *Endocrinology* **2019**, *160*, 1234–1246. [CrossRef]
53. Kendziorski, J.A.; Belcher, S.M. Strain-specific induction of endometrial periglandular fibrosis in mice exposed during adulthood to the endocrine disrupting chemical bisphenol A. *Reprod. Toxicol.* **2015**, *58*, 119–130. [CrossRef]
54. Li, Q.; Davila, J.; Kannan, A.; Flaws, J.A.; Bagchi, M.K.; Bagchi, I.C. Chronic Exposure to Bisphenol A Affects Uterine Function During Early Pregnancy in Mice. *Endocrinology* **2016**, *157*, 1764–1774. [CrossRef]
55. Mallozzi, M.; Leone, C.; Manurita, F.; Bellati, F.; Caserta, D. Endocrine Disrupting Chemicals and Endometrial Cancer: An Overview of Recent Laboratory Evidence and Epidemiological Studies. *Int. J. Environ. Res. Public Health* **2017**, *14*, 334. [CrossRef]
56. Adu-Gyamfi, E.A.; Rosenfeld, C.S.; Tuteja, G. The impact of bisphenol A on the placenta. *Biol. Reprod.* **2022**, *106*, 826–834. [CrossRef] [PubMed]
57. Tait, S.; Tassinari, R.; Maranghi, F.; Mantovani, A. Bisphenol A affects placental layers morphology and angiogenesis during early pregnancy phase in mice. *J. Appl. Toxicol.* **2015**, *35*, 1278–1291. [CrossRef]
58. Lee, J.H.; Ahn, C.; Kang, H.Y.; Hong, E.J.; Hyun, S.H.; Choi, K.C.; Jeung, E.B. Effects of Octylphenol and Bisphenol A on the Metal Cation Transporter Channels of Mouse Placentas. *Int. J. Environ. Res. Public Health* **2016**, *13*, 965. [CrossRef]
59. Lan, X.; Fu, L.J.; Zhang, J.; Liu, X.Q.; Zhang, H.J.; Zhang, X.; Ma, M.F.; Chen, X.M.; He, J.L.; Li, L.B.; et al. Bisphenol A exposure promotes HTR-8/SVneo cell migration and impairs mouse placentation involving upregulation of integrin-β1 and MMP-9 and stimulation of MAPK and PI3K signaling pathways. *Oncotarget* **2017**, *8*, 51507–51521. [CrossRef] [PubMed]
60. Mao, J.; Kinkade, J.A.; Bivens, N.J.; Rosenfeld, C.S. miRNA changes in the mouse placenta due to bisphenol A exposure. *Epigenomics* **2021**, *13*, 1909–1919. [CrossRef] [PubMed]
61. Cao, Y.; Chen, S.; Lu, J.; Zhang, M.; Shi, L.; Qin, J.; Lv, J.; Li, D.; Ma, L.; Zhang, Y. BPA induces placental trophoblast proliferation inhibition and fetal growth restriction by inhibiting the expression of SRB1. *Environ. Sci. Pollut. Res. Int.* **2023**, *30*, 60805–60819. [CrossRef] [PubMed]
62. Strakovsky, R.S.; Wang, H.; Engeseth, N.J.; Flaws, J.A.; Helferich, W.G.; Pan, Y.X.; Lezmi, S. Developmental bisphenol A (BPA) exposure leads to sex-specific modification of hepatic gene expression and epigenome at birth that may exacerbate high-fat diet-induced hepatic steatosis. *Toxicol. Appl. Pharmacol.* **2015**, *284*, 101–112. [CrossRef]

63. Shi, M.; Whorton, A.E.; Sekulovski, N.; MacLean, J.A.; Hayashi, K. Prenatal Exposure to Bisphenol A, E, and S Induces Transgenerational Effects on Female Reproductive Functions in Mice. *Toxicol. Sci.* **2019**, *170*, 320–329. [CrossRef]
64. Wu, F.; Zhao, J.; Zhang, E.; Wu, Q.; Wu, X.; Zhang, D.; Liu, Y.; Wang, R.; Li, W. Bisphenol A affects ovarian development in adolescent mice caused by genes expression change. *Gene* **2020**, *740*, 144535. [CrossRef]
65. Snijder, C.A.; Heederik, D.; Pierik, F.H.; Hofman, A.; Jaddoe, V.W.; Koch, H.M.; Longnecker, M.P.; Burdorf, A. Fetal growth and prenatal exposure to bisphenol A: The generation R study. *Environ. Health Perspect.* **2013**, *121*, 393–398. [CrossRef]
66. Pinney, S.E.; Mesaros, C.A.; Snyder, N.W.; Busch, C.M.; Xiao, R.; Aijaz, S.; Ijaz, N.; Blair, I.A.; Manson, J.M. Second trimester amniotic fluid bisphenol A concentration is associated with decreased birth weight in term infants. *Reprod. Toxicol.* **2017**, *67*, 1–9. [CrossRef]
67. Burstyn, I.; Martin, J.W.; Beesoon, S.; Bamforth, F.; Li, Q.; Yasui, Y.; Cherry, N.M. Maternal exposure to bisphenol-A and fetal growth restriction: A case-referent study. *Int. J. Environ. Res. Public Health* **2013**, *10*, 7001–7014. [CrossRef] [PubMed]
68. Xu, X.; Chiung, Y.M.; Lu, F.; Qiu, S.; Ji, M.; Huo, X. Associations of cadmium, bisphenol A and polychlorinated biphenyl co-exposure in utero with placental gene expression and neonatal outcomes. *Reprod. Toxicol.* **2015**, *52*, 62–70. [CrossRef] [PubMed]
69. Hu, C.Y.; Li, F.L.; Hua, X.G.; Jiang, W.; Mao, C.; Zhang, X.J. The association between prenatal bisphenol A exposure and birth weight: A meta-analysis. *Reprod. Toxicol.* **2018**, *79*, 21–31. [CrossRef]
70. Troisi, J.; Mikelson, C.; Richards, S.; Symes, S.; Adair, D.; Zullo, F.; Guida, M. Placental concentrations of bisphenol A and birth weight from births in the Southeastern U.S. *Placenta* **2014**, *35*, 947–952. [CrossRef]
71. Susiarjo, M.; Xin, F.; Bansal, A.; Stefaniak, M.; Li, C.; Simmons, R.A.; Bartolomei, M.S. Bisphenol a exposure disrupts metabolic health across multiple generations in the mouse. *Endocrinology* **2015**, *156*, 2049–2058. [CrossRef]
72. Cantonwine, D.E.; Ferguson, K.K.; Mukherjee, B.; McElrath, T.F.; Meeker, J.D. Urinary Bisphenol A Levels during Pregnancy and Risk of Preterm Birth. *Environ. Health Perspect.* **2015**, *123*, 895–901. [CrossRef]
73. Weinberger, B.; Vetrano, A.M.; Archer, F.E.; Marcella, S.W.; Buckley, B.; Wartenberg, D.; Robson, M.G.; Klim, J.; Azhar, S.; Cavin, S.; et al. Effects of maternal exposure to phthalates and bisphenol A during pregnancy on gestational age. *J. Matern.-Fetal Neonatal Med.* **2014**, *27*, 323–327. [CrossRef]
74. Smarr, M.M.; Grantz, K.L.; Sundaram, R.; Maisog, J.M.; Kannan, K.; Louis, G.M. Parental urinary biomarkers of preconception exposure to bisphenol A and phthalates in relation to birth outcomes. *Environ. Health* **2015**, *14*, 73. [CrossRef]
75. Behnia, F.; Peltier, M.; Getahun, D.; Watson, C.; Saade, G.; Menon, R. High bisphenol A (BPA) concentration in the maternal, but not fetal, compartment increases the risk of spontaneous preterm delivery. *J. Matern.-Fetal Neonatal Med.* **2016**, *29*, 3583–3589. [CrossRef]
76. Barberio, L.; Paulesu, L.; Canesi, L.; Grasselli, E.; Mandalà, M. Bisphenol a Interferes with Uterine Artery Features and Impairs Rat Feto-Placental Growth. *Int. J. Mol. Sci.* **2021**, *22*, 6912. [CrossRef]
77. Guida, M.; Troisi, J.; Ciccone, C.; Granozio, G.; Cosimato, C.; Di SpiezioSardo, A.; Ferrara, C.; Guida, M.; Nappi, C.; Zullo, F.; et al. Bisphenol A and congenital developmental defects in humans. *Mutat. Res.* **2015**, *774*, 33–39. [CrossRef] [PubMed]
78. Christiansen, S.; Axelstad, M.; Boberg, J.; Vinggaard, A.M.; Pedersen, G.A.; Hass, U. Low-dose effects of bisphenol A on early sexual development in male and female rats. *Reproduction* **2014**, *147*, 477–487. [CrossRef] [PubMed]
79. Ullah, A.; Pirzada, M.; Jahan, S.; Ullah, H.; Turi, N.; Ullah, W.; Siddiqui, M.F.; Zakria, M.; Lodhi, K.Z.; Khan, M.M. Impact of low-dose chronic exposure to bisphenol A and its analogue bisphenol B, bisphenol F and bisphenol S on hypothalamo-pituitary-testicular activities in adult rats: A focus on the possible hormonal mode of action. *Food Chem. Toxicol.* **2018**, *121*, 24–36. [CrossRef] [PubMed]
80. Fernández, M.F.; Arrebola, J.P.; Jiménez-Díaz, I.; Sáenz, J.M.; Molina-Molina, J.M.; Ballesteros, O.; Kortenkamp, A.; Olea, N. Bisphenol A and other phenols in human placenta from children with cryptorchidism or hypospadias. *Reprod. Toxicol.* **2016**, *59*, 89–95. [CrossRef] [PubMed]
81. Mammadov, E.; Uncu, M.; Dalkan, C. High Prenatal Exposure to Bisphenol A Reduces Anogenital Distance in Healthy Male Newborns. *J. Clin. Res. Pediatr. Endocrinol.* **2018**, *10*, 25–29. [CrossRef] [PubMed]
82. Dobrzyńska, M.M.; Gajowik, A.; Jankowska-Steifer, E.A.; Radzikowska, J.; Tyrkiel, E.J. Reproductive and developmental F1 toxicity following exposure of pubescent F0 male mice to bisphenol A alone and in a combination with X-rays irradiation. *Toxicology* **2018**, *410*, 142–151. [CrossRef] [PubMed]
83. Chianese, R.; Troisi, J.; Richards, S.; Scafuro, M.; Fasano, S.; Guida, M.; Pierantoni, R.; Meccariello, R. Bisphenol A in Reproduction: Epigenetic Effects. *Curr. Med. Chem.* **2018**, *25*, 748–770. [CrossRef]
84. Zhang, G.L.; Zhang, X.F.; Feng, Y.M.; Li, L.; Huynh, E.; Sun, X.F.; Sun, Z.Y.; Shen, W. Exposure to bisphenol A results in a decline in mouse spermatogenesis. *Reprod. Fertil. Dev.* **2013**, *25*, 847–859. [CrossRef]
85. Lan, H.C.; Wu, K.Y.; Lin, I.W.; Yang, Z.J.; Chang, A.A.; Hu, M.C. Bisphenol A disrupts steroidogenesis and induces a sex hormone imbalance through c-Jun phosphorylation in Leydig cells. *Chemosphere* **2017**, *185*, 237–246. [CrossRef] [PubMed]
86. Li, N.; Mruk, D.D.; Lee, W.M.; Wong, C.K.; Cheng, C.Y. Is toxicant-induced Sertoli cell injury in vitro a useful model to study molecular mechanisms in spermatogenesis? *Semin. Cell. Dev. Biol.* **2016**, *59*, 141–156. [CrossRef]
87. Kotwicka, M.; Skibinska, I.; Jendraszak, M.; Jedrzejczak, P. 17β-estradiol modifies human spermatozoa mitochondrial function in vitro. *Reprod. Biol. Endocrinol.* **2016**, *14*, 50. [CrossRef] [PubMed]
88. Ji, H.; Miao, M.; Liang, H.; Shi, H.; Ruan, D.; Li, Y.; Wang, J.; Yuan, W. Exposure of environmental Bisphenol A in relation to routine sperm parameters and sperm movement characteristics among fertile men. *Sci. Rep.* **2018**, *8*, 17548. [CrossRef] [PubMed]

89. Vitku, J.; Chlupacova, T.; Sosvorova, L.; Hampl, R.; Hill, M.; Heracek, J.; Bicikova, M.; Starka, L. Development and validation of LC-MS/MS method for quantification of bisphenol A and estrogens in human plasma and seminal fluid. *Talanta* **2015**, *140*, 62–67. [CrossRef]
90. Manfo, F.P.; Jubendradass, R.; Nantia, E.A.; Moundipa, P.F.; Mathur, P.P. Adverse effects of bisphenol A on male reproductive function. *Rev. Environ. Contam. Toxicol.* **2014**, *228*, 57–82. [CrossRef]
91. Sun, X.; Li, D.; Liang, H.; Miao, M.; Song, X.; Wang, Z.; Zhou, Z.; Yuan, W. Maternal exposure to bisphenol A and anogenital distance throughout infancy: A longitudinal study from Shanghai, China. *Environ. Int.* **2018**, *121*, 269–275. [CrossRef]
92. Barrett, E.S.; Sathyanarayana, S.; Mbowe, O.; Thurston, S.W.; Redmon, J.B.; Nguyen, R.H.N.; Swan, S.H. First-Trimester Urinary Bisphenol A Concentration in Relation to Anogenital Distance, an Androgen-Sensitive Measure of Reproductive Development, in Infant Girls. *Environ. Health Perspect.* **2017**, *125*, 077008. [CrossRef]
93. Liu, D.; Shen, L.; Tao, Y.; Kuang, Y.; Cai, L.; Wang, D.; He, M.; Tong, X.; Zhou, S.; Sun, J.; et al. Alterations in gene expression during sexual differentiation in androgen receptor knockout mice induced by environmental endocrine disruptors. *Int. J. Mol. Med.* **2019**, *44*, 1183, Erratum for: *Int. J. Mol. Med.* **2015**, *35*, 399–404. [CrossRef]
94. Chen, Y.; Xu, H.S.; Guo, T.L. Modulation of cytokine/chemokine production in human macrophages by bisphenol A: A comparison to analogues and interactions with genistein. *J. Immunotoxicol.* **2018**, *15*, 96–103. [CrossRef]
95. Berger, K.; Eskenazi, B.; Kogut, K.; Parra, K.; Lustig, R.H.; Greenspan, L.C.; Holland, N.; Calafat, A.M.; Ye, X.; Harley, K.G. Association of Prenatal Urinary Concentrations of Phthalates and Bisphenol A and Pubertal Timing in Boys and Girls. *Environ. Health Perspect.* **2018**, *126*, 97004. [CrossRef]
96. Perera, F.; Nolte, E.L.R.; Wang, Y.; Margolis, A.E.; Calafat, A.M.; Wang, S.; Garcia, W.; Hoepner, L.A.; Peterson, B.S.; Rauh, V.; et al. Bisphenol A exposure and symptoms of anxiety and depression among inner city children at 10–12 years of age. *Environ. Res.* **2016**, *151*, 195–202. [CrossRef]
97. Jensen, T.K.; Mustieles, V.; Bleses, D.; Frederiksen, H.; Trecca, F.; Schoeters, G.; Andersen, H.R.; Grandjean, P.; Kyhl, H.B.; Juul, A.; et al. Prenatal bisphenol A exposure is associated with language development but not with ADHD-related behavior in toddlers from the Odense Child Cohort. *Environ. Res.* **2019**, *170*, 398–405. [CrossRef]
98. Kanlayaprasit, S.; Thongkorn, S.; Panjabud, P.; Jindatip, D.; Hu, V.W.; Kikkawa, T.; Osumi, N.; Sarachana, T. Autism-Related Transcription Factors Underlying the Sex-Specific Effects of Prenatal Bisphenol A Exposure on Transcriptome-Interactome Profiles in the Offspring Prefrontal Cortex. *Int. J. Mol. Sci.* **2021**, *22*, 13201. [CrossRef] [PubMed]
99. Zhang, H.; Wang, Z.; Meng, L.; Kuang, H.; Liu, J.; Lv, X.; Pang, Q.; Fan, R. Maternal exposure to environmental bisphenol A impairs the neurons in hippocampus across generations. *Toxicology* **2020**, *432*, 152393. [CrossRef] [PubMed]
100. Bi, N.; Ding, J.; Zou, R.; Gu, X.; Liu, Z.H.; Wang, H.L. Developmental exposure of bisphenol A induces spatial memory deficits by weakening the excitatory neural circuits of CA3-CA1 and EC-CA1 in mice. *Toxicol. Appl. Pharmacol.* **2021**, *426*, 115641. [CrossRef]
101. Wang, Z.; Alderman, M.H.; Asgari, C.; Taylor, H.S. Fetal Bisphenol-A Induced Changes in Murine Behavior and Brain Gene Expression Persisted in Adult-aged Offspring. *Endocrinology* **2020**, *161*, bqaa164. [CrossRef] [PubMed]
102. Ni, Y.; Hu, L.; Yang, S.; Ni, L.; Ma, L.; Zhao, Y.; Zheng, A.; Jin, Y.; Fu, Z. Bisphenol A impairs cognitive function and 5-HT metabolism in adult male mice by modulating the microbiota-gut-brain axis. *Chemosphere* **2021**, *282*, 130952. [CrossRef]
103. Heredia-García, G.; Elizalde-Velázquez, G.A.; Gómez-Oliván, L.M.; Islas-Flores, H.; García-Medina, S.; Galar-Martínez, M.; Dublán-García, O. Realistic concentrations of Bisphenol-A trigger a neurotoxic response in the brain of zebrafish: Oxidative stress, behavioral impairment, acetylcholinesterase inhibition, and gene expression disruption. *Chemosphere* **2023**, *330*, 138729. [CrossRef]
104. Schirmer, E.; Schuster, S.; Machnik, P. Bisphenols exert detrimental effects on neuronal signaling in mature vertebrate brains. *Commun. Biol.* **2021**, *4*, 465. [CrossRef]
105. Kochmanski, J.J.; Marchlewicz, E.H.; Cavalcante, R.G.; Perera, B.P.U.; Sartor, M.A.; Dolinoy, D.C. Longitudinal Effects of Developmental Bisphenol A Exposure on Epigenome-Wide DNA Hydroxymethylation at Imprinted Loci in Mouse Blood. *Environ. Health Perspect.* **2018**, *126*, 077006. [CrossRef]
106. Perrot-Applanat, M.; Kolf-Clauw, M.; Michel, C.; Beausoleil, C. Alteration of mammary gland development by bisphenol and evidence of a mode of action mediated through endocrine disruption. *Mol. Cell. Endocrinol.* **2018**, *475*, 29–53. [CrossRef]
107. Wolstenholme, J.T.; Goldsby, J.A.; Rissman, E.F. Transgenerational effects of prenatal bisphenol A on social recognition. *Horm. Behav.* **2013**, *64*, 833–839. [CrossRef]
108. Bhandari, R.K.; Deem, S.L.; Holliday, D.K.; Jandegian, C.M.; Kassotis, C.D.; Nagel, S.C.; Tillitt, D.E.; Vom Saal, F.S.; Rosenfeld, C.S. Effects of the environmental estrogenic contaminants bisphenol A and 17α-ethinyl estradiol on sexual development and adult behaviors in aquatic wildlife species. *Gen. Comp. Endocrinol.* **2015**, *214*, 195–219. [CrossRef]
109. Alonso-Magdalena, P.; Rivera, F.J.; Guerrero-Bosagna, C. Bisphenol-A and metabolic diseases: Epigenetic, developmental, and transgenerational basis. *Environ. Epigenet.* **2016**, *2*, dvw022. [CrossRef] [PubMed]
110. Bansal, A.; Li, C.; Xin, F.; Duemler, A.; Li, W.; Rashid, C.; Bartolomei, M.S.; Simmons, R.A. Transgenerational effects of maternal bisphenol: An exposure on offspring metabolic health. *J. Dev. Orig. Health Dis.* **2019**, *10*, 164–175, Erratum in: *J. Dev. Orig. Health Dis.* **2019**, *10*, 138. [CrossRef] [PubMed]
111. Mahalingam, S.; Ther, L.; Gao, L.; Wang, W.; Ziv-Gal, A.; Flaws, J.A. The effects of in utero bisphenol A exposure on ovarian follicle numbers and steroidogenesis in the F1 and F2 generations of mice. *Reprod. Toxicol.* **2017**, *74*, 150–157. [CrossRef] [PubMed]

112. Rahman, M.S.; Pang, W.K.; Ryu, D.Y.; Park, Y.J.; Pang, M.G. Multigenerational and transgenerational impact of paternal bisphenol A exposure on male fertility in a mouse model. *Hum. Reprod.* **2020**, *35*, 1740–1752. [CrossRef] [PubMed]
113. Molina, A.; Abril, N.; Morales-Prieto, N.; Monterde, J.; Ayala, N.; Lora, A.; Moyano, R. Hypothalamic-pituitary-ovarian axis perturbation in the basis of bisphenol A (BPA) reproductive toxicity in female zebrafish (*Danio rerio*). *Ecotox. Environ. Safe.* **2018**, *156*, 116–124. [CrossRef]
114. Sharma, S.; Ahmad, S.; Afjal, M.A.; Habib, H.; Parvez, S.; Raisuddin, S. Dichotomy of bisphenol A-induced expression of peroxisome proliferator-activated receptors in hepatic and testicular tissues in mice. *Chemosphere* **2019**, *236*, 124264, Erratum in *Chemosphere* **2020**, *249*, 126601. [CrossRef]
115. Shi, M.; Whorton, A.E.; Sekulovski, N.; MacLean, J.A.; Hayashi, K. Prenatal Exposure to Bisphenol A, E, and S Induces Transgenerational Effects on Male Reproductive Functions in Mice. *Toxicol. Sci.* **2019**, *172*, 303–315. [CrossRef]
116. Wolstenholme, J.T.; Drobná, Z.; Henriksen, A.D.; Goldsby, J.A.; Stevenson, R.; Irvin, J.W.; Flaws, J.A.; Rissman, E.F. Transgenerational Bisphenol A Causes Deficits in Social Recognition and Alters Postsynaptic Density Genes in Mice. *Endocrinology* **2019**, *160*, 1854–1867. [CrossRef]
117. García-Arevalo, M.; Alonso-Magdalena, P.; Rebelo Dos Santos, J.; Quesada, I.; Carneiro, E.M.; Nadal, A. Exposure to bisphenol-A during pregnancy partially mimics the effects of a high-fat diet altering glucose homeostasis and gene expression in adult male mice. *PLoS ONE* **2014**, *9*, e100214. [CrossRef] [PubMed]
118. Marmugi, A.; Lasserre, F.; Beuzelin, D.; Ducheix, S.; Huc, L.; Polizzi, A.; Chetivaux, M.; Pineau, T.; Martin, P.; Guillou, H.; et al. Adverse effects of long-term exposure to bisphenol A during adulthood leading to hyperglycaemia and hypercholesterolemia in mice. *Toxicology* **2014**, *325*, 133–143. [CrossRef] [PubMed]
119. Lejonklou, M.H.; Dunder, L.; Bladin, E.; Pettersson, V.; Rönn, M.; Lind, L.; Waldén, T.B.; Lind, P.M. Effects of Low-Dose Developmental Bisphenol A Exposure on Metabolic Parameters and Gene Expression in Male and Female Fischer 344 Rat Offspring. *Environ. Health Perspect.* **2017**, *125*, 067018. [CrossRef]
120. Moon, M.K.; Jeong, I.K.; Jung, O.T.; Ahn, H.Y.; Kim, H.H.; Park, Y.J.; Jang, H.C.; Park, K.S. Long-term oral exposure to bisphenol A induces glucose intolerance and insulin resistance. *J. Endocrinol.* **2015**, *226*, 35–42. [CrossRef]
121. Oliveira, K.M.; Figueiredo, L.S.; Araujo, T.R.; Freitas, I.N.; Silva, J.N.; Boschero, A.C.; Ribeiro, R.A. Prolonged bisphenol-A exposure decreases endocrine pancreatic proliferation in response to obesogenic diet in ovariectomized mice. *Steroids* **2020**, *160*, 108658. [CrossRef]
122. Legeay, S.; Faure, S. Is bisphenol A an environmental obesogen? *Fundam. Clin. Pharmacol.* **2017**, *31*, 594–609. [CrossRef]
123. Errico, S.; Portaccio, M.; Nicolucci, C.; Meccariello, R.; Chianese, R.; Scafuro, M.; Lepore, M.; Diano, N. A novel experimental approach for liver analysis in rats exposed to Bisphenol A by means of LC-mass spectrometry and infrared spectroscopy. *J. Pharm. Biomed. Anal.* **2019**, *165*, 207–212. [CrossRef]
124. Roepke, T.A.; Yang, J.A.; Yasrebi, A.; Mamounis, K.J.; Oruc, E.; Zama, A.M.; Uzumcu, M. Regulation of arcuate genes by developmental exposures to endocrine-disrupting compounds in female rats. *Reprod. Toxicol.* **2016**, *62*, 18–26. [CrossRef]
125. Desai, M.; Ferrini, M.G.; Jellyman, J.K.; Han, G.; Ross, M.G. In vivo and in vitro bisphenol A exposure effects on adiposity. *J. Dev. Orig. Health Dis.* **2018**, *9*, 678–687. [CrossRef]
126. Aktağ, E.; Yurdakök, K.; Yalçın, S.S.; Kandemir, N. Urinary bisphenol A levels in prepubertal children with exogenous obesity according to presence of metabolic syndrome. *J. Pediatr. Endocrinol. Metab.* **2021**, *34*, 495–502. [CrossRef]
127. Shu, X.; Tang, S.; Peng, C.; Gao, R.; Yang, S.; Luo, T.; Cheng, Q.; Wang, Y.; Wang, Z.; Zhen, Q.; et al. Bisphenol A is not associated with a 5-year incidence of type 2 diabetes: A prospective nested case-control study. *Acta Diabetol.* **2018**, *55*, 369–375. [CrossRef] [PubMed]
128. Yang, Y.J.; Hong, Y.P.; Chae, S.A. Reduction in semen quality after mixed exposure to bisphenol A and isobutylparaben in utero and during lactation periods. *Hum. Exp. Toxicol.* **2016**, *35*, 902–911. [CrossRef] [PubMed]
129. Shu, L.; Meng, Q.; Diamante, G.; Tsai, B.; Chen, Y.W.; Mikhail, A.; Luk, H.; Ritz, B.; Allard, P.; Yang, X. Prenatal Bisphenol A Exposure in Mice Induces Multi tissue Multiomics Disruptions Linking to Cardiometabolic Disorders. *Endocrinology* **2019**, *160*, 409–429. [CrossRef]
130. Wehbe, Z.; Nasser, S.A.; El-Yazbi, A.; Nasreddine, S.; Eid, A.H. Estrogen and Bisphenol A in Hypertension. *Curr. Hypertens. Rep.* **2020**, *22*, 23. [CrossRef]
131. Moon, S.; Yu, S.H.; Lee, C.B.; Park, Y.J.; Yoo, H.J.; Kim, D.S. Effects of bisphenol A on cardiovascular disease: An epidemiological study using National Health and Nutrition Examination Survey 2003–2016 and meta-analysis. *Sci. Total Environ.* **2021**, *763*, 142941. [CrossRef]
132. Agas, D.; Lacava, G.; Sabbieti, M.G. Bone and bone marrow disruption by endocrine-active substances. *J. Cell. Physiol.* **2018**, *234*, 192–213. [CrossRef]
133. Thent, Z.C.; Froemming, G.R.A.; Muid, S. Bisphenol A exposure disturbs the bone metabolism: An evolving interest towards an old culprit. *Life Sci.* **2018**, *198*, 1–7. [CrossRef]
134. Wang, Y.; Aimuzi, R.; Nian, M.; Zhang, Y.; Luo, K.; Zhang, J. Bisphenol A substitutes and sex hormones in children and adolescents. *Chemosphere* **2021**, *278*, 130396. [CrossRef]
135. Molina, A.M.; Abril, N.; Lora, A.J.; Huertas-Abril, P.V.; Ayala, N.; Blanco, C.; Moyano, M.R. Proteomic profile of the effects of low-dose bisphenol A on zebrafish ovaries. *Food Chem. Toxicol.* **2021**, *156*, 112435. [CrossRef]

136. Park, J.C.; Lee, M.C.; Yoon, D.S.; Han, J.; Kim, M.; Hwang, U.K.; Jung, J.H.; Lee, J.S. Effects of bisphenol A and its analogs bisphenol F and S on life parameters, antioxidant system, and response of defensome in the marine rotifer Brachionuskoreanus. *Aquat. Toxicol.* **2018**, *199*, 21–29. [CrossRef]
137. Xu, J.; Huang, G.; Guo, T.L. Developmental Bisphenol A Exposure Modulates Immune-Related Diseases. *Toxics* **2016**, *4*, 23. [CrossRef]
138. Xu, J.; Huang, G.; Nagy, T.; Teng, Q.; Guo, T.L. Sex-dependent effects of bisphenol A on type 1 diabetes development in non-obese diabetic (NOD) mice. *Arch. Toxicol.* **2019**, *93*, 997–1008. [CrossRef] [PubMed]
139. Olukole, S.G.; Lanipekun, D.O.; Ola-Davies, E.O.; Oke, B.O. Maternal exposure to environmentally relevant doses of bisphenol A causes reproductive dysfunction in F1 adult male rats: Protective role of melatonin. *Environ. Sci. Pollut. Res Int.* **2019**, *26*, 28940–28950. [CrossRef]
140. Kaur, K.; Chauhan, V.; Gu, F.; Chauhan, A. Bisphenol A induces oxidative stress and mitochondrial dysfunction in lymphoblasts from children with autism and unaffected siblings. *Free Radic. Biol. Med.* **2014**, *76*, 25–33. [CrossRef] [PubMed]
141. Kazemi, S.; Mousavi, S.N.; Aghapour, F.; Rezaee, B.; Sadeghi, F.; Moghadamnia, A.A. Induction Effect of Bisphenol A on Gene Expression Involving Hepatic Oxidative Stress in Rat. *Oxid. Med. Cell. Longev.* **2016**, *2016*, 6298515. [CrossRef] [PubMed]
142. Yuan, J.; Kong, Y.; Ommati, M.M.; Tang, Z.; Li, H.; Li, L.; Zhao, C.; Shi, Z.; Wang, J. Bisphenol A-induced apoptosis, oxidative stress and DNA damage in cultured rhesus monkey embryo renal epithelial Marc-145 cells. *Chemosphere* **2019**, *234*, 682–689. [CrossRef]
143. Abedelhaffez, A.S.; El-Aziz, E.A.A.; Aziz, M.A.A.; Ahmed, A.M. Lung injury induced by Bisphenol A: A food contaminant, is ameliorated by selenium supplementation. *Pathophysiology* **2017**, *24*, 81–89. [CrossRef]
144. Shirani, M.; Alizadeh, S.; Mahdavinia, M.; Dehghani, M.A. The ameliorative effect of quercetin on bisphenol A-induced toxicity in mitochondria isolated from rats. *Environ. Sci. Pollut. Res. Int.* **2019**, *26*, 7688–7696. [CrossRef]
145. Silva, M.M.D.; Xavier, L.L.F.; Gonçalves, C.F.L.; Santos-Silva, A.P.; Paiva-Melo, F.D.; Freitas, M.L.; Fortunato, R.S.; Alves, L.M.; Ferreira, A.C.F. Bisphenol A increases hydrogen peroxide generation by thyrocytes both in vivo and in vitro. *Endocr. Connect.* **2018**, *7*, 1196–1207. [CrossRef]
146. Da Silva, M.M.; Gonçalves, C.F.L.; Miranda-Alves, L.; Fortunato, R.S.; Carvalho, D.P.; Ferreira, A.C.F. Inhibition of Type 1 Iodothyronine Deiodinase by Bisphenol A. *Horm. Metab. Res.* **2019**, *51*, 671–677. [CrossRef]
147. Silva, B.S.; Bertasso, I.M.; Pietrobon, C.B.; Lopes, B.P.; Santos, T.R.; Peixoto-Silva, N.; Carvalho, J.C.; Claudio-Neto, S.; Manhães, A.C.; Cabral, S.S.; et al. Effects of maternal bisphenol A on behavior, sex steroid and thyroid hormones levels in the adult rat offspring. *Life Sci.* **2019**, *218*, 253–264. [CrossRef] [PubMed]
148. Xu, X.; Lu, Y.; Zhang, G.; Chen, L.; Tian, D.; Shen, X.; Yang, Y.; Dong, F. Bisphenol A promotes dendritic morphogenesis of hippocampal neurons through estrogen receptor-mediated ERK1/2 signal pathway. *Chemosphere* **2014**, *96*, 129–137. [CrossRef] [PubMed]
149. Sadowski, R.N.; Park, P.; Neese, S.L.; Ferguson, D.C.; Schantz, S.L.; Juraska, J.M. Effects of perinatal bisphenol A exposure during early development on radial arm maze behavior in adult male and female rats. *Neurotoxicol. Teratol.* **2014**, *42*, 17–24. [CrossRef]
150. Sanlidag, B.; Dalkan, C.; Yetkin, O.; Bahçeciler, N.N. Evaluation of Dose Dependent Maternal Exposure to Bisphenol A on Thyroid Functions in Newborns. *J. Clin. Med.* **2018**, *7*, 119. [CrossRef] [PubMed]
151. Li, S.; Jin, Y.; Zhao, H.; Jiang, Y.; Cai, Z. Evaluation of bisphenol A exposure induced oxidative RNA damage by liquid chromatography-mass spectrometry. *Chemosphere* **2019**, *222*, 235–242. [CrossRef]

animals

MDPI

Brief Report

In Vitro Lethality of Fenbendazole to the Eyeworm *Oxyspirura petrowi*

Jeremiah Leach, Hannah N. Suber, Emilynn Banks, Ashley Kaskocsak, Henry Valencia, Benjamin Hames, Regan Rivera, Sarah Colette and Ronald J. Kendall *

Wildlife Toxicology Laboratory, Texas Tech University, 1234 Davis Dr., Lubbock, TX 79416, USA
* Correspondence: ron.kendall@ttu.edu

Simple Summary: There are growing concerns about wildlife and livestock interactions and the impacts of those interactions on the sustainability of livestock. One of those concerns is the spillover of wildlife pathogens, including helminths, into livestock. This concern will likely become realized as the demand for free-range animal products increases. One such helminth with spillover potential is the eyeworm *Oxyspirura petrowi*. This eyeworm is common in many wild birds, and particularly common in Northern bobwhite quail. Related helminths are already commonly found in poultry raised in free-range conditions in developing nations. The purpose of this research was to investigate the lethality of fenbendazole, a widely available drug for treating parasites, to these eyeworms. The lethality estimates were similar to estimates of lethality to other roundworm parasites. However, studies that have investigated concentrations in host blood following administration of the drug indicate that it does not stay in the system long enough to achieve elimination of the parasite after a single dose. This indicates that in order to effectively treat eyeworm, fenbendazole must be delivered in a repeated or continuous manner.

Abstract: *Oxyspirura petrowi* is a heteroxenous nematode that infects the harderian gland and other ocular tissues in birds. High-intensity infections often cause damage to the infected tissues. Due to the nature of the infection sites, treatment of *O. petrowi* in these hosts can be difficult. Fenbendazole (FBZ) is a common anthelmintic used to treat birds for helminth infections; however, little information exists as to the efficacy of the drug on *O. petrowi* infections. The present study aims to estimate lethal concentrations of FBZ to *O. petrowi*. Adult *O. petrowi* were maintained in vitro and exposed to doses of 5, 50, 100, and 200 μM concentrations of FBZ and included both negative and vehicle controls. Exposure lasted 7.5 days and lethality was determined for each treatment. Negative and vehicle controls did not differ, and both had 75% survival at the end of the treatment period. The percentage survivorship in ascending order of concentration, corrected for the controls, was 66.67%, 44.44%, 33.33%, and 0%. LC_{10}, LC_{50}, and LC_{90} estimates were 7.5 ± 0.26, 49.1 ± 1.69, and 163.2 ± 5.63 μM, respectively. In the context of known pharmacokinetics of FBZ in birds, a single oral dose of FBZ can achieve exposure levels that are lethal to *O. petrowi*, but the drug does not stay in the system long enough. Thus, treatment of *O. petrowi* infections will require multiple oral doses over several days.

Keywords: *Oxyspirura petrowi*; fenbendazole; lethality; in vitro; LC_{50}; nematode; benzimidazole

1. Introduction

Fenbendazole (FBZ), a member of the benzimidazole class of drugs, is a broad-spectrum anthelmintic approved for treating gastrointestinal helminth infections in various types of livestock. This anthelmintic is also used to treat helminth infections in people. The drug works by interacting with β-tubulin molecules and preventing the formation of microtubules in the cell [1]. This results in a collapse of cell structure and subsequent death of the target parasite [2]. Since exposure is often through ingestion, the consequence of benzimidazole action on nematode intestinal cells has been well studied and has been shown to impair digestion and excretion in *Haemonchus contortus*, a nematode that infects the rumen of many ungulates [3]. The effectiveness of FBZ as a nematicide and its relative safety in vertebrates has made FBZ an important anthelmintic [4].

Oxyspirura petrowi is a heteroxenous nematode commonly found to infect wild birds in North America [5–9]. This eyeworm can be highly prevalent in quail and passerines in endemic areas. Surveys in West Texas revealed an 89–100% prevalence and a mean abundance of 44 worms in wild quail [10–13]. These high-intensity infections in quail were also correlated with cell atrophy, eye inflammation, edema, and damage to the cornea and eye ducts [13,14]. *Oxyspirura petrowi* has also been found in songbirds at prevalences of 42.9%, 85.7%, and 100% in Northern cardinals (*Cardinalis cardinalis*), Northern mockingbirds (*Mimus polyglottus*), and Curve-billed thrashers (*Toxostoma curvirostre*), respectively [6]. The prevalence and abundance of *O. petrowi* in wild birds is so great that concern of spillover into domestic poultry in Michigan was expressed in 1935 [15]. These concerns will likely be realized with increasing demand for free-range poultry products as *Oxyspirura* spp. infections have already been found in poultry kept in free-ranging conditions [16–18].

The global distribution and epidemic potential of *O. petrowi* and congenerics make understanding control methods a priority, especially if pharmaceutical interventions become more relevant in their control. The goal of this research was to explore the pharmacodynamics of FBZ to *O. petrowi* and put it in the context of known pharmacokinetics. Knowing the concentrations at which anthelmintics cause lethality to *O. petrowi* is important and will allow for more effective control of *O. petrowi* populations in hosts and can inform future work of the in vivo efficacy of FBZ to *O. petrowi* and its congeners. The objective of this study is to assess the dose-response of *O. petrowi* to the anthelmintic FBZ via in vitro methods to quantify survivorship. FBZ was selected as the anthelmintic for this study because it is widely available and already approved in several nations for use in many domestic bird species.

2. Methods

2.1. Chemical Source and Quality

FBZ was obtained from Sigma-Aldrich® (Darmstadt, Germany) (≥98% purity, lot number MKBR9907V). Dimethyl sulfoxide (DMSO) was obtained from Fisher Chemical® (Pittsburgh, Pennsylvania, USA) (ACS Grade, lot number 187334). Sodium phosphate monobasic (NaH_2PO_4) and potassium phosphate monobasic (KH_2PO_4) were both obtained from Sigma-Aldrich® (Darmstadt, Germany), lot numbers BCBL2768V and SLBD9446V, respectively. Sodium chloride (NaCl) was obtained from Fisher Chemical® (Pittsburgh, Pennsylvania, USA) (lot number 135570). NaH_2PO_4, KH_2PO_4, and NaCl were all ≥99% purity. Egg whites were obtained from a local market.

2.2. Solution Preparation and Treatment Groups

Worms were split into a total of six groups for FBZ lethality testing. The groups were control, vehicle control, and four treatment groups. Each of the treatment and control solutions were made based on Dunham et al. [19]. The control solution consisted of physiological saline, as described in Corba et al. [20], mixed with egg white at a 1:1 ratio. The physiological saline was made using distilled water and sterilized by autoclave. The physiological saline for vehicle controls and all treatments was made using 3% DMSO. Vehicle controls and all treatments consisted of 50% drug solution and 50% egg white to obtain a final concentration of 1.5% DMSO for the vehicle control and 1.5% DMSO with 5 μM (1.5 ppm) concentration, 50 μM (15 ppm) concentration, 100 μM (30 ppm) concentration, and 200 μM (60 ppm) concentration.

2.3. Eyeworm Collection

Eyeworms were collected from hunter-harvested wild *Colinus virginianus* from Fisher County, Texas. A researcher would follow along during the hunt and collect birds as they were harvested. The researcher would place the whole carcass in a resealable plastic bag and place the bag in a portable insulated box. The temperature of the box was maintained between 21 and 27 °C using Hothands™ single-use warmers (Kobayashi Healthcare, Dalton, Georgia, USA). The warmers were placed under a cloth towel in the bottom of the box and temperature was monitored using a digital thermometer. Temperature was checked at least once an hour and whenever the box was opened. The researcher would remove the heads of the birds and return them to the resealable bag and insulated box once the hunt was completed. The heads were then transported to the Wildlife Toxicology Laboratory at Texas Tech University where the eyes and associated tissues were inspected for eyeworms according to Dunham et al. [7]. Once removed from the host tissue, eyeworms were placed in 0.01 M PBS or control solution for assessment. Worms were considered suitable for use in this experiment if there was no visible damage and they demonstrated unprompted activity within 24 h of being collected.

2.4. Experimental Design

The experimental protocol was carried out in six-well cell culture plates with six replicates. The wells of each plate were randomly assigned one of the six experimental conditions and 10 mL of the appropriate solution was added to the well. Four worms were placed in each well, beginning with well number 1, once all wells had the appropriate solution. Worms were maintained in a cell incubator at 40 C with 5% CO_2. Worms were checked 12 h later, and then checked at 24-h intervals for a total of 7.5 days under 10× magnification and assessed as live or moribund. While not a definitive confirmation, the worms were deemed moribund if they failed to respond to gentle prodding with a metal probe. Percent mortality was assessed for each treatment and statistical analysis was completed using the R package drc in R Studio® version 2023.06.0 Build 421 [21]. The model was fitted using the exponential decay function with the lower limit set at 0. Controls were then removed from the data, the model was run again, and the resulting model was used to estimate benchmark concentrations [22].

3. Results

A total of 29 *C. virginianus* heads were donated and examined for eyeworm infection. Prevalence of eyeworms was 86.2% and mean abundance was 11.7 worms/bird. In total, 144 worms were used to test the lethality of FBZ, with 24 worms in each treatment and control. Estimated parameters were statistically significant, with the plateau d = 0.695 ($p < 0.0001$) and k = 69.04 ($p < 0.0001$). Table 1 shows the survival of worms at each time point for the concentrations used in this study. The dose–response curve in relation to FBZ concentration at 7.5 days post-treatment with 95% confidence intervals is shown in Figure 1. The percent mortality relative to control and DMSO treatments are displayed in Table 2 and the mortality curve corrected for the control groups is shown in Figure 2. Estimates of LC_{10}, LC_{50}, and LC_{90} and their standard errors are 7.5 ± 0.26 µM (2.47 ± 0.079 ppm), 49.1 ± 1.69 µM (14.7 ± 0.51 ppm), and 163.2 ± 5.63 µM (48.65 ± 1.69 ppm), respectively.

Table 1. Percent survivorship of *O. petrowi* at increasing concentrations of FBZ. Sample size is denoted after the treatment group with the letter n.

Treatment	12 h	36 h	60 h	84 h	108 h	132 h	156 h	180 h
Con (n = 24)	100.00%	100.00%	91.67%	95.83%	91.67%	79.17%	75.00%	75.00%
DMSO (n = 24)	100.00%	100.00%	95.83%	87.50%	87.50%	79.17%	66.67%	75.00%
5 µM (n = 24)	100.00%	100.00%	100.00%	87.50%	87.50%	66.67%	50.00%	50.00%
50 µM (n = 24)	87.50%	83.33%	79.17%	79.17%	75.00%	66.67%	41.67%	33.33%
100 µM (n = 24)	100.00%	100.00%	95.83%	95.83%	91.67%	66.67%	41.67%	25.00%
200 µM (n = 24)	95.83%	95.83%	91.67%	87.50%	70.83%	54.17%	8.33%	0.00%

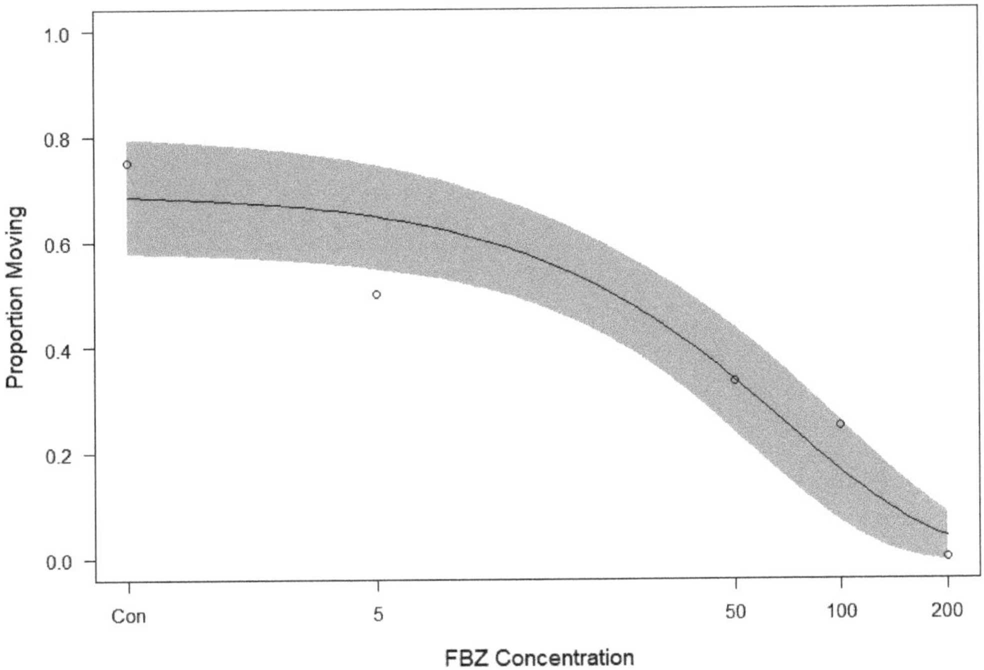

Figure 1. Proportion of worms found moribund when placed in a solution containing FBZ after 180 h with observed proportion moribund (circles) and 95% confidence interval (shaded area). Concentrations are in μM and control and vehicle control groups were pooled. Con = controls.

Table 2. Percent survivorship of FBZ-exposed worms relative to controls and DMSO-exposed worms combined.

Dose	Percent Control
Control and DMSO	100
5 μM	66.67
50 μM	44.44
100 μM	33.33
200 μM	0

4. Discussion

This represents the first report of the in vitro lethality of FBZ on the eyeworm *O. petrowi*. The percentage of control worms surviving to the end of this experiment was similar to the percent surviving in other in vitro studies of *O. petrowi*. Dunham et al. [19] reported 75% survival after 10 days, reflected here in the survival of control and vehicle control worms after 7.5 days. Survivability of worms was reduced even at low concentrations of FBZ and all worms were dead after 7.5 days in a solution containing 200 μM FBZ. The effect of FBZ on *O. petrowi* reported here is similar to reports in other nematodes. In the free-living nematode *Caenorhabditis elegans*, a concentration of 100 μM was sufficient to achieve 100% mortality in an albendazole susceptible strain [23]. FBZ concentrations of about 6.7 μM were sufficient to reduce populations of *Pristionchus maupasi*, a soil nematode, by over 50% relative to controls [24]. Substantial reduction of the viability of *Trichinella spiralis*, an intestinal worm that is transmitted through the ingestion of raw or undercooked meat, was observed at concentrations of 1.88 μM albendazole solution, a benzimidazole-class anthelmintic that is more lethal to *C. elegans* than FBZ [23,25]. Concentrations of 500 μg/mL (1.67 mM) of FBZ, greater than eight times the maximum dose used in this study, were sufficient to obtain nearly 90% lethality in *Ascaridia galli* after 36 h [26]. Based on the results of this study, the lethality of FBZ to *O. petrowi* is within the range of lethality to other nematodes.

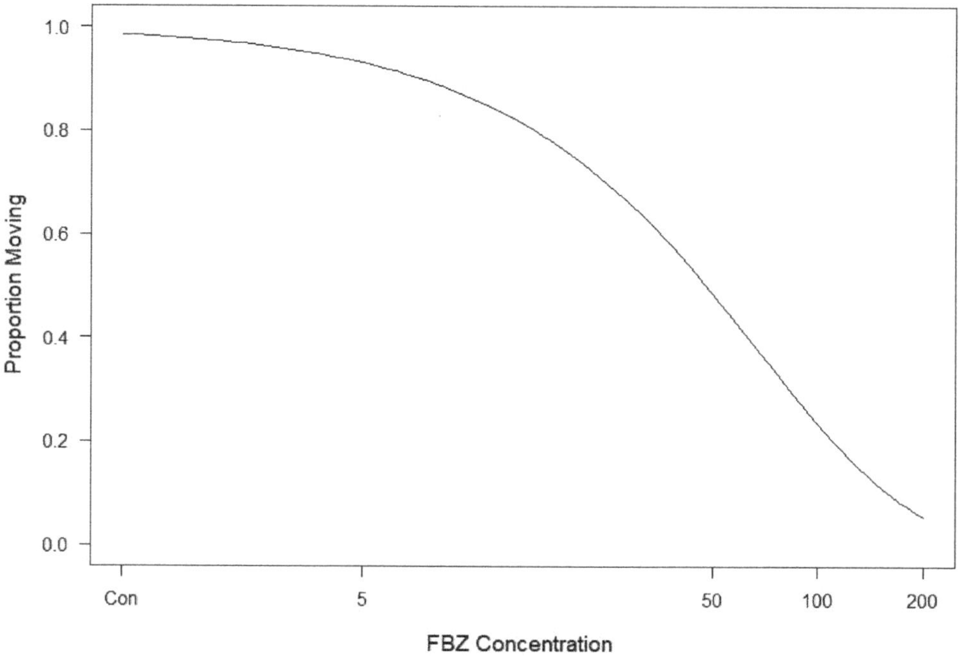

Figure 2. Dose–response curve of *O. petrowi* corrected for control groups after 7.5 days of exposure to FBZ. Con = controls.

Interpreting these results in the context of naturally infected hosts is difficult. Studies of the pharmacokinetics of FBZ in livestock show substantial diversity in the absorption and secretion rate of the anthelmintic. FBZ is absorbed more slowly and tends to have longer systemic residence than other benzimidazoles [27], further increasing the difficulty of interpreting these data in the context of naturally occurring infections. A comparative study of FBZ in Droughtmaster cattle (*Bos indicus* and *B. taurus* cross) and Swamp buffalo (*Bubalus bubalis*) found higher FBZ concentrations in blood plasma and greater retention time in cattle [28]. Beagle dogs given a dose of 20 mg/kg body weight had concentrations of FBZ in their plasma greater than 0.1 μg/mL for nearly 24 h, with an area under the curve (AUC) of 9.74 μg·h/mL [29]. Plasma concentrations in goats were similar to that of the Beagle, with max concentrations of 0.19 μg/mL and concentrations greater than 0.01 μg/mL for nearly 24 h [30]. The AUC in goats administered an oral dose of FBZ at 7.5 mg/kg body weight was 4.76 μg·h/mL [30]. Metabolism and excretion of FBZ and its metabolites was more similar between domestic chickens (*Gallus gallus domesticus*) and domestic ducks (*Anas platyrhyncos domesticus*) than chickens and domestic turkeys (*Meleagris gallopavo f. domesticus*) [31]. While information on the pharmacokinetics of FBZ in birds is lacking, it appears to be highly variable, even within birds of the same order. Despite the variability in the available pharmacokinetic data, blood plasma concentrations of FBZ are below the concentrations used in this study. However, the AUCs reported suggest that while the expected FBZ exposure in vivo should be high enough to have lethal effects on *O. petrowi*, the drug simply does not have a long enough residency time. This suggests that the use of anthelmintics to treat *O. petrowi* infections should consist of multiple or continuous doses over time and is consistent with in vivo studies of oxfendazole and albendazole in poultry [32]. However, while the benchmark concentrations reported here should be attainable in the blood plasma, only an in vivo study conducted with the target host can verify efficacy of FBZ against *O. petrowi*. It is also worth considering that one of the major metabolites of FBZ is oxfendazole. Thus, any worm exposed to FBZ is also being exposed to oxfendazole, which is a potent anthelmintic in its own right [33]. As the detrimental effects of heavy parasite burdens in wildlife are being realized, an increase in anthropogenic intervention is likely, including drug treatment. Future research studying the pharmacokinetics of FBZ in the wildlife hosts would be extremely beneficial, especially if used in conjunction with the results of this study. It would allow for a prediction of the efficacy of FBZ in treating wildlife species for *O. petrowi*, which in turn would allow for the implementation of more efficient management plans for the wildlife of concern.

5. Conclusions

Epidemics and spillover events will become more common as the world continues to change. This will very likely include an increase in the detrimental effects of helminths on wildlife and helminths common to wildlife finding their way into livestock and poultry. Understanding the response of enzootic helminths to available anthelmintics will become ever more imperative to controlling outbreaks. Here we demonstrated the use of an in vitro assay for measuring the effects of a common anthelmintic on *O. petrowi*, a helminth that is likely to occur in free-range poultry and is common in wild birds. The benchmark doses reported here are similar to those of other in vitro studies with nematodes; however, in vivo studies must be conducted in order to determine effective treatment plans and efficacy of fenbendazole against *O. petrowi* and its congeners. In vivo studies using other benzimidazole class anthelmintics suggest single-dose treatment regimens using recommended doses may not be suitable for treating *O. petrowi*. Furthermore, pharmacokinetic information indicates the FBZ does not have an appropriate residual time in the host. Thus, in vivo studies and treatment plans should focus on the use of medicated feeds with continuous or near continuous access for at least 7 days. Another alternative would be the co-administration of cytochrome P450 inhibitors, which have been shown to increase the concentration of FBZ in the blood plasma and the residual time [29]. Lastly, FBZ may have a wide margin of safety, but it can be toxic to vertebrates and particularly so at high doses. Future work investigating the efficacy of FBZ against *O. petrowi* should consider this during research planning. There is clearly still work to be done and it is our hope that this work will stimulate further investigations into best practices for treating helminths found outside of the host gastrointestinal tract.

Author Contributions: J.L., H.N.S. and R.J.K. were equally involved in the conceptualization and design of the experiment. J.L. and H.N.S. contributed equally to field collections of *C. virginianus*. All authors contributed equally to the laboratory work. Specifically, B.H., J.L. and S.C. contributed equally to solution preparation. E.B., A.K., R.R., S.C., B.H. and H.V. contributed equally to necropsies identifying candidate worms this study. J.L. and H.N.S. contributed equally to daily checks and recording the daily status of the worms. Formal analysis, data curation, and the original draft were done by J.L. All authors contributed equally to manuscript revisions. Project administration, supervision, funding, and material acquisition were all done by R.J.K. All authors have read and agreed to the published version of the manuscript.

Funding: Funding was provided by a generous donation by Park Cities Quail Coalition donation number 24A.

Institutional Review Board Statement: The researchers involved did not handle any live vertebrates and the hunter-harvested *C. virginianus* were not collected for scientific purposes. However, to the best of our knowledge, all donated *C. virginianus* were harvested ethically and in compliance with state and local law.

Informed Consent Statement: Not applicable.

Data Availability Statement: Data are available upon reasonable request to the corresponding author.

Acknowledgments: The authors would like to thank the staff at the Rolling Plains Quail Research Ranch and those who hunted there in the 2023–2024 quail season for their participation in collecting worms. We would also like to thank Park Cities Quail Coalition for their generosity in funding this study.

Conflicts of Interest: The authors report no conflicts of interest with regards to this work.

References

1. Friedman, P.A.; Platzer, E.G. Interaction of anthelmintic benzimidazoles and benzimidazole derivatives with bovine brain tubulin. *Biochim. Biophys. Acta Gen. Subj.* **1978**, *544*, 605–614. [CrossRef] [PubMed]
2. Abongwa, M.; Martin, R.J.; Robertson, A.P. A brief review on the mode of action of antinematodal drugs. *Acta Vet.* **2017**, *67*, 137–152. [CrossRef] [PubMed]
3. Jasmer, D.P.; Yao, C.; Rehman, A.; Johnson, S. Multiple lethal effects induced by a benzimidazole anthelmintic in the anterior intestine of the nematode *Haemonchus contortus*. *Mol. Biochem. Parasitol.* **2000**, *105*, 81–90. [CrossRef] [PubMed]
4. Danaher, M.; Howells, L.C.; Crooks, S.R.; Cerkvenik-Flajs, V.; O'Keeffe, M. Review of methodology for the determination of macrocyclic lactone residues in biological matrices. *J. Chromatogr. B* **2006**, *844*, 175–203. [CrossRef]
5. Dunham, N.R.; Kendall, R.J. Evidence of *Oxyspirura petrowi* in migratory songbirds found in the rolling plains of West Texas, USA. *J. Wildl. Dis.* **2014**, *50*, 711–712. [CrossRef] [PubMed]
6. Herzog, J.L.; Lukashow-Moore, S.P.; Brym, M.Z.; Kalyanasundaram, A.; Kendall, R.J. A Helminth Survey of Northern Bobwhite Quail (*Colinus virginianus*) and Passerines in the Rolling Plains Ecoregion of Texas. *J. Parasitol.* **2021**, *107*, 132–137. [CrossRef] [PubMed]
7. Dunham, N.R.; Soliz, L.A.; Fedynich, A.M.; Rollins, D.; Kendall, R.J. Evidence of an *Oxyspirura petrowi* epizootic in northern bobwhites (*Colinus virginianus*), Texas, USA. *J. Wildl. Dis.* **2014**, *50*, 552–558. [CrossRef] [PubMed]
8. Villareal, S.M.; Bruno, A.; Fedynich, A.M.; Brennan, L.A.; Rollins, D. Helminth Infections Across a Northern Bobwhite (*Colinus virginianus*) Annual Cycle in Fisher County, Texas. *West. N. Am. Nat.* **2016**, *76*, 275–280. [CrossRef]
9. Pence, D.B. The Genus *Oxyspirura* (Nematoda: Thelaziidae) from Birds in Louisiana. *Proc. Helminthol. Soc. Wash.* **1972**, *39*, 23–28.
10. Brym, M.Z.; Henry, C.; Kendall, R.J. Potential Parasite Induced Host Mortality in Northern Bobwhite (*Colinus virginianus*) from the Rolling Plains Ecoregion of West Texas. *Arch. Parasitol.* **2018**, *2*, 115.
11. Henry, C.; Brym, M.; Kendall, R. *Oxyspirura petrowi* and *Aulonocephalus pennula* infection in wild northern bobwhite quail in the Rolling Plains ecoregion, Texas: Possible evidence of a die-off. *Arch. Parasitol.* **2017**, *1*, 109.
12. Henry, C.; Brym, M.Z.; Skinner, K.; Blanchard, K.R.; Henry, B.J.; Hay, A.L.; Herzog, J.L.; Kalyanasundaram, A.; Kendall, R.J. "Weight of evidence" as a tool for evaluating disease in wildlife: An example assessing parasitic infection in Northern bobwhite (*Colinus virginianus*). *Int. J. Parasitol. Parasites Wildl.* **2020**, *13*, 27–37. [CrossRef]
13. Dunham, N.R.; Reed, S.; Rollins, D.; Kendall, R.J. *Oxyspirura petrowi* infection leads to pathological consequences in Northern bobwhite (*Colinus virginianus*). *Int. J. Parasitol. Parasites Wildl.* **2016**, *5*, 273–276. [CrossRef]
14. Bruno, A.; Fedynich, A.M.; Smith-Herron, A.; Rollins, D. Pathological response of northern bobwhites to *Oxyspirura petrowi* infections. *J. Parasitol.* **2015**, *101*, 364–368. [CrossRef] [PubMed]
15. Saunders, G. Michigan's studies of sharp-tailed grouse. In Proceedings of the Transactions of the American Game Conference, New York, NY, USA, 21–23 January 1935; pp. 342–344.
16. Mathew, D.P.; Priya, M.; Deepa, C.; Syamala, K.; Ajithkumar, K.; Ravindran, R. *Oxyspirura mansoni* in backyard poultry of Kerala. *J. Indian Vet. Assoc.* **2012**, *10*, 43.
17. Santoyo-De-Estéfano, F.A.; Espinoza-Leija, R.R.; Zárate-Ramos, J.J.; Hernández-Velasco, X. Identification of *Oxyspirura mansoni* (Spirurida: Thelaziidae) in a free-range hen (*Gallus gallus domesticus*) and its intermediate host, *Surinam cockroach* (*Pycnoscelus surinamensis*) in Monterrey, Nuevo Leon, Mexico. *Acta Zoológica Mex.* **2014**, *30*, 106–113. [CrossRef]
18. Hassan, N.; Awang, A.; Rahman, M.S. Parasitic burden and Its relation with the body weight of free range chicken in oil palm dominated Sandakan District of Malaysian Borneo. *Int. J. Livest. Res.* **2015**, *5*, 10–20. [CrossRef]
19. Dunham, N.R.; Soliz, L.A.; Brightman, A.; Rollins, D.; Fedynich, A.M.; Kendall, R. Live eyeworm (*Oxyspirura petrowi*) extraction, in vitro culture, and transfer for experimental studies. *J. Parasitol.* **2015**, *101*, 98–101. [CrossRef] [PubMed]
20. Corba, J.; Scales, B.; Froyd, G. The effect of dl-tetramisole on *Thelazia rhodesii* (eye-worm) in cattle. *Trop. Anim. Health Prod.* **1969**, *1*, 19–22. [CrossRef]
21. Ritz, C.; Baty, F.; Streibig, J.C.; Gerhard, D. Dose-Response Analysis Using R. *PLoS ONE* **2016**, *10*, e0146021. [CrossRef]
22. Kappenberg, F.; Brecklinghaus, T.; Albrecht, W.; Blum, J.; van der Wurp, C.; Leist, M.; Hengstler, J.G.; Rahnenführer, J. Handling deviating control values in concentration-response curves. *Arch. Toxicol.* **2020**, *94*, 3787–3798. [CrossRef] [PubMed]
23. Enos, A.; Coles, G. Effect of benzimidazole drugs on tubulin in benzimidazole resistant and susceptible strains of *Caenorhabditis elegans*. *Int. J. Parasitol.* **1990**, *20*, 161–167. [CrossRef] [PubMed]
24. Grønvold, J.; Svendsen, T.S.; Kraglund, H.-O.; Bresciani, J.; Monrad, J. Effect of the antiparasitic drugs fenbendazole and ivermectin on the soil nematode *Pristionchus maupasi*. *Vet. Parasitol.* **2004**, *124*, 91–99. [CrossRef] [PubMed]

25. Navarrete-Vazquez, G.; Yepez, L.; Hernandez-Campos, A.; Tapia, A.; Hernandez-Luis, F.; Cedillo, R.; Gonzalez, J.; Martınez-Fernandez, A.; Martınez-Grueiro, M.; Castillo, R. Synthesis and antiparasitic activity of albendazole and mebendazole analogues. *Bioorganic Med. Chem.* **2003**, *11*, 4615–4622. [CrossRef] [PubMed]
26. Aziz, A.R.A.; AbouLaila, M.R.; Aziz, M.; Omar, M.A.; Sultan, K. In vitro and in vivo anthelmintic activity of pumpkin seeds and pomegranate peels extracts against *Ascaridia galli*. *Beni-Suef Univ. J. Basic Appl. Sci.* **2018**, *7*, 231–234.
27. Prichard, R.K. The pharmacology of anthelmintics in livestock. *Int. J. Parasitol.* **1987**, *17*, 473–482. [CrossRef] [PubMed]
28. Knox, M.; Kennedy, P.; Hennessy, D.; Steel, J.; Le Jambre, L. Comparative pharmacokinetics of fenbendazole in buffalo and cattle. *Vet. Res. Commun.* **1994**, *18*, 209–216. [CrossRef] [PubMed]
29. McKellar, Q.; Harrison, P.; Galbraith, E.; Inglis, H. Pharmacokinetics of fenbendazole in dogs. *J. Vet. Pharmacol. Ther.* **1990**, *13*, 386–392. [CrossRef] [PubMed]
30. Benchaoui, H.; McKellar, Q. Interaction between fenbendazole and piperonyl butoxide: Pharmacokinetic and pharmacodynamic implications. *J. Pharm. Pharmacol.* **1996**, *48*, 753–759. [CrossRef]
31. Short, C.; Barker, S.; Hsieh, L.; Ou, S.P.; Pedersoli, W.; Krista, L.; Spanoh, J. The elimination of fenbendazole and its metabolites in the chicken, turkey and duck. *J. Vet. Pharmacol. Ther.* **1988**, *11*, 204–209. [CrossRef]
32. Manuel, M.; Gale, L. The efficacy of oxfendazole and albendazole against *Oxyspirura mansoni* and other helminths of chickens. *Philipp. J. Anim. Ind.* **1985**, *38*, 1–13.
33. Gonzalez, A.E.; Codd, E.E.; Horton, J.; Garcia, H.H.; Gilman, R.H. Oxfendazole: A promising agent for the treatment and control of helminth infections in humans. *Expert Rev. Anti-Infect. Ther.* **2019**, *17*, 51–56. [CrossRef] [PubMed]

MDPI AG
Grosspeteranlage 5
4052 Basel
Switzerland
Tel.: +41 61 683 77 34

Animals Editorial Office
E-mail: animals@mdpi.com
www.mdpi.com/journal/animals

www.ingramcontent.com/pod-product-compliance
Lightning Source LLC
Chambersburg PA
CBHW062031220926
51850CB00010B/2513
* 9 7 8 3 7 2 5 8 6 3 5 2 5 *